BASIC AND CLINICAL SCIENCE COURSE

Refractive Surgery

Section 13

2005–2006

(First edition 2004–2005)

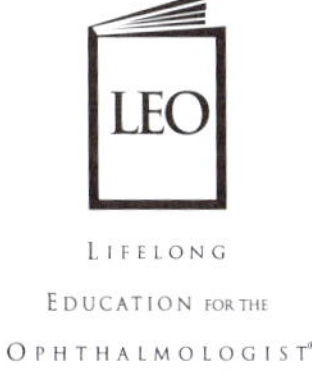

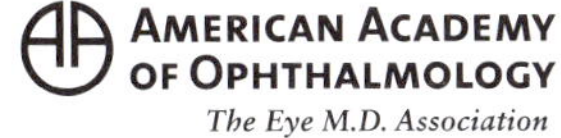

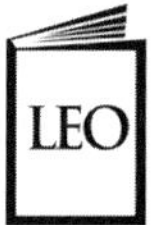

The Basic and Clinical Science Course is one component of the Lifelong Education for the Ophthalmologist (LEO) framework, which assists members in planning their continuing medical education. LEO includes an array of clinical education products that members may select to form individualized, self-directed learning plans for updating their clinical knowledge. Active members or fellows who use LEO components may accumulate sufficient CME credits to earn the LEO Award. Contact the Academy's Clinical Education Division for further information on LEO.

The American Academy of Ophthalmology is accredited by the Accreditation Council for Continuing Medical Education to provide continuing medical education for physicians.

The American Academy of Ophthalmology designates this educational activity for a maximum of 30 category 1 credits toward the AMA Physician's Recognition Award. Each physician should claim only those hours of credit that he/she actually spent in the activity.

The American Medical Association has determined that non-US licensed physicians who participate in this CME activity are eligible for AMA PRA category 1 credit.

The Academy provides this material for educational purposes only. It is not intended to represent the only or best method or procedure in every case, nor to replace a physician's own judgment or give specific advice for case management. Including all indications, contraindications, side effects, and alternative agents for each drug or treatment is beyond the scope of this material. All information and recommendations should be verified, prior to use, with current information included in the manufacturers' package inserts or other independent sources, and considered in light of the patient's condition and history. Reference to certain drugs, instruments, and other products in this course is made for illustrative purposes only and is not intended to constitute an endorsement of such. Some material may include information on applications that are not considered community standard, that reflect indications not included in approved FDA labeling, or that are approved for use only in restricted research settings. The FDA has stated that it is the responsibility of the physician to determine the FDA status of each drug or device he or she wishes to use, and to use them with appropriate patient consent in compliance with applicable law. The Academy specifically disclaims any and all liability for injury or other damages of any kind, from negligence or otherwise, for any and all claims that may arise from the use of any recommendations or other information contained herein.

Printed in the United States of America

Basic and Clinical Science Course

Section 13

Faculty Responsible for This Edition

Jayne S. Weiss, MD, *Chair,* Detroit, Michigan
Dimitri T. Azar, MD, Boston, Massachusetts
Michael W. Belin, MD, Slingerlands, New York
Robert S. Feder, MD, Chicago, Illinois
Christopher J. Rapuano, MD, Philadelphia, Pennsylvania
Steven C. Schallhorn, MD, San Diego, California
Roger F. Steinert, MD, Boston, Massachusetts
William S. Clifford, MD, Garden City, Kansas
Practicing Ophthalmologists Advisory Committee for Education

The authors state the following financial relationships:
Dr Azar: Alcon, consultant and meeting support; Bausch & Lomb, consultant and travel and meeting support; Thermal Vision, consultant

Dr Steinert: Advanced Medical Optics, consultant; Alcon, consultant and medical advisory board; VISX, national advisory board

Dr Weiss: Alcon, speaker

The other authors state that they have no significant financial interest or other relationship with the manufacturer of any commercial product discussed in the chapters that they contributed to this publication or with the manufacturer of any competing commercial product.

American Academy of Ophthalmology Staff

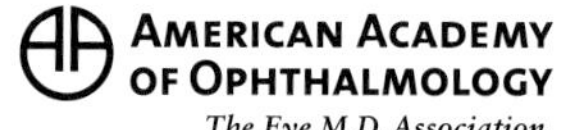

655 Beach Street
Box 7424
San Francisco, CA 94120-7424

Contents

General Introduction

The Basic and Clinical Science Course (BCSC) is designed to meet the needs of residents and practitioners for a comprehensive yet concise curriculum of the field of ophthalmology. The BCSC has developed from its original brief outline format, which relied heavily on outside readings, to a more convenient and educationally useful self-contained text. The Academy updates and revises the course annually, with the goals of integrating the basic science and clinical practice of ophthalmology and of keeping ophthalmologists current with new developments in the various subspecialties.

The BCSC incorporates the effort and expertise of more than 80 ophthalmologists, organized into 13 section faculties, working with Academy editorial staff. In addition, the course continues to benefit from many lasting contributions made by the faculties of previous editions. Members of the Academy's Practicing Ophthalmologists Advisory Committee for Education serve on each faculty and, as a group, review every volume before and after major revisions.

Organization of the Course

The Basic and Clinical Science Course comprises 13 volumes, incorporating fundamental ophthalmic knowledge, subspecialty areas, and special topics:

1. Update on General Medicine
2. Fundamentals and Principles of Ophthalmology
3. Clinical Optics
4. Ophthalmic Pathology and Intraocular Tumors
5. Neuro-Ophthalmology
6. Pediatric Ophthalmology and Strabismus
7. Orbit, Eyelids, and Lacrimal System
8. External Disease and Cornea
9. Intraocular Inflammation and Uveitis
10. Glaucoma
11. Lens and Cataract
12. Retina and Vitreous
13. Refractive Surgery

In addition, a comprehensive Master Index allows the reader to easily locate subjects throughout the entire series.

References

Readers who wish to explore specific topics in greater detail may consult the journal references cited within each chapter and the Basic Texts listed at the back of the book.

These references are intended to be selective rather than exhaustive, chosen by the BCSC faculty as being important, current, and readily available to residents and practitioners.

Related Academy educational materials are also listed in the appropriate sections. They include books, audiovisual materials, self-assessment programs, clinical modules, and interactive programs.

Study Questions and CME Credit

Each volume of the BCSC is designed as an independent study activity for ophthalmology residents and practitioners. The learning objectives for this volume are given on page 1. The text, illustrations, and references provide the information necessary to achieve the objectives; the study questions allow readers to test their understanding of the material and their mastery of the objectives. Physicians who wish to claim CME credit for this educational activity may do so by mail, by fax, or online. The necessary forms and instructions are given at the end of the book.

Conclusion

The Basic and Clinical Science Course has expanded greatly over the years, with the addition of much new text and numerous illustrations. Recent editions have sought to place a greater emphasis on clinical applicability, while maintaining a solid foundation in basic science. As with any educational program, it reflects the experience of its authors. As its faculties change and as medicine progresses, new viewpoints are always emerging on controversial subjects and techniques. Not all alternate approaches can be included in this series; as with any educational endeavor, the learner should seek additional sources, including such carefully balanced opinions as the Academy's Preferred Practice Patterns.

The BCSC faculty and staff are continuously striving to improve the educational usefulness of the course; you, the reader, can contribute to this ongoing process. If you have any suggestions or questions about the series, please do not hesitate to contact the faculty or the editors.

The authors, editors, and reviewers hope that your study of the BCSC will be of lasting value and that each section will serve as a practical resource for quality patient care.

Objectives

Upon completion of BCSC Section 13, *Refractive Surgery*, the reader should be able to:

- Explain the contribution of the cornea's shape and tissue layers to the optics of the eye and how these components are affected biomechanically by different types of keratorefractive procedures
- Outline the basic concepts of wavefront analysis and its relationship to different types of optical aberrations
- Review the general types of lasers used in refractive surgeries
- Describe the role of the FDA in the development and approval of ophthalmic devices used in refractive surgery
- Outline the steps—including medical and social history, ocular examination, and ancillary testing—in evaluating whether a patient is an appropriate candidate for refractive surgery
- For incisional keratorefractive surgery (radial keratotomy, transverse keratotomy, arcuate keratotomy, and limbal relaxing incisions), review the history, patient selection, surgical techniques, outcomes, and complications
- List the various types of corneal onlays and inlays that have been used for refractive correction
- For photorefractive keratotomy (PRK) and laser subepithelial keratomileusis (LASEK), review patient selection, epithelial debridement, laser calibration and techniques, refractive outcomes, and complications
- Describe the different methods for creating a LASIK flap using a microkeratome or a femtosecond laser as well as instrumentation and possible complications associated with each
- Review patient selection, surgical techniques, outcomes, and complications for laser in situ keratomileusis (LASIK)
- Explain recent developments in the application of wavefront technology to PRK and LASIK
- For conductive keratoplasty, provide a brief overview of history, patient selection, and safety issues

- Discuss how intraocular surgical procedures, including clear lens extraction with IOL implantation or phakic IOL implantation, can be used in refractive correction, with or without corneal intervention
- Discuss the different types of IOLs used for refractive correction
- Explain the leading theories of accommodation and how they relate to potential treatment of presbyopia
- Describe nonaccommodative and accommodative approaches to the treatment of presbyopia
- Discuss considerations for, and possible contraindications to, refractive surgery in the setting of preexisting ocular and systemic disease
- List some of the effects of prior refractive procedures on later IOL calculations, contact lens wear, and ocular surgery

PART I

Underlying Concepts of Refractive Surgery

CHAPTER 1

The Science of Refractive Surgery

Refractive surgical procedures can be categorized as *corneal* or *lenticular.* Keratorefractive (corneal) procedures include radial keratotomy (RK), astigmatic keratotomy (arcuate keratotomy [AK], limbal relaxing incisions [LRIs], and transverse keratotomy), photorefractive keratectomy (PRK), laser in situ keratomileusis (LASIK), laser subepithelial keratomileusis (LASEK), epikeratoplasty, implantation of plastic intrastromal corneal ring segments (ICRS, or Intacs), keratophakia, laser thermal keratoplasty (LTK), and conductive, or radiofrequency, keratoplasty (CK). Lenticular refractive procedures include cataract surgery and clear lens extraction with intraocular lens (IOL) implantation, phakic IOL implantation, accommodative IOL implantation, and piggyback IOL implantation. Although all of these techniques alter the optical properties of the eye, current keratorefractive procedures may be more likely than lenticular refractive surgery to produce unwanted optical aberrations. In this chapter, we review the optical principles discussed in BCSC Section 3 *(Clinical Optics)* as they apply to keratorefractive surgery.

Contribution of the Corneal Layers and Shape to the Optics of the Eye

The air–tear film interface provides the major optical power of the eye. The tear film itself has a relatively small optical effect unless an abnormality is present. For instance, in patients with epiphora, the tear meniscus may partially cover the pupil and cause blurred vision. In addition, an uneven tear meniscus may result in deterioration of the quality of vision.

The optical power of the eye derives primarily from the anterior corneal curvature, which produces approximately two thirds of the eye's refractive power, accounting for approximately +48.0 diopters (D). The overall corneal power is less (approximately +43.0 D) as a result of the negative power (−5.8 D) of the posterior corneal surface. Standard keratometers and corneal topography instruments measure the anterior corneal radius of curvature. Because the back corneal surface curvature and the exact refractive index are not measured, these instruments *estimate* total corneal power from front surface measurements.

By altering corneal shape, keratorefractive surgical procedures change the refractive status of the eye. The tolerances involved in altering corneal dimensions are relatively small. For instance, changing the refractive status of the eye by 2 D may require a shape change of less than 30 µm. Thus, achieving predictable results is sometimes problematic because minuscule changes in the shape of the cornea may produce large changes in refraction.

Another factor in corneal shape is that the central cornea is not spherical. The aspheric shape of the cornea generally reduces spherical aberration, minimizing refractive error fluctuations as the pupil changes size. When the central cornea is steeper than its periphery, the corneal shape is *prolate.* When the central cornea is flatter than its periphery, the corneal shape is *oblate.* Prolate corneas reduce spherical aberrations, while oblate corneas increase spherical aberrations.

Although most of the corneal optical zone is outside of the paraxial (central) region, this paraxial region may be the most optically important part of the cornea in patients undergoing refractive surgery. Flattening of the paraxial region of the cornea in conventional myopic excimer laser surgery may reverse its shape (from prolate to oblate), and steepening the paraxial region in hyperopia increases its prolateness.

Another consideration relating to corneal shape after conventional keratorefractive surgery is that while the surgery may reduce spherical refractive error and regular astigmatism, it often does so at the cost of increasing corneal surface irregularities. Keratorefractive surgery moves the location of the best focus closer to the retina but, at the same time, the rays do not necessarily meet at one point. This can be seen as irregular astigmatism by topography and as higher-order aberrations by wavefront analysis. Such irregular astigmatism causes many of the optical complications following keratorefractive surgery.

Computerized Corneal Topography

Corneal topography can be determined using keratoscopic images or using corneal elevation data. Keratoscopy images can be digitally captured and analyzed. Placido disk–based computerized topographers are the most commonly used. These units assume that the angle of incidence is nearly perpendicular to the corneal surface and that the radius of curvature is the distance from the surface to the intersection with the line of sight or visual axis of the patient *(axial distance).* Elevation-based topography instruments determine the initial shape using triangulation or other methods and then calculate the power map from the shape. Some topographers provide information regarding posterior corneal curvature, which may be especially useful in identifying patients with keratoconus and in the follow-up of patients with, or at risk of developing, corneal ectasia after LASIK surgery. For a more extensive discussion of other uses of computerized corneal topography, refer to BCSC Section 3 *(Clinical Optics)* and Section 8 *(External Disease and Cornea).*

Axial Power and Curvature

The curvature and power of the central 1 to 2 mm of the cornea can be closely approximated by the axial power and curvature indices. These indices, however, fail to describe the true shape and power of the peripheral cornea. Most normal corneas show decreasing dioptric power toward the periphery, as displayed by the Placido disk. Topographic maps displaying axial power and curvature provide an intuitive sense of the physiologic flattening of the cornea but do not represent the true refractive power or the true curvature of peripheral regions of the cornea.

Instantaneous Power and Curvature

A second method of describing the corneal curvature on Placido disk–based topography is to use the *instantaneous radius of curvature* (also called *tangential power*). This radius is determined by taking a perpendicular path through the point in question from a plane that intersects the point and the visual axis but allowing the radius to be the length necessary to correspond to a sphere with the same curvature at that point. The instantaneous radius of curvature, with curvature given in diopters, is estimated by the difference between the corneal index of refraction and 1.000 divided by this tangentially determined radius. The tangential map typically shows better sensitivity to peripheral changes with less "smoothing" of the curvature than the axial maps (Fig 1-1). (In these maps, diopters are relative units of curvature and not the equivalent of diopters of corneal power.)

Mean Curvature

A third map, the *mean curvature map,* does not require the perpendicular ray to cross the visual axis, allowing for an infinite number of spheres to fit the curvature at that point. The algorithm determines a minimum-size and maximum-size best-fit sphere and from their radii determines an average curvature (arithmetic mean of principal curvatures) known as the *mean curvature* for that point. These powers are then mapped using standard colors to represent diopter changes, allowing even more sensitivity to peripheral changes of curvature.

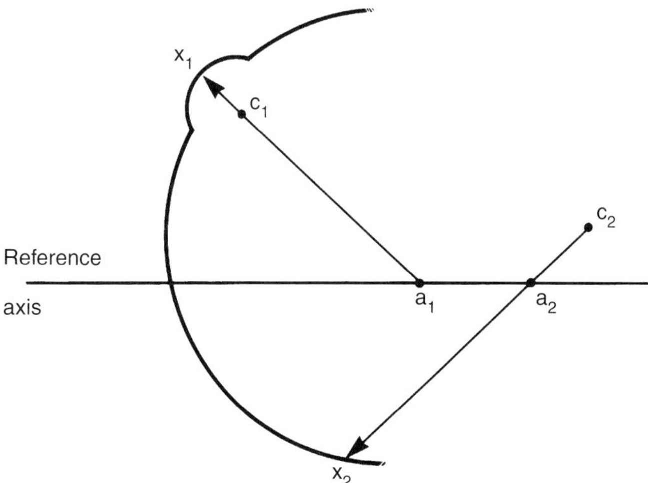

Figure 1-1 Axial and instantaneous corneal power (two dimensional). Axial curvature at points x_1 and x_2 is based on axial distances x_1 to a_1 and x_2 to a_2. Instantaneous curvature at points x_1 and x_2 is based on radii of curvature from x_1 to c_1 and x_2 to c_2. *(Illustration by Christine Gralapp.)*

Corneal Shape

Corneal shape can be indirectly described from Placido disk–based topography. A more direct approach is to derive corneal shape by means of scanning slits or rectangular grids and then to determine power from that shape.

In order to represent shape directly, maps may display a *z-height* from an arbitrary plane (iris plane, limbal plane, or frontal plane) using color maps. Just as viewing the curvature of the earth from beyond a certain scale fails to show details of mountains and basins, these *z* maps do not show clinically important variations. Geographic maps show land elevation relative to sea level. Similarly, corneal surface maps are plotted to show differences from best-fit spheres or other objects that closely mimic the normal corneal shape (Fig 1-2).

Elevation-based topography is especially helpful in refractive surgery for depicting the anterior and posterior surface shapes of the cornea and lens. Ray tracing can be used to plot an accurate refractive map of the corneal and lens surfaces. With such information, alterations to the shape of the eye structures can be determined with greater accuracy. The American National Standards Institute (ANSI) in the United States has developed standards for the corneal topography industry to make the comparison of maps more uniform and to clarify the confusion of terminology.

Other Features

In addition to power and elevation maps, computerized topographic systems may display other data: pupil size and location, indices estimating regular and irregular astigmatism, estimates of the probability of having keratoconus, simulated keratometry, and corneal asphericity. The asphericity of the cornea can be quantified by determining the Q value,

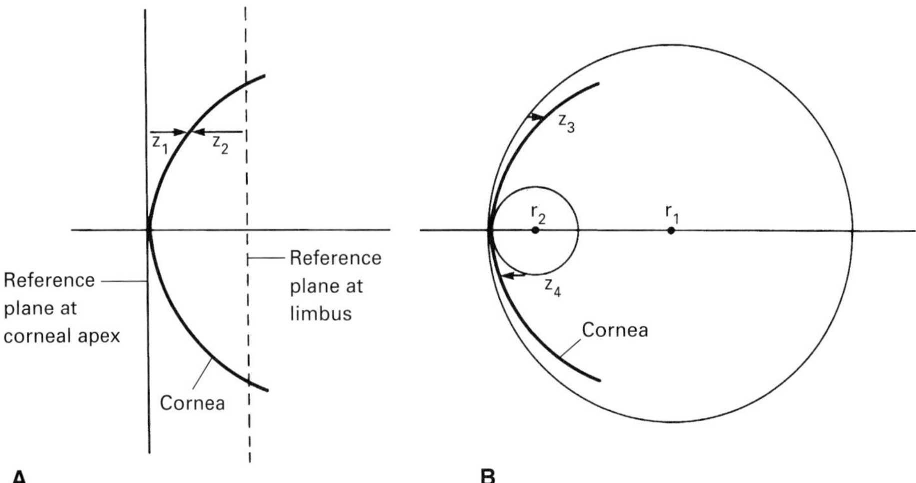

Figure 1-2 Height maps (typically in μm). **A,** Height is relative to plane surface; z_1 is below surface parallel to corneal apex; z_2 is above surface parallel to corneal limbus. **B,** Height relative to reference sphere; z_3 is below a flat sphere of radius r_1; z_4 is above a steep sphere of radius r_2. *(Illustration by Christine Gralapp.)*

with $Q = 0$ for spherical corneas, $Q < 0$ for prolate corneas, and $Q > 0$ for oblate corneas. Prolate corneas minimize the problem of spherical aberrations by virtue of the relatively flat peripheral curve. Conversely, oblate corneal contours, in which the peripheral cornea is steeper than the center, increase the problem of spherical aberrations. Following conventional refractive surgery for myopia, corneal asphericity increases in the oblate direction, which may cause degradation of the optics of the eye.

Indications for Corneal Topography in Refractive Surgery

Corneal topography is helpful in the preoperative evaluation of potential refractive surgical candidates. About two thirds of patients with normal corneas have a symmetric pattern that is round, oval, or bowtie-shaped (Fig 1-3). Asymmetric patterns include inferior steepening, superior steepening, asymmetric bowtie pattern, or other nonspecific irregularities.

Corneal topography detects irregular astigmatism, which may result from contact lens warpage, keratoconus and other thinning disorders, corneal surgery, trauma, and postinflammatory and degenerative conditions. Repeated topographic examinations may be helpful in clarifying the underlying etiology. Different values obtained at subsequent examinations can signal a change in corneal contour (if the eye and the instrument are aligned). Patients with corneal warpage (irregular astigmatism and/or peripheral steepening, distorted keratoscopic mires) benefit from discontinuation of contact lens wear to allow the corneal map and refraction to stabilize prior to refractive surgery. Patients with keratoconus are not routinely considered for refractive surgery, because the thin cornea has an unpredictable response and reducing its thickness may lead to progression of the keratoconus. Forme fruste, or subclinical, keratoconus recognized by Placido disk–based and elevation topography requires caution on the part of the ophthalmologist and is now considered to be a contraindication to certain refractive surgical procedures (eg, LASIK). Studies are under way to determine the suitability of other keratorefractive procedures (eg, intrastromal corneal ring segments) as an alternative therapeutic modality for these patients.

Corneal topography can also be used to demonstrate the effects of keratorefractive procedures. Pre- and postoperative maps may be compared to determine the achieved

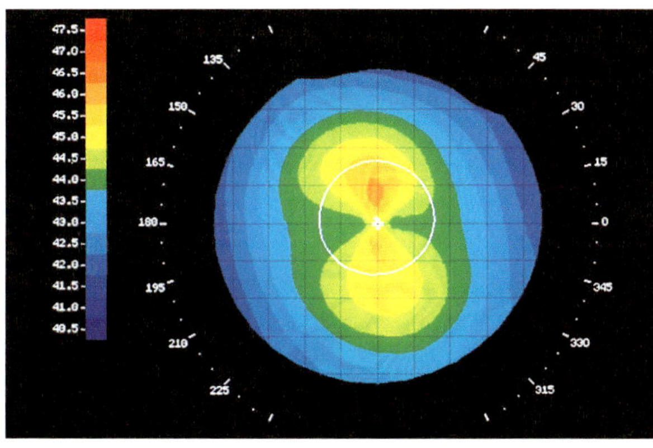

Figure 1-3 Keratography of normal cornea with regular astigmatism. White circle indicates pupil. *(Keratograph courtesy of Kirk R. Wilhelmus, MD.)*

refractive effect (difference map). Corneal mapping may help to explain unexpected results, including undercorrections, aberrations, induced astigmatism, or glare and haloes, by detecting decentered surgery or inadequate surgery such as shallow incisions in radial keratotomy. Corneal topography also confirms the expected physiologic effects of refractive surgery. For example, in radial keratotomy, difference maps may demonstrate the effect of peripheral incisions that lead to flattening of the central cornea associated with peripheral steepening (Fig 1-4).

Corneal Topography and Irregular Astigmatism

Regular astigmatism is correctable with spherocylindrical lenses. The traditional definition of irregular astigmatism is a form of astigmatism that is not correctable by spherocylindrical lenses. Irregular astigmatism can decrease the patient's best-corrected visual acuity and may cause contrast sensitivity loss. Depending on the magnitude of the irregularities, patients may have only vague complaints.

Irregular astigmatism can be diagnosed clinically, by corneal topography, or by wavefront analysis. Unlike glasses, which can only correct regular astigmatism, gas-permeable and hard contact lenses can correct visual acuity reductions resulting from corneal irregular astigmatism.

Clinically one important sign of postsurgical irregular astigmatism is a refraction inconsistent with the uncorrected acuity. Another clinical sign is when the refractionist is unable to determine the axis of astigmatism in a patient with a large cylinder. In contrast to patients with regular astigmatism, in whom it is easy to accurately determine the axis, a patient with irregular astigmatism following keratorefractive surgery may achieve nearly the same acuity with large powers of cylinder at markedly different axes.

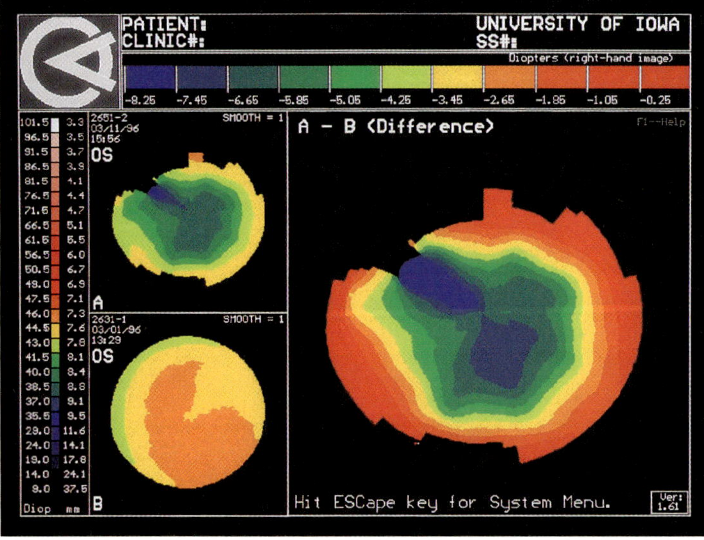

Figure 1-4 Difference map in radial keratotomy. Both central and peripheral flattening are seen in the postoperative image **(A)** and in the difference map on the right. **B** is the preoperative image.

Corneal topography is very helpful in the diagnosis of irregular astigmatism. Topographic changes include nonorthogonality of the steep and flat axes and hemimeridional asymmetry. Wavefront analysis (discussed later in chapter) often confirms the topographic findings in patients with irregular astigmatism, showing evidence of higher-order aberrations (such as coma, trefoil, tetrafoil, or secondary astigmatism). Wavefront analysis has the advantage of measuring various forms of higher-order aberration, thus allowing the clinician to quantitate irregular astigmatism in much the same way as we quantitate regular astigmatism.

The ability to differentiate regular and irregular astigmatism has clinical significance. There is presently no definitive refractive surgical treatment that effectively treats irregular astigmatism. In addition, astigmatic enhancements (such as by astigmatic keratotomy or LASIK) are rather unpredictable in patients with irregular astigmatism. While it is tempting to perform astigmatic enhancement on patients who had little preexisting astigmatism but have significant postoperative astigmatism, it may be prudent to avoid further intervention in patients who are satisfied with their postoperative uncorrected visual acuity. This is especially important after incisional surgery, where astigmatic enhancements may cause the axis to change dramatically (without much change in cylinder power) and may potentially worsen the uncorrected visual acuity.

Limitations of Corneal Topography

In addition to the limitations of the specific algorithms and the variations in terminology of various manufacturers, the accuracy of corneal topography may be affected by various potential problems:

- Tear film effects
- Distortions
- Misalignment (misaligned corneal topography may give a false impression of corneal apex decentration, suggestive of keratoconus)
- Stability (test-to-test variation)
- Sensitivity to focus errors
- Area of coverage (central and limbal)
- Nonstandardized data maps
- Map colors (may be absolute or varied [normalized])
- Decreased accuracy of corneal power simulation measurements (Sim K) after refractive surgical procedures

Clinical Situations Illustrating the Role of Corneal Topography in Refractive Surgery

Pellucid marginal degeneration

Pellucid marginal degeneration is an uncommon, nonhereditary, bilateral disease in which clear, inferior, peripheral corneal thinning is found in the absence of inflammation. Protrusion of the cornea occurs above the band of thinning. At times, a clear distinction between pellucid marginal degeneration and keratoconus is not possible. A cornea with keratoconus will show protrusion at the point of maximal thinning, but pellucid marginal degeneration can be superior or inferior and will show protrusion above the area of maximum thinning. No vascularization or lipid deposition occurs in pellucid marginal degeneration, but posterior stromal scarring has been noted within the thinned area. Decreased vision results from high irregular astigmatism. Corneal topography classically demonstrates high against-the-rule irregular astigmatism, with steepening nasally and temporally and circling inferiorly (see Figure 3-5). Refractive surgery should be avoided in this condition.

Keratoconus

Keratoconus (KC) is a progressive condition in which corneal thinning occurs in the central or paracentral cornea, resulting in asymmetrical corneal steepening and reduced spectacle-corrected visual acuity. The topography of keratoconic eyes typically shows two principal and unrelated shapes: a steep ectatic paracentral area that is disease dependent and a flatter superior paralimbal surface that is less affected by the disease. Refractive surgery is typically contraindicated in KC, although intrastromal corneal ring segments (Intacs) are being investigated in select cases of KC as an alternative to penetrating keratoplasty. The mainstay of treatment remains the rigid gas-permeable lens designed for KC.

It is the patient who will ultimately develop KC but has no obvious clinical signs of KC who poses the greatest difficulty in refractive surgical preoperative evaluations. Corneal topography may reveal subtle abnormalities that should alert the surgeon to this problem. The difference between inferior and superior corneal curvature can be measured by comparing the average curvature of 5 points below the horizontal and 5 equidistant points above the horizontal. This is known as the *I–S number.* The I–S number (normal <1.4 D; KC >1.9 D), central power (normal <47.2 D; KC >48.7 D), and corneal thinning, especially if the cornea is thin in the steep area on corneal topography, are helpful in estimating the likelihood of KC. Corneal thinning corresponding to the steepest zone on Placido disk–based topography and to the area of anterior bulging of the endothelial surface on Orbscan topography is also suggestive of KC. Several investigators obtain posterior float measurements to quantitate the extent of anterior bulging of the endothelial surface and use a measurement above 50 to 75 μm as suggestive of KC. LASIK surgery, when performed in patients having topographic features of KC, carries the risk of progressive keratectasia, which may be detrimental to the visual outcomes after surgery.

Post–penetrating keratoplasty

Corneal topography is very helpful in the management of postoperative astigmatism following penetrating keratoplasty. Complex peripheral patterns may result in a refractive axis of astigmatism that is not aligned with the topographic axis. Failure to correct the underlying shape by removing appropriate sutures or by operating on the appropriate axis may lead to unexpected results. The appropriate axis depends on the type of surgery (incisional surgery is done on the steep axis, compression sutures are placed on the flat axis, and minus cylinder surgery is done on the flat axis).

Wavefront Analysis

The wave theory of light has one of its major applications in wavefront analysis. Currently, wavefront analysis can be performed clinically by four methods: Hartmann-Shack, Tscherning, thin-beam single ray tracing, and optical path difference (Nidek), which combines retinoscopy with corneal topography. Each of these methods results in a detailed report of higher-order aberrations (the majority of which are associated with irregular astigmatism). This information is useful in refractive surgery both in explaining patients' symptoms and in aiding the calculation of custom ablations to correct problems or enhance vision.

Wavefront Analysis and Irregular Astigmatism

As discussed above, irregular astigmatism is usually caused by irregularities of corneal shape resulting from such factors as keratoconus, refractive surgery, penetrating keratoplasty, and scars following traumatic injury. Although irregular astigmatism follows no simple geometric form, it can still be described mathematically by the process of analytic extension (see BCSC Section 3, *Clinical Optics*, for more details).

For rotationally symmetrical corneas, paraxial rays focus at one point on the retina. Regular astigmatism results when paraxial rays are focused by toric optical systems. However, most of the rays passing through a lens are not paraxial. Whether or not the optical system is symmetrical, rays outside the paraxial region do not focus at one point on the retina.

Visually significant irregular astigmatism is a relatively uncommon problem typically associated with corneal grafts or scars requiring a gas-permeable contact lens for visual rehabilitation. Spectacles do not correct irregular astigmatism. Conventional (non–wavefront-guided) refractive surgery does not address higher-order aberrations; rather, it induces visually significant irregular astigmatism. Wavefront-guided keratorefractive surgery may, in principle, be able to treat preexisting optical aberrations. However, several obstacles need to be overcome before surgically induced optical aberration can be treated or prevented with high predictability.

Fermat's Principle and Wavefront Analysis

The most effective method developed to date for describing irregular astigmatism quantitatively is wavefront analysis. An optically perfect imaging system brings all rays from a single object point to a point focus. Fermat's principle states that this is possible only when the amount of time required for light to travel from the object point to the image point is identical for all possible paths the light might take. The light waves travel at the same speed in air and at the same (but slower) speed in glass or other homogeneous medium. If the rays do not reach the image point simultaneously, the image is astigmatic. Light waves going through the center of a biconvex (plus) lens, for instance, travel a short distance in air, but they are slowed down by moving through the thickest part of the lens. Light waves going through the edge of the lens travel a longer distance in air, but slow down only briefly when they traverse a thin section of glass. The shape of the ideal optical system precisely balances each path so that no matter what path the light travels, it reaches the image at the same time. Otherwise the focus is astigmatic.

Wavefront analysis measures the relative location of the light waves based on an arbitrary reference sphere. As the light waves converge to the focal point in an ideal optical system, they cross the reference sphere simultaneously. If the image is astigmatic, the light waves will cross the reference sphere at slightly different times. The *geometric wavefront* represents the position of the light waves relative to the reference sphere. In other words, in an optically perfect system, the reference sphere and the wavefront coincide so the wavefront aberration is zero.

Measurement of Wavefront Aberrations and Graphical Representations

There are several techniques for measuring wavefront aberrations clinically, but the most popular is based on the Hartmann-Shack wavefront sensor. In this device, a low-power laser beam is focused on the retina. A point on the retina then acts as a point source. In a perfect eye, all the rays would emerge in parallel and the wavefront would be a flat plane. In reality, the wavefront is not flat. An array of lenses samples parts of the wavefront and focuses light on a detector (Fig 1-5). The wavefront shape can be determined from the position of the focus on each detector.

There are different ways to represent wavefront aberrations. One approach is to represent the wavefront aberrations as three-dimensional shapes. This is currently the approach most commonly adopted for refractive surgery. Two-dimensional contour plots may become more popular in the future. In both systems, optical aberrations can be resolved into a variety of basic shapes, the combination of which represents the total aberration of the system, just as conventional refractive error is a combination of sphere and cylinder. Optical aberrations consisting of sphere and cylinder are considered lower-order (second-order) aberrations. Other optical aberrations are called higher-order ab-

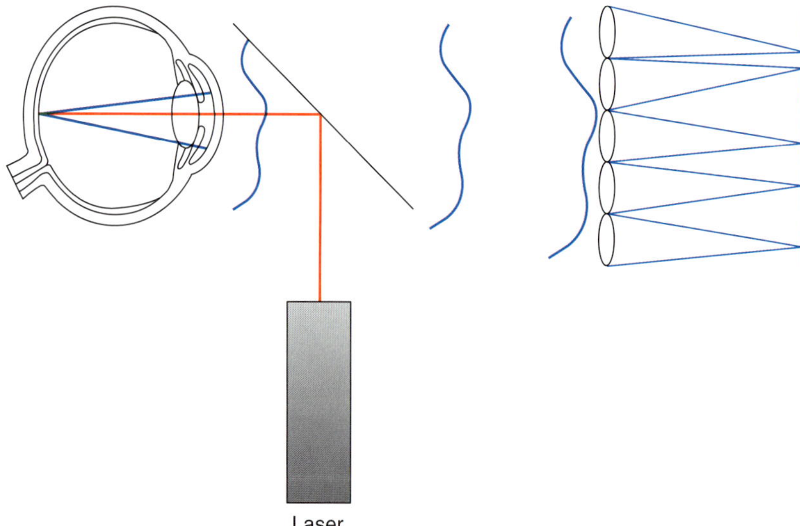

Figure 1-5 Schematic of a Hartmann-Shack wavefront sensor.

errations. By specifying the amount of each basic optical aberration, the total refractive error can be computed. Once we are familiar with the basic forms of optical aberration, there will be little need for three-dimensional graphs and two-dimensional contour plots. We will simply specify the amount of each basic form of optical aberration that is present in a given patient.

Currently, wavefront aberrations are specified by Zernike polynomials. Zernike polynomials are simply the mathematical formulas used to describe surfaces. The wavefront aberration surfaces are represented by three-dimensional graphs generated using Zernike polynomials and mathematical graphing software. Each aberration can induce a predictable reduction in the quality of the image (such as that of a Snellen E chart). It is estimated that a root mean square (RMS) error of 0.30 µm for an average aberration may result in a clinically significant reduction of Snellen acuity.

Lower-Order Aberrations

Myopia, hyperopia, and regular astigmatism can be expressed as wavefront aberrations. Myopia produces an aberration that optical engineers call *positive defocus* (Fig 1-6). Hyperopia is called *negative defocus.* Regular (cylindrical) astigmatism produces a wavefront aberration that has orthogonal and oblique components (Fig 1-7). Defocus and astigmatism are second-order aberrations. Other lower-order aberrations are non–visually significant aberrations known as first-order aberrations, such as vertical and horizontal prisms (Fig 1-8), and zero-order aberrations (piston).

Higher-Order Aberrations

Spherical aberrations

Wavefront aberration is a function of pupil position. When peripheral rays focus in front of more central rays, the effect is called *spherical aberration* (Fig 1-9). Clinically, this

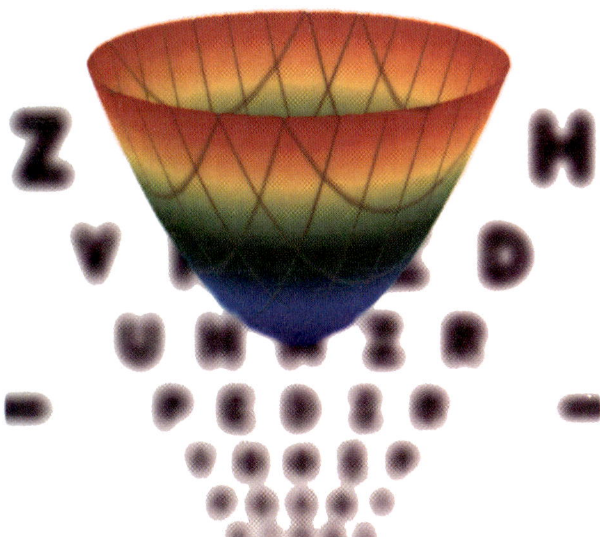

Figure 1-6 Zernike polynomial representation of defocus. *(Used with permission, Alcon Laboratories.)*

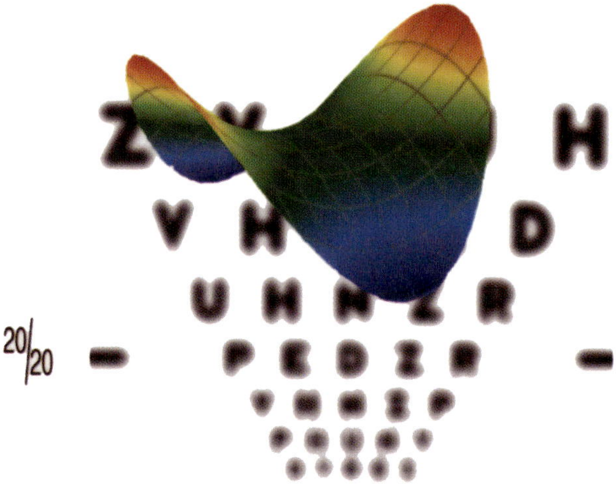

Figure 1-7 Representation of astigmatism using Zernike polynomials. *(Used with permission, Alcon Laboratories.)*

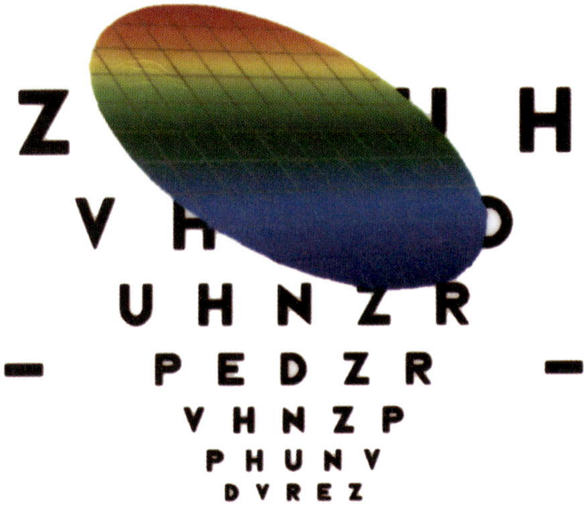

Figure 1-8 Representation of vertical prism using Zernike polynomials. *(Used with permission, Alcon Laboratories.)*

radially symmetrical fourth-order aberration is the cause of night myopia and is commonly seen after myopic LASIK and PRK.

Coma and trefoil

A common aberration after refractive surgery is called *coma*. In this third-order aberration, rays at one edge of the pupil cross the finish line first, while rays at the opposite edge of the pupil cross the finish line last. The effect is that the image of each object point resembles a comet, having vertical and horizontal components (Fig 1-10). Coma is common in patients with decentered corneal grafts, keratoconus, and decentered laser ablation.

Trefoil is another third-order aberration seen after refractive surgery. It seems to be less detrimental to the quality of the image as compared with coma of similar root mean square (RMS) magnitude (Fig 1-11).

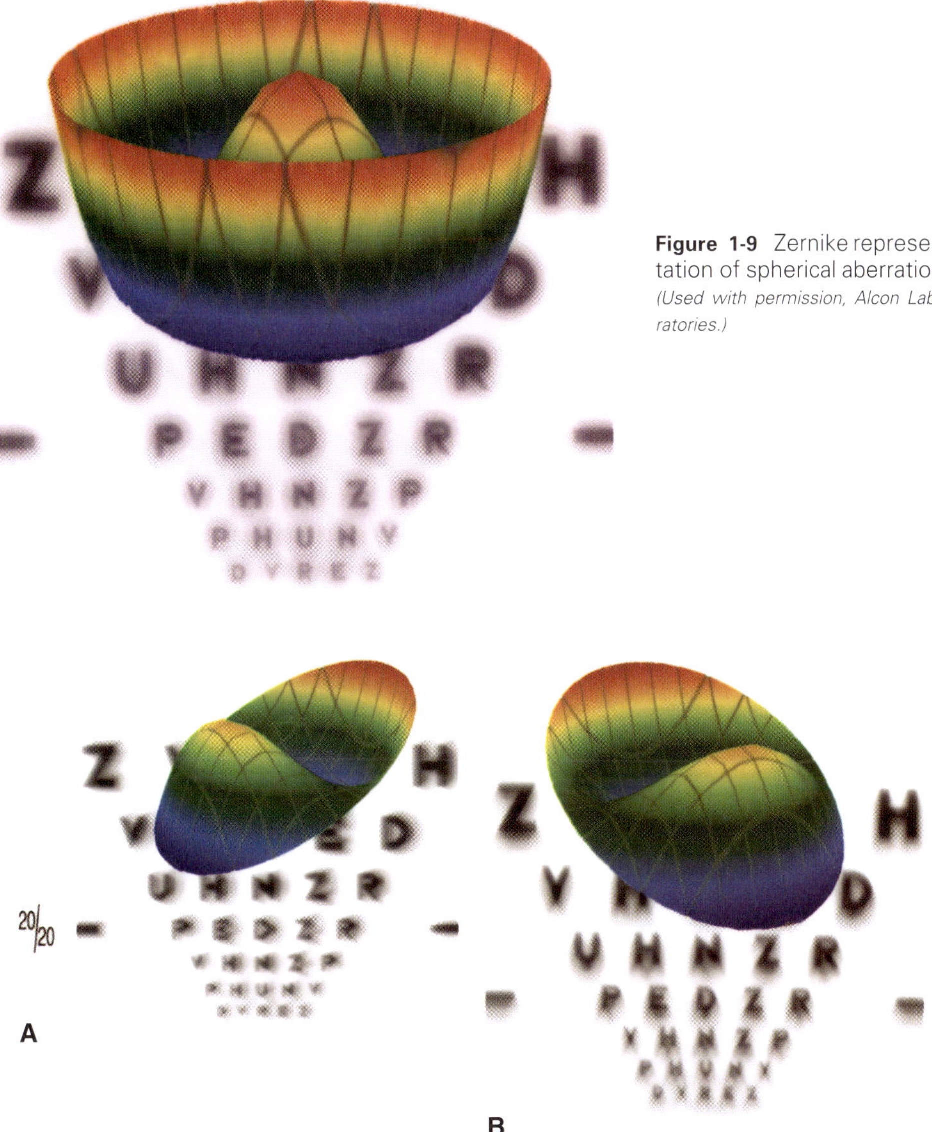

Figure 1-9 Zernike representation of spherical aberration. *(Used with permission, Alcon Laboratories.)*

Figure 1-10 Representation of horizontal coma **(A)** and vertical coma **(B)** using Zernike polynomials. *(Used with permission, Alcon Laboratories.)*

Other higher-order aberrations

Optical engineers have found that there are numerous basic types of astigmatism, of which only a small number are of clinical interest. Most patients after refractive surgery have a combination of these aberrations. *Secondary astigmatism* (Fig 1-12) and *quadrafoil* (Fig 1-13) are forms of fourth-order aberration with dramatically different effects on vision. As our knowledge of surgically induced aberration increases, more of the basic types of aberration may become clinically relevant.

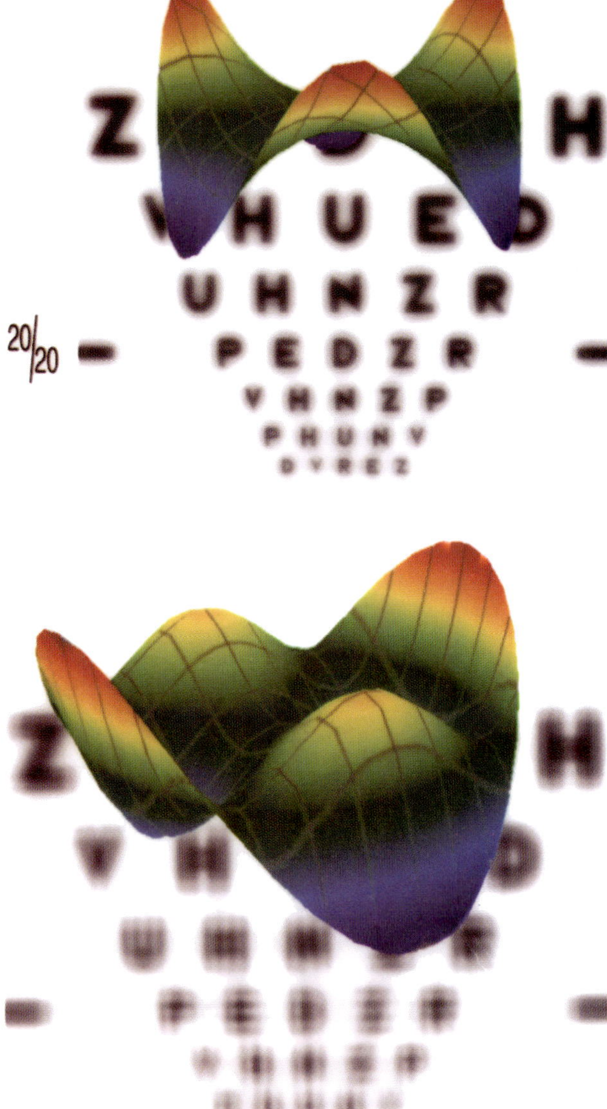

Figure 1-11 Zernike representation of trefoil. *(Used with permission, Alcon Laboratories.)*

Figure 1-12 Zernike representation of secondary astigmatism. *(Used with permission, Alcon Laboratories.)*

Biomechanics of the Cornea

The cornea is a composite material consisting of collagen fibrils that stretch from limbus to limbus, packaged in lamellae that are arranged in parallel fashion and embedded in an extracellular matrix of glycosaminoglycans. The layers slide easily over each other, indicating a very low shear resistance, but the stroma itself is an inelastic, anisotropic structure that distributes tensile stress unequally throughout its thickness, depending on the corneal hydration.

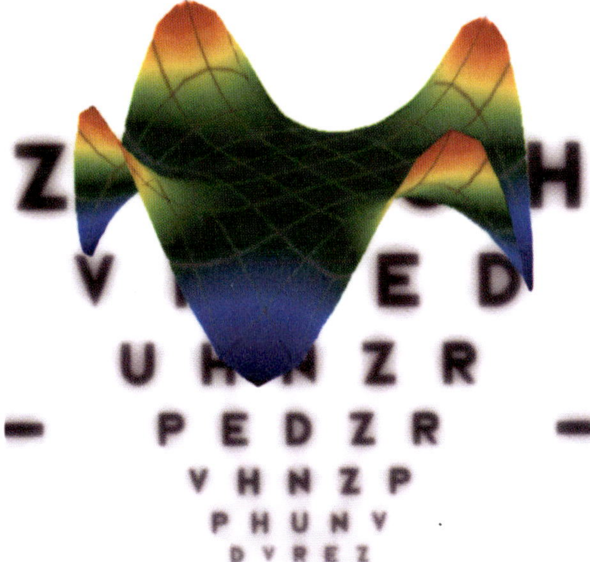

Figure 1-13 Zernike representation of quadrafoil. *(Used with permission, Alcon Laboratories.)*

When the cornea is in a dehydrated state, stress is distributed either principally to the posterior layers or uniformly over the entire structure. When the cornea is healthy or edematous, the anterior lamellae take up the strain. Stress within the tissue is partly related to IOP but not in a linear manner under physiologic conditions (normal IOP range).

Effects of Keratorefractive Surgery

Corneal refractive procedures can be classified as lamellar, keratotomy, keratectomy, collagen shrinkage, or penetrating keratoplasty (Table 1-1). These procedures can alter the corneal biomechanics in several ways:

- Incisional effect
- Tissue addition or subtraction
- Alloplastic material addition
- Laser effect
- Collagen shrinkage

Incisional effect

Incisions perpendicular to the corneal surface will predictably alter its shape, depending on direction, depth, location, and number. (See Chapter 4.) All incisions cause a local flattening of the cornea. Radial incisions lead to flattening in both the meridian of the incision and 90° away. Tangential (arcuate or linear) incisions (Fig 1-14) lead to flattening in the meridian of the incision, and steepening in the meridian 90° away that may be equal to or less than the magnitude of the decrease in the primary meridian; this phenomenon is known as *coupling* (see Figure 4-6).

The closer that radial incisions approach the visual axis (ie, the smaller the optical zone), the greater their effect; similarly, the closer that tangential incisions are placed to

Table 1-1 Classification of Corneal Refractive Surgery

Type of Refractive Surgery	Basic Surgical Technique	Variations of Surgical Technique or Material	Refractive Error Treated	Comment
Lamellar	Keratomileusis (cutting corneal disc with microkeratome)	Microkeratome techniques	Myopia, hyperopia, aphakia	
		• Manual or mechanical advance		
		• Oscillating or femtosecond laser		
		Method of making refractive stromal cut		
		• Barraquer's cryolathe		Historical
		• Excimer laser (ArF, 193 nm)		
		Source of tissue for disc		
		• Patient (autoplastic)		
		• Donor (homoplastic)		
	Laser in situ keratomileusis	Excimer laser	Myopia, hyperopia, astigmatism, high-order aberrations	FDA approved for −15.0 to +6.0 D; astigmatism to 6.0 D; most surgeons do not use for highest limits
	Epikeratoplasty	Human donor lenticule	Aphakia, hyperopia, astigmatism, myopia, keratoconus	Rarely used
		• Cryolathe		
		• Lyophilized		
		Synthetic (eg, collagen and coated hydrogel)		
	Intracorneal lens or ring	Microkeratome (lamellar bed)		
		• Hydrogel lenticule	Myopia, hyperopia	Clinical trials for hyperopia
		Lamellar pocket		
		• High index of refraction (eg, fenestration polysulfone)	Aphakia	
		Intracorneal ring segments (Intacs)	Myopia	FDA approved for −1.0 to −3.0 D
			Keratoconus, ectasia	FDA approved under HDE

(Continued)

Table 1-1 Classification of Corneal Refractive Surgery (Continued)

Type of Refractive Surgery	Basic Surgical Technique	Variations of Surgical Technique or Material	Refractive Error Treated	Comment
Keratotomy	Radial	Nomogram-based Staged with repeated adjustments	Myopia	Rarely used
	Astigmatic (transverse keratotomy, arcuate keratotomy, limbal relaxing incisions)	Straight (T cuts)	Astigmatism: primary (naturally occurring); compound myopic astigmatism	Incision made in the steep corneal meridian (axis of plus refractive cylinder); rarely used
		Modification of penetrating keratoplasty (arcuate keratotomy) • Wound separation or incision in wound • Arcuate incision in donor	Postoperative astigmatism	Often staged under keratoscopic or keratometric control
	Astigmatic	Modification of cataract surgery • Intraoperative ▪ Limbal relaxing incision	Astigmatism	Limbal or corneal, cataract incision acts like arcuate keratotomy
Keratectomy	Laser	Photorefractive keratectomy • Excimer laser (ArF, 193 nm) • Wavefront-guided • 5th harmonic Nd:YAG laser (213 nm)	Myopia, astigmatism, hyperopia • Primary (naturally occurring) • Secondary (eg, after radial keratotomy, epikeratoplasty, penetrating keratoplasty)	FDA approved for −13.0 to +6.0 D; astigmatism to −4.0 D; most surgeons do not use for highest limits
		Intrastromal photodisruption • Picosecond • Femtosecond	Myopia	In laboratory development

(Continued)

Table 1-1 Classification of Corneal Refractive Surgery (Continued)

Type of Refractive Surgery	Basic Surgical Technique	Variations of Surgical Technique or Material	Refractive Error Treated	Comment
Keratectomy *(continued)*	Mechanical	Crescentic wedge • Wedge resection after penetrating keratoplasty	Astigmatism	Limited use
Collagen shrinkage	Noncontact: holmium YAG laser (2.06 μm)	Radial or circular pattern	Hyperopia	FDA approved for +0.75 to +2.5 D
		Treatment in flat meridian with or without concurrent treatment for hyperopia	Astigmatism	In clinical trials
	Contact	Peripheral, intrastromal, radial pattern	Hyperopia	Seldom used
	Conductive keratoplasty	Radio frequency	Hyperopia	FDA approved for +0.75 to +3.25 D
Penetrating keratoplasty (refractive aspects)	Donor–host size disparity	Donor oversized	Hyperopia, aphakia	
		Donor undersized	Myopia, keratoconus	
	Suture adjustment during or after surgery	Selective removal or interrupted sutures in steep meridian Adjustment of running suture Early opening of wound in steep meridian Early placement of interrupted sutures in flat meridian		
		Endothelial replacement only (with flap or from posterior)	Reduced anterior curvature	In clinical trials

(Updated from Waring GO III. Making sense of keratospeak IV: classification of refractive surgery. *Arch Ophthalmol.* 1992;110:1385–1391. For IOL implants, see BCSC Section 11, *Lens and Cataract.*)

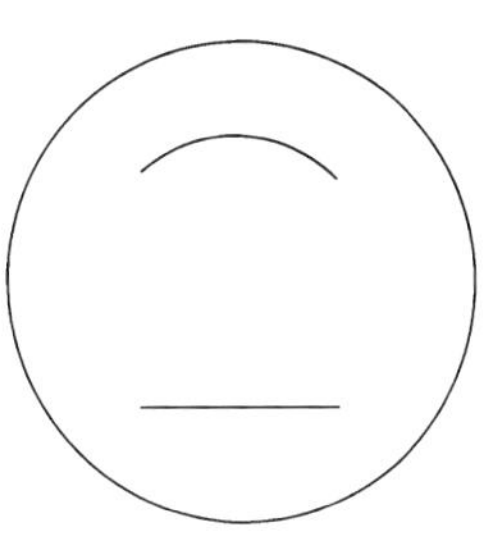

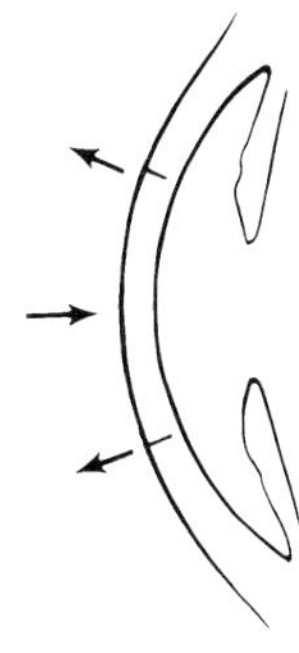

Figure 1-14 Tangential incisions (astigmatic keratotomy): schematic arcuate *(above)* and transverse *(below)* incision. The peripheral cornea bulges in the axis perpendicular to the keratotomy.

the visual axis, the greater the effect. The longer a radial incision, the greater its effect until approximately an 11 mm diameter is achieved, and then the effect reverses. The larger the angle severed by the tangential incision, the greater the effect.

For optimum effect, an incision should be 85%–90% deep to allow an intact posterior lamellae and maximum anterior bowing of the other lamellae. Nomograms for numbers of incisions and optical zone size can be calculated based on finite element analysis, but they are typically generated empirically. The important variables for radial and astigmatic surgery include patient age and number, depth, and length of incisions. IOP and preoperative corneal curvature are not significant predictors of effect.

The effect of incisional surgery is dependent to a great extent on the hydration of the stroma and less on the IOP (Fig 1-15). A hyperopic refractive shift can occur in patients exposed to high altitude or low pO_2 following radial keratotomy as a result of swelling in the vicinity of the wound. Daily fluctuation in refraction (typically hyperopic in the morning) in patients with radial keratotomy may also be related to stromal hydration effects rather than to diurnal variation in IOP.

Tissue addition or subtraction

Lamellar surgery also alters the biomechanics of the cornea. *Keratomileusis* was originated by Barraquer as "carving" of the anterior surface of the cornea. It is defined as a method of modifying the spherical or meridional surfaces of a healthy cornea by tissue subtraction. Tissue subtraction may be performed on the surface, by PRK (Fig 1-16), or intrastromally, by LASIK (Fig 1-17). (See Chapter 6.) The critical uncut depth of the cornea necessary to maintain normal integrity has not been determined but is presumed to be at least 250 to 300 µm or 50% of the stromal depth.

Epikeratoplasty (sometimes called epikeratophakia) adds carved donor tissue to the surface to cause hyperopic or myopic changes (Fig 1-18). *Keratophakia* requires the addition of a tissue lenticule or synthetic inlay intrastromally. (See Chapter 5.)

Alloplastic material addition

The biomechanics of the cornea can be altered by adding alloplastic material such as hydrogel on the surface or into the corneal stroma to effect a change in the anterior shape or the refractive index of the cornea (Fig 1-19). For example, the two arc segments of an *intrastromal corneal ring* can be placed in two pockets of the stroma to directly alter the surface contour based on the profile of the individual rings (Fig 1-20). These rings

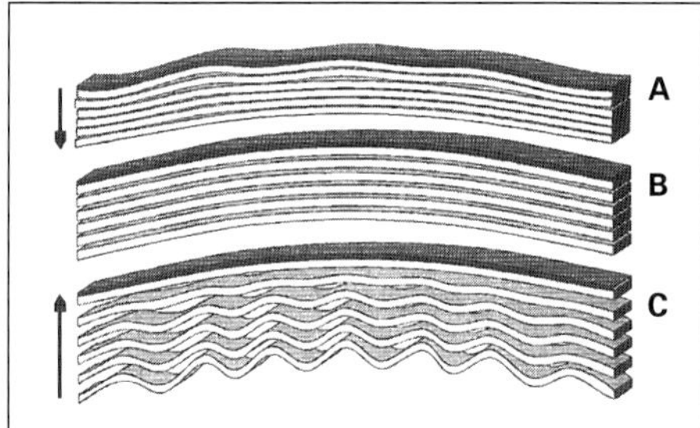

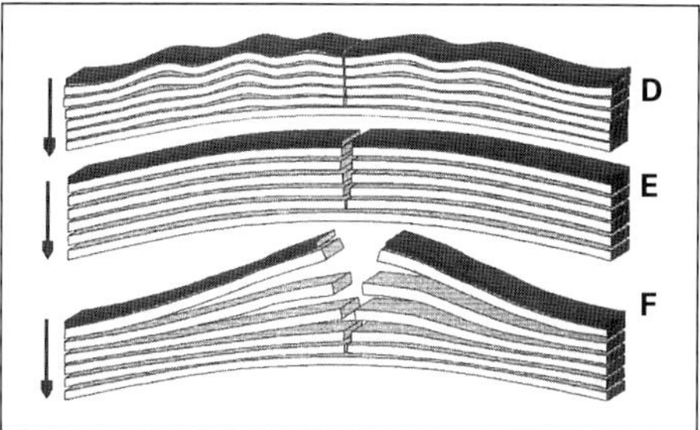

Figure 1-15 Diagram of the corneal stress model. For unoperated eyes, the anterior curvature is not affected by IOP or corneal hydration as a result of the inelasticity of the cornea. However, the stress in the cornea is displaced posteriorly **(A)** or uniformly **(B)** when dehydrated and is anteriorly displaced in a normal or hydrated cornea **(C)**. After radial keratotomy, the anterior curvature remains either unchanged or mildly affected when in dehydrated **(D)** or normally hydrated **(E)** states. The anterior lamellae remain closely packed, and the inelastic nature of the intact posterior lamellae prevents changes in the shape of the cornea. When hydration increases, the loose anterior stroma absorbs water (swells) and the stress attempts to move anteriorly. However, since these layers have been cut, the cornea flattens its curvature and the posterior lamellae retain their shape by holding the stresses **(F)**. *(Reprinted with permission from Simon G, Ren Q. Biomechanical behavior of the cornea and its response to radial keratotomy.* J Refract Corneal Surg. *1994;10:349.)*

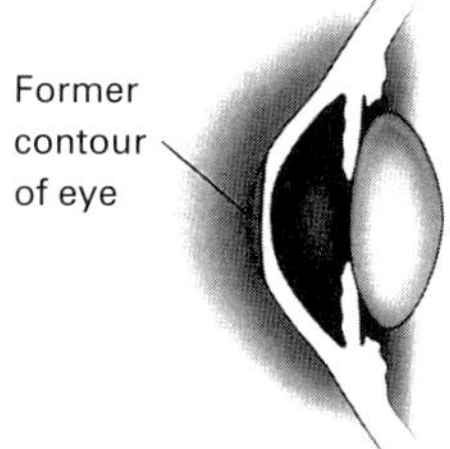

Figure 1-16 PRK for myopia.

do not work by changing the circumferential measurement of the cornea (ie, by spreading the peripheral cornea to flatten the center); rather, the manufacturer suggests that the rings work by stiffening or stretching the cornea, much as a hammock spreader tightens and gives shape to the sagging mesh. (See Chapter 5.)

Laser effect

PRK of the anterior surface is limited in the depth that can be removed while still avoiding the complications of forward bowing and scarring. For low amounts of correction (<7 D), the amount of tissue to remove centrally is estimated by Munnerlyn's formula:

> Ablation depth in micrometers (μm) approximately equals diopters (D) of myopia multiplied by the square of the optical zone (mm), divided by 3.

Clinical experience has confirmed that the effective change is independent of the initial curvature of the cornea, although other formulas have been proposed that take into account preoperative curvature. Munnerlyn's formula also highlights some of the problems and limitations of PRK. The amount of ablation increases by the square of the

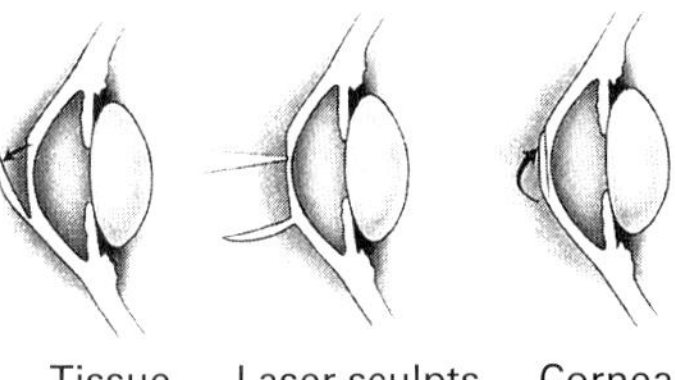

Figure 1-17 LASIK for myopia.

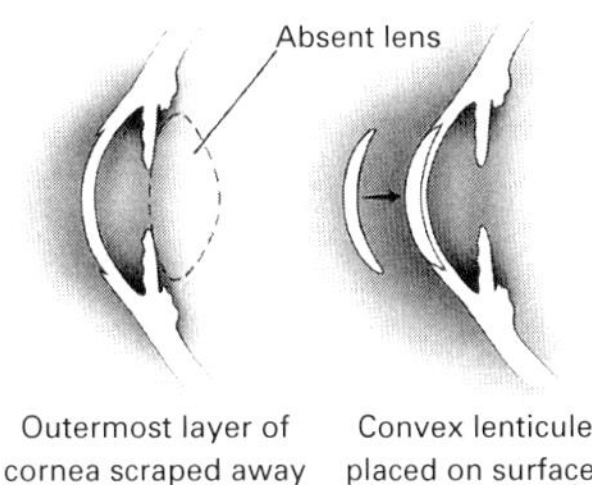

Figure 1-18 Epikeratoplasty for aphakia or hyperopia.

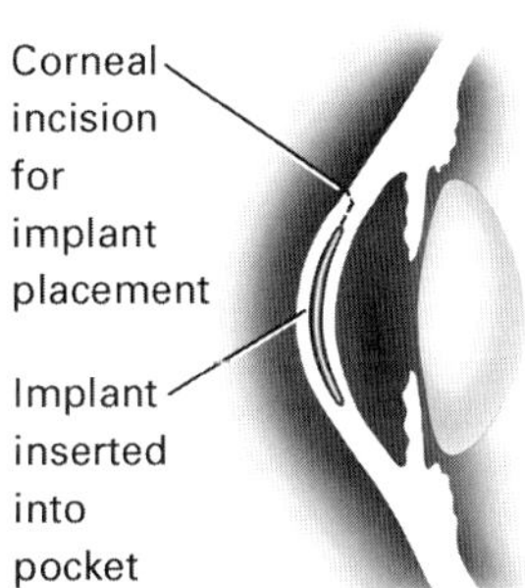

Figure 1-19 Intrastromal hydrogel implant. *(Illustration by Jeanne Koelling.)*

optical zone, but the complications of glare, haloes, and regression increase when the optical zone decreases. To reduce these side effects, the optical zone should be 6 mm or larger.

Multizone keratectomies use several concentric optical zones to generate the total refraction required. This method can provide the full correction centrally, while the tapering peripheral zones reduce symptoms and allow higher degrees of myopia to be treated. For example, 12 D of myopia can be treated as follows: 6 D are corrected with a 4.5 mm optical zone, 3 D with a 5.5 mm optical zone, and 3 D with a 6.5 mm optical zone (Fig 1-21). Thus, the total 12 D correction is achieved in the center using a

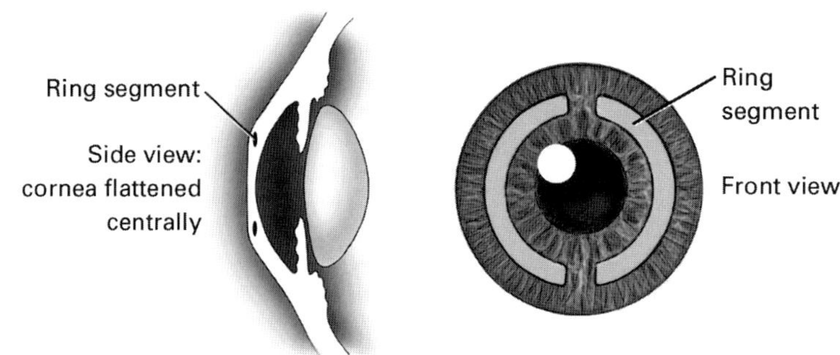

Figure 1-20 Intrastromal corneal ring segments. *(Illustration by Jeanne Koelling.)*

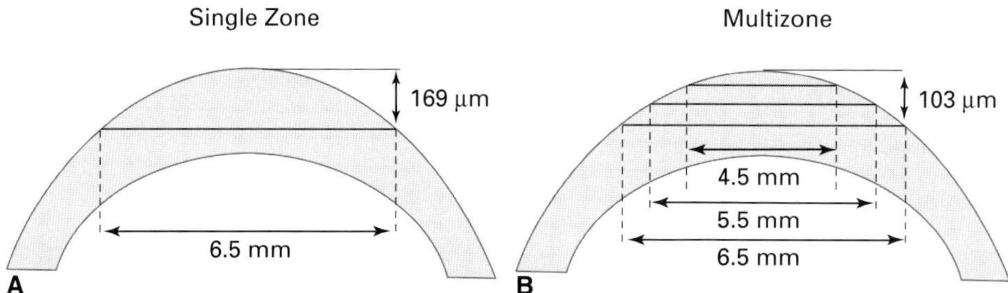

Figure 1-21 Multizone keratectomies. **A,** Depth of ablation required to correct 12 D of myopia in a single pass. **B,** Figure demonstrates how use of multiple zones reduces the ablation depth required. *(Illustration by C. H. Wooley.)*

shallower ablation depth than would be necessary for a single pass (103 μm instead of 169 μm). Similarly, *bitoric ablations* (combining a myopic with a hyperopic ablation profile) can minimize ablation depth and provide a more physiologic postoperative topography (Fig 1-22).

LASIK combines a lamellar incision with ablation of the cornea, typically in the stromal bed (see Figure 1-17). The same theoretical limits for residual posterior cornea apply as with PRK, and the calculated effect is based on a modification of Munnerlyn's formula empirically. To reduce the complications of surface irregular astigmatism, the flap is typically cut 130 to 180 μm thick. The thickness and diameter of the LASIK flap depend on instrumentation, corneal diameter, corneal curvature, and corneal thickness. Flatter corneas require smaller diameter and thinner flaps.

Hyperopic PRK and LASIK use a similar formula for determining the maximum ablation depth, but the ablation zone is much larger than the optical zone (Fig 1-23). The zone of maximal ablation coincides with the outer edge of the optical zone. A transition zone of ablated cornea is necessary to blend the edge of the optical zone to the peripheral cornea.

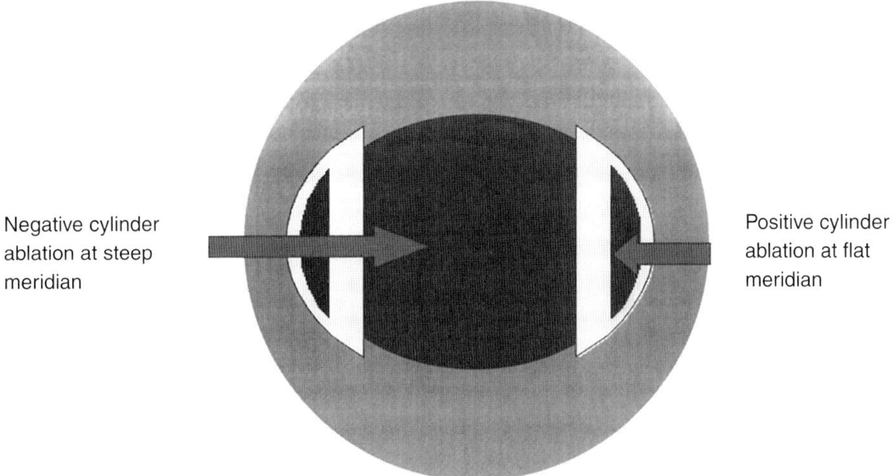

Figure 1-22 Bitoric ablation. *(From Chayet AS, Montes M, Gomez L. Bitoric laser in situ keratomileusis for the correction of simple myopic and mixed astigmatism.* Ophthalmology. *2001;108:304.)*

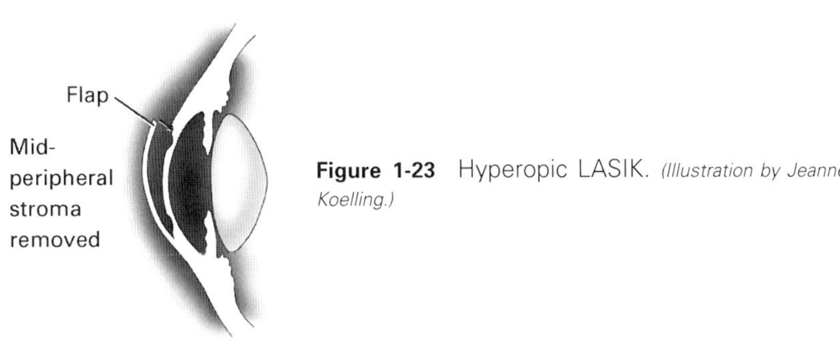

Figure 1-23 Hyperopic LASIK. *(Illustration by Jeanne Koelling.)*

Collagen shrinkage

Alteration in corneal biomechanics can also be achieved by shrinkage of collagen. Heating collagen to a critical temperature of 55° to 60° C will cause it to shrink, inducing changes in the corneal curvature. *Thermokeratoplasty* and *conductive keratoplasty* are avoided in the central cornea because of scarring but can be used in the midperiphery (Fig 1-24). (See Chapter 7.) Collagen can be heated ab externo with a holmium laser in thermokeratoplasty (Sunrise Hyperion) or directly with a radiofrequency diathermy probe in conductive keratoplasty (Refractec).

Shrinkage can also be performed in a linear manner to induce central flattening and correct myopia, but no clinical trials have been conducted. If the temperature is too high,

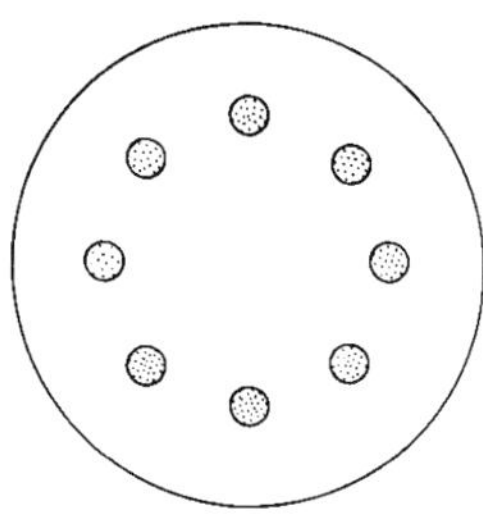

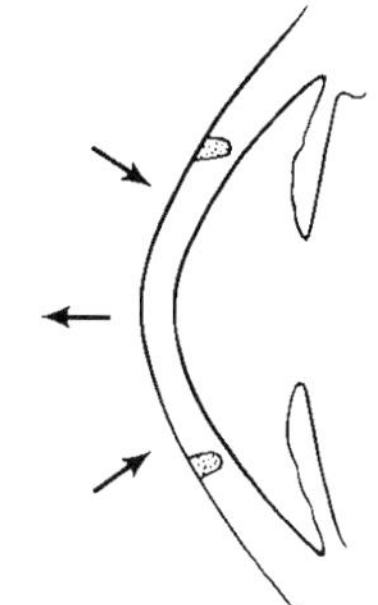

Figure 1-24 Thermokeratoplasty and conductive keratoplasty: heat shrinks the peripheral cornea, causing central steepening.

local necrosis will occur, and if the source of heat is nonuniform or nonuniformly applied, irregular astigmatism will be induced.

Corneal Wound Healing

All forms of keratorefractive surgery are exquisitely dependent on the process of corneal wound healing. Satisfactory results after refractive surgery require either modifying or reducing wound healing or exploiting normal wound healing for the benefit of the patient. For example, astigmatic keratotomy requires initial weakening followed by permanent healing with replacement of the epithelial plugs with collagen and remodeling of the collagen to ensure stability and to avoid long-term hyperopic drift. PRK requires the epithelium to heal quickly with minimal stimulation of the underlying keratocytes, to avoid corneal scar and haze. Lamellar keratoplasty requires intact epithelium and healthy endothelium early in the postoperative period to sear the flap; later, the cornea must heal in the periphery to secure the carp in place and to avoid late-term displacement while minimizing irregular astigmatism.

Our understanding of corneal wound healing has advanced tremendously with recognition of the multiple factors involved in a cascade of events initiated by corneal wounding. The cascade is somewhat dependent on the nature of the injury. Injury to the epithelium can lead to loss of underlying keratocytes from apoptosis. The remaining keratocytes respond by generating new glycosaminoglycans and collagen, to a degree dependent on the duration of the epithelial defect and the depth of the stromal injury. The tendency toward haze formation is greater with deeper ablations and prolonged absence of the epithelium. Despite loss of Bowman's layer, normal or even enhanced numbers of hemidesmosomes and anchoring fibrils form to secure the epithelium to the stroma.

Controversy persists over the value of different agents for modulating wound healing in PRK. Typically, clinicians in the United States use corticosteroids in a tapering manner following surgery to reduce inflammation. Other anti-inflammatory agents have also been tried with no established effect. Mitomycin has been applied to the stromal bed after excimer ablation to attempt to decrease haze formation (see Chapter 6). Other agents, such as transforming growth factor-β have been proposed, but no information on their value is yet available.

Haze formation does not seem to occur following lamellar keratoplasty, which may be related either to lack of significant epithelial injury and the consequent subcellular signaling or to the maintenance of some intact surface neurons. Lamellar surgery shows very little long-term evidence of healing between the disrupted lamellae and only typical stromal healing at the peripheral wound. The lamellae are initially held in position by negative stromal pressure generated by the endothelial cells aided by an intact epithelial surface. Even at 1 year, the lamellar interface can be broken and the flap lifted, indicating that only a minimal amount of healing occurs.

Aberrant healing can occur if the flap is placed with wrinkles (striae) or if epithelium grows into the interface. Epithelium in the interface acts as a barrier to nutrient flow and must be removed at any sign of thinning, inflammation, or obstruction of the visual axis. Interface debris can lead to inflammation or light scattering and should be minimized at the time of surgery. Epikeratoplasty from donor stroma will slowly repopulate host keratocytes.

Laser Biophysics

Laser–Tissue Interactions

Three laser–tissue interactions are exploited for keratorefractive surgery. *Photothermal* effects are achieved by focusing a holmium:YAG laser with a wavelength of 2.13 µm into the anterior stroma. The laser beam is absorbed by water, causing collagen shrinkage from heat. This technique is approved by the FDA for treating low hyperopia.

Photodisruption uses picosecond Nd:YAG or Nd:YLF lasers to perform intrastromal ablations by means of optical breakdown within the corneal stroma and vaporization of tissue. The laser–tissue interaction is entirely intrastromal, and its refractive effect depends on collapse of the tissue above it. The picosecond lasers, however, create large cavities of photodisruption. This disadvantage can be avoided by using the femtosecond laser (IntraLase), in which the cavities of photodisruption are microscopic. The femtosecond laser is also approved by the FDA for creating corneal flaps for LASIK.

Photoablation, the most important laser–tissue interaction in refractive surgery, breaks chemical bonds using excimer (for "excited dimer") lasers or other lasers of the appropriate wavelength. Laser energy of more than 4 eV per photon is sufficient to break carbon-nitrogen or carbon-carbon tissue bonds. Argon-fluoride (ArF) lasers are excimer lasers that use electrical energy to stimulate argon to form dimers with the caustic fluorine gas. They generate a wavelength of 193 nm with 6.4 eV per photon. The 193 nm light is in the ultraviolet C (high ultraviolet) range, approaching the wavelength of x-rays. In addition to having high energy per photon, light at this end of the electromagnetic spectrum also has very low tissue penetrance and thus is suitable for operating on the surface of tissue. Not only is the laser energy capable of great precision, with little thermal spread in tissue, but its lack of penetrance or lethality to cells makes the 193 nm laser nonmutagenic, enhancing its safety. (DNA mutagenicity occurs in the range of 250 nm.) Solid-state lasers have been designed to generate wavelengths of light near 193 nm without the need for toxic gas, but the technical difficulties in manufacturing these lasers have limited their clinical use.

Types of Photoablating Lasers

Photoablating lasers can be divided into broad-beam lasers, scanning-slit lasers, and flying-spot lasers. *Broad-beam lasers* rely on internal optics to create a smooth and homogeneous multimode laser beam of up to approximately 7 mm in diameter. They have very high energy per pulse and require a small number of pulses to ablate the cornea. *Scanning-slit lasers* use excimer technology to generate a narrower slit beam that is scanned over the surface of the tissue to alter the photoablation profile, improving the smoothness of the ablated cornea and allowing for larger-diameter ablation zones. *Flying-spot lasers* use smaller-diameter beams (0.9 to 2.0 mm) that are scanned at a higher rate but require a tracking mechanism for precise placement to create the desired pattern of ablation. Broad-beam lasers and some scanning-slit lasers require an iris or other masking device to create the desired shape in the cornea. The flying-spot lasers and some of the scanning-slit lasers use the pattern projected onto the surface to create the desired laser ablation profile without masking.

Wavefront-Guided Laser Ablation

In wavefront-guided laser ablation, information obtained from a wavefront-sensing aberrometer (which quantifies the aberrations) is transferred electronically to the treatment laser in order to program the laser ablation. This is distinct from conventional excimer lasers in which the subjective refraction is used to program the laser ablation. The wavefront-guided laser uses an active tracking system, which stabilizes the eye during treatment and allows the delivery of the customized ablation profile. The wavefront-guided laser attempts to treat both the lower-order (myopia or hyperopia and/or astigmatism) and the higher-order aberrations.

Wavefront-guided lasers apply complex ablation patterns to the cornea to correct wavefront deviations from a desired final corneal shape. The correction of higher-order aberrations requires non–radially symmetric patterns of ablation (which are often much smaller in magnitude than ablations needed to correct defocus and astigmatism). Based on the difference between the desired and the actual wavefront, a three-dimensional map of the ablation is generated. Until the surgically induced wavefront changes can be predicted with certainty, wavefront-guided treatments will remain predominantly limited to the correction of preexisting higher-order aberrations.

Gatinel D, Hoang-Xuan T, Azar DT. Determination of corneal asphericity after myopia surgery with the excimer laser: a mathematical model. *Invest Ophthalmol Vis Sci.* 2001;42: 1736–1742.

Krueger R, Applegate R, MacRae S. *Wavefront Customized Visual Correction: The Quest for Super Vision.* 2nd ed. Thorofare, NJ: Slack, Inc; 2003.

CHAPTER 2

The Role of the FDA in Refractive Surgery

The field of refractive surgery is uniquely dependent on rapidly changing technology that dictates surgical technique. Many of the investigational devices discussed in the following chapters will receive Food and Drug Administration (FDA) approval by the time this book is published. Other "promising" devices or techniques may have already fallen out of favor.

Because of the continual introduction of new devices to the U.S. market, the FDA approval process has particular influence in refractive surgery. Therefore we have included this brief introduction to the FDA approval process. Table 2-1 gives a list of FDA-approved lasers for refractive surgery, as of December 2003. The most current list can be found on the Web at www.fda.gov/cdrh/LASIK/lasers.htm.

The FDA

The scope of the FDA's work is established by legislation. The Food, Drug, and Cosmetic Act passed by Congress in 1938 required for the first time that companies prove the safety of new drugs before putting them on the market and required regulation of cosmetics and therapeutic devices. The Medical Device Amendments of 1976 authorized the FDA to ensure that medical devices are safe and effective before they come to market in the United States. This Amendment also provided for classification of medical devices into three categories depending on potential risk of the device, established three pathways to market, and established advisory panels to assist the FDA in the review of devices. The Ophthalmic Devices Panel reviews, and votes on approval of, marketing applications for ophthalmic devices with new technologies, devices with new indications for use, or those devices that raise significant issues of safety and effectiveness, before such devices are granted FDA approval.

Device Classification

Class I devices (eg, refractometers, perimeters, wavefront aberrometers, sunglasses) are usually considered minimal-risk devices. These devices are subject to general controls by the FDA, such as current good manufacturing practice regulations and prohibitions

Table 2-1 Refractive Laser PMA/HDE Approvals as of November 21, 2003

Doc #	Sponsor	Ap'd Date	Device	Indications (Range)
P9 10062	**VISX**	9-29-1995	Mdl B & C (Star & Star S2)	PTK procedures indicated for subjects with decreased BCVA and/or with disabling pain that are the result of superficial corneal irregularities or stromal scars. For examples of those conditions that may warrant PTK, see the SSED.
P930016	VISX	3-27-1996	Mdl B & C (Star & Star S2)	PRK, myopia: 0 to −6.00 D SPH
P930016/S3	VISX	4-24-1997	Mdl B & C (Star & Star S2)	PRK, myopia: 0 to −6.00 D SPH and −0.75 to −4.00 D CYL
P930016/S5	VISX	1-29-1998	Mdl B & C (Star & Star S2)	PRK, myopia: 0 to −12.00 D SPH and 0 to −4.00 D CYL
P930016/S7	VISX	11-2-1998	Star S2	PRK, hyperopia: +1.00 to +6.00 D
P990010	CRS/VISX	11-19-1999	Star S2	LASIK, myopia: *(See CRS/VISX P990010):* 0.00 to −14.00 D SPH and −0.5 to −5.0 D CYL. NLO
P990010/S1	VISX	04-20-2000	Star S3 (EyeTracker)	Same as S2, except with eye tracker
P930016/S10	VISX	10-18-2000	Star S2 & S3	PRK, hyperopia +0.5 to +5.0 D SPH and +0.5 to +4.0 D CYL with ≤ +6.0 D MRSE
P930016/S13	VISX	03-19-2001	Star S2 & S3	Add myopia blend zone: 6.5 mm to 8.0 mm
P930016/S12	VISX	04-27-2001	Star S2 & S3	**LASIK-Hyperopic Astigmatism**: hyperopia +0.5 to +5.0 D SPH w/ or w/o astig up to +3.0 D, with ≤6.0 D MRSE. NLO
P930016/S14	VISX	11-06-2001	Star S2 & S3	**LASIK-Mixed Astigmatism**: magnitude of cylinder (≤6.0 D at the spectacle plane) is greater than the magnitude of sphere, and the cylinder and sphere have opposite signs.
P930016/S16	VISX	05-23-2003	S4 & WaveScan Syst	**Wavefront-guided LASIK**: myopic astig up to −6.00 D MRSE w/Cyl ≤ −3.00 D. LO > −6 D. 6.0 mm OZ; 8.0 mm TZ.
H000002	VISX	12-19-2001	Star S3	C-CAP (Custom Contoured Ablation Pattern) Method ™ for the treatment of certain patients (see SSED) with symptomatic decentered ablations from previous laser surgery as viewed on the Zeiss Humphrey® topography unit

(Continues)

Notes: NLO—No Lock-Out for range of treatment; SPH—Sphere; CYL—Cylinder

Table 2-1 Refractive Laser PMA/HDE Approvals as of November 21, 2003 (Continued)

Doc #	Sponsor	Ap'd Date	Device	Indications (Range)
P910067	**Summit**	3-10-1995	Apex	PTK procedures which treat superficial corneal pathologies where other less invasive treatments have failed or are not possible. Limited to patients with decreased visual acuity or symptoms of pain and discomfort causing disability for patients with certain conditions (see SSED)
P930034	Summit	10-25-1995	Apex & Apex Plus	PRK, myopia: −1.50 to −7.00 D
P930034/S9	Summit	3-11-1998	Apex Plus	PRK, myopia: −1.00 to < −6.00 D SPH w/−1.00 to < −4.00 D CYL, and max combined spherical equiv (SE) < −6.00 D
P930034/S12	Summit	10-21-1999	Apex Plus	PRK, hyperopia: +1.5 to +4.0 D SPH with < −1.00 D CYL
P930034/S13	Summit	10-21-1999	Apex Plus	**LASIK-Myopic Astigmatism**: myopia: 0.00 to −14.00 D SPH and 0.5 to 5.0 D CYL. NLO
P970043	**ATC**	11-2-1998	**LADARVision**	PRK, myopia: −1.00 to −10.00 D SPH and ≤ −4.00 D CYL
P970043/S5	ATC	5-9-2000	LADARVision	LASIK, myopia: < −9.00 D SPH with or without CYL ≥ −0.5 D and < −3.00 D; NLO ≤ −11 D SPH & < −6 D CYL
P970043	Summit Autonomous		LADARVision	Name Change Only
P970043/S7	Alcon	9-22-2000	LADARVision	**LASIK-Hyperopic Astigmatism & Mixed Astigmatism**: hyperopia: ≤6.00 D SPH and ≤ −6.00 D CYL for hyperopia with & without astigmatism and mixed astigmatism.
P970043/S10	Alcon	10-18-2002	LADARVision	**Wavefront-guided LASIK**: myopia up to −7.00 D SPH w/<0.50 D CYL. LO > −7 D. 6.5 mm OZ; 9.0 mm TZ.
P970053	**Nidek**	12-17-1998	EC-5000	PRK, myopia: −0.75 to −13.00 D of SPH
P970053/S1	Nidek	9-29–1999	EC-5000	PRK, myopia: −1.00 to −8.00 SE and −0.50 to −4.00 CYL
P970053/S2	Nidek	4-14-2000	EC-5000	**LASIK-Myopic Astigmatism**: myopia: −1.00 to −14.00 SE and ≤4.00 CYL
P970056	**B & L**	9-28-1999	KERACOR 116	PRK, myopia: −1.50 to −7.00 D of SPH and ≤ −4.50 D CYL

(Continues)

Notes: NLO—No Lock-Out for range of treatment; SPH—Sphere; CYL—Cylinder

Table 2-1 Refractive Laser PMA/HDE Approvals as of November 21, 2003 (Continued)

Doc #	Sponsor	Ap'd Date	Device	Indications (Range)
P990027	B & L	2-23-2000	Technolas 217A	**LASIK-Myopic Astigmatism**: myopia: −1.00 to −7.00 D of SPH and up to < −3.00 D CYL.
P990027/S2	B & L	5-15-2002	Technolas 217A	**LASIK-High Myopic Astigmatism**: up to −12 D MRSE w/SPH up to −10.99 and CYL up to < −3.00 D.
P990027/S4	B & L	2-25-2003	Technolas 217A	**LASIK-Hyperopic Astigmatism**: up to +4D MRSE, w/SPH 1.00 to 4.00 D w/ or w/o CYL up to +2.00 D. OZ: 5–6 mm; Blend: 1.90 mm spherical hyper; 1.75 mm hyperopic astig. LO for sphere >4.00 D and CYL >2.00 D.
P990027/S6	B & L	10-10-2003	Technolas 217Z	**Wavefront-guided LASIK**: myopia up to −7.00 D SPH w/≤3.00 D CYL, MRSE ≥ −7.50 D. LO > −7 D SPH. 6.5 mm OZ; 9.0 mm TZ
P980008	**LaserSight**	11-12-1999	LaserScan LSX	**PRK-Myopia**: myopia: −1.00 to < −6.00 D of SPH and ≤1.00 D CYL.
P980008/S5	LaserSight	09-28-2001	LaserScan LSX	**LASIK-Myopic Astigmatism**: myopia: −0.5 to < −6.00 D of SE and up to ≤4.50 D CYL. LO −6 D SE & above.
P990010	CRS/VISX	11-19-1999	VISX Star S2	LASIK, myopia: −1.00 to −14.00 D SPH and 0.5 to 5.0 D CYL. NLO
P020050	WaveLight	10-07-03	Allegretto Wave	**LASIK-Myopic Astigmatism**: myopia: up to −12.00 D SPH and up to −6.0 D CYL. OZ: 6.0 & 6.50 mm; TZ: up to 9.0 mm
P030008	WaveLight	10-10-03	Allegretto Wave	**LASIK-Hyperopic Astigmatism**: hyperopia: up to +6.00 D SPH and up to 5.0 D CYL w/MRSE up to +6.0 D. OZ: 6.0 & 6.50 mm; TZ: up to 9.0 mm
Single Site PMAs				
P970005	Kremer	7-30-1998	Kremer Laser	LASIK, myopia: −1.00 to −15.00 D SPH and ≤ −5.00 D CYL. NLO
P970049	Dishler	12-16-1999	Dishler Excimer	LASIK, myopia: −0.50 to −13.00 D SPH and −0.50 to −4.00 CYL. NLO
Non-Excimer PMAs				
P990078	**Sunrise**	6-30-2000	Hyperion LTK	**Hyperopia LTK**: +0.75 to +2.5 D SPH with ≤0.75 D CYL
P010018	Refractec	4-11-2002	ViewPoint CK System	Hyperopia, CK: +0.75 to +3.25 D SPH with ≤0.75 D CYL

Notes: NLO—No Lock-Out for range of treatment; SPH—Sphere; CYL—Cylinder

against adulteration and misbranding (eg, false and misleading labeling). Most Class I devices are exempt from premarket review by the FDA. With few exceptions, manufacturers can go directly to market with their Class I device.

Class II devices (eg, phacoemulsification units, glaucoma shunts, tonometers, daily wear contact lenses) are usually considered moderate-risk devices. These devices, in addition to general controls, are subject to special controls, which may include the requirement for submission of performance data (clinical and/or bench testing) to the FDA. With few exceptions, Class II devices require premarket review by the FDA before they can go to market.

Class III devices (eg, excimer lasers, IOLs, extended-wear contact lenses, intraocular fluids and gases) are considered significant-risk devices that present a potential unreasonable risk of illness or injury. Class III devices cannot be marketed in the United States until the FDA determines that there is a reasonable assurance that the device is safe and effective. Most Class III devices come to market through the Premarket Approval (PMA) process and require an extensive review by the FDA before approval is granted for marketing.

Class III devices with new technologies, devices with new indications for use, or those devices that raise significant issues of safety and effectiveness are brought before the advisory panel for a review and recommendation before the FDA makes a decision on the application. Class III devices that have been modified and that do not raise new issues of safety or effectiveness, or devices that are similar to other Class III devices that have already been reviewed by the panel, do not require a review and recommendation by the advisory panel before the FDA makes its marketing decision. With rare exceptions, Class I and Class II devices do not need a review and recommendation by the advisory panel.

Pathways to Market

Premarket Notification 510(k)

Manufacturers of Class I and Class II devices that are not otherwise exempt from premarket review must submit a Premarket Notification, commonly referred to as a 510(k) application, to the FDA before going to market. In the 510(k) application, a manufacturer must demonstrate that its device is substantially equivalent to a legally marketed device (commonly referred to as the predicate device) of the same type and for the same intended use. The FDA must make its determination of substantial equivalence within 90 days. If a device is not found to be substantially equivalent, it is placed into Class III.

Humanitarian Device Exemption (HDE)

Devices marketed under an HDE are intended for the treatment or diagnosis of diseases or conditions that affect or are manifested in fewer than 4000 individuals per year in the United States. The sponsor is required to provide an HDE application to the FDA containing a reasonable assurance of safety. Efficacy information is limited to a demonstration of "probable benefits to health" rather than the higher standard of "reasonable assurance of effectiveness" as would otherwise be required for a PMA. These devices must be used in a facility with an Institutional Review Board (IRB) for treatment. The FDA has 75 days to review and make a decision on an HDE application.

Product Development Protocol (PDP)

This pathway to market is rarely used in ophthalmology and involves early interaction between the sponsor and the FDA, with Ophthalmic Devices Panel review of the Preclinical and Clinical Development Plan.

Premarket Approval (PMA)

The PMA process is the primary pathway to market for Class III devices. The first step is the granting of an investigational device exemption (IDE) by the FDA for the clinical study to support the PMA and to allow the beginning of systematic collection of safety and effectiveness data on the investigational device. The FDA has 30 days to review and grant approval of an IDE application. Applications containing deficiencies in such areas as bench testing, study design, or informed consent documents are denied or conditionally approved. During the IDE process, the sponsor often meets with the FDA to discuss the details of the clinical trial in order to facilitate effective data collection for eventual review. After IRB approval is received, investigators at different sites can begin the systematic collection of safety and effectiveness data on the investigational device. Clinical data from the IDE study, along with manufacturing information, preclinical bench testing, animal data (if needed), and labeling wording, is submitted to the FDA as a PMA application. The FDA must make a decision on the application within 180 days. The time for making the decision is extended when the application lacks the required information or contains information that is incomplete or insufficient for the FDA to reach its decision.

Ophthalmic Devices Panel

The Ophthalmic Devices Panel consists of seven voting members, one nonvoting consumer representative, and one nonvoting industry representative. Panel consultants are included on the panel as the need for their expertise dictates. The panel includes ophthalmologists as well as other experts, such as vision scientists, biostatisticians, and optometrists. All panel members are considered "special government employees" and are subject to conflict of interest rules and ethics requirements for government employees.

First-of-a-kind medical devices and PMA applications that raise new issues of safety and effectiveness are reviewed by the panel. The actual meeting is a public forum in which the sponsor, the FDA, and all panel attendees discuss the data from the PMA application. The sponsor submits clinical study data from the PMA study as well as labeling information for doctors and sometimes for patients. The panel also discusses changes that should be made to the labeling that is included in these documents.

After deliberation, the panel members decide whether the PMA application demonstrates a reasonable assurance of safety and effectiveness by voting a recommendation either for approval, approvable with conditions, or not approvable. An approvable with conditions vote indicates that the PMA has been found to be approvable subject to specified conditions, such as physician or patient education, labeling changes, or further analysis of existing data. The summary minutes and complete transcript of the meeting are placed on the FDA website.

Labeling

The sponsor defines the inclusion and exclusion criteria for the clinical trial. The Ophthalmic Devices Panel reviews and makes recommendations for changes in the device labeling using the data from the population studied. For example, if dry eyes are an exclusion criteria for the PMA study, there will be no data on subjects with dry eyes. Consequently, the device is not approved in this subset of patients, and the labeling will indicate that dry eyes are an exclusion criteria. This does not mean that the device is contraindicated in dry eye patients, but that the safety and efficacy of the device cannot be evaluated in this population because there are no data. Some exclusion criteria may be contraindications to treatment. For example, keratoconus could be an exclusion criterion as well as a contraindication to LASIK.

The clinical trial is performed for a limited range of refractive errors. Safety and effectiveness data guide the range of refractive error that is approved for use in the PMA labeling.

If the treating clinician does not follow the labeling recommendations for the device, he or she is using the device "off-label." Some off-label uses reflect the PMA's lack of data on safety and efficacy (eg, use of the device in a patient listed within the exclusion criteria), while other off-label uses reflect decreased safety or efficacy (eg, use of the device beyond the refractive range of the labeling).

In the United States, ophthalmologists are permitted to use a device off-label because the FDA does not control the practice of medicine. Use of an FDA-approved device in an off-label fashion, however, may place an ophthalmologist at increased risk of legal scrutiny, particularly if there is a poor result. Consequently, if off-label use is anticipated, the patient should be informed, and an ancillary signed consent should be considered.

Delays in FDA Approval

At times the clinical trials of a PMA application may have deficiencies that result in delays before the application can come to a vote before the Ophthalmic Devices Panel. Alternatively, a PMA application may be recommended for approval by the panel and yet may have to wait for final FDA approval before marketing. Usually, a panel recommendation for approval is granted with conditions that must be met before final FDA approval is granted. For example, the panel may request that data obtained on study subjects with certain ophthalmic characteristics be submitted to the FDA to determine if visual results in this subset of patients demonstrate efficacy.

When delays occur, the public naturally wants information as to the cause. The FDA is legally bound to keep the result of the PMA application process confidential and is prohibited by law from revealing any information about the PMA, favorable or unfavorable. However, the company is not bound by these same rules and is not restricted in what it chooses to tell the public. The dissemination of information about the PMA has financial implications because it can affect public perception of a product, which can affect the stock price of the company. The agency does not comment on statements made by the company, which does not indicate an FDA endorsement of any representation by the company. Even if a company releases incorrect information about the reasons for delay in FDA approval, the FDA is still prohibited from discussing details of the PMA application, which could include evidence contrary to statements made by the company. It is only in the public sessions of the Ophthalmic Devices Panel that information about the PMA process is legally allowed to be released to the public before a final decision on the application is made by the FDA. All other deliberations regarding the application, before and after the panel meeting, remain subject to the FDA confidentiality rules. Consequently, the panel meeting is the best forum for the public to actually observe the true data from the PMA clinical trial before the FDA reaches its decision.

CHAPTER 3

Patient Evaluation

A thorough preoperative patient evaluation is of critical importance in achieving a successful outcome following refractive surgery. It is during this encounter that the physician begins to develop an impression as to whether the patient is or is not a good candidate for refractive surgery.

Preoperative Evaluation

The evaluation actually begins before the physician sees the patient. Receptionists or refractive surgical coordinators who speak with the patient prior to the visit may get a sense of the patient's goals and expectations regarding refractive surgery. If the patient is quarrelsome about the time or date of the appointment or argues about cost, the surgeon should be informed. Such a patient may be too demanding to be a good candidate for surgery.

Important parts of the preoperative evaluation include an assessment of the patient's expectations, the history, the manifest and cycloplegic refractions, a complete ophthalmologic evaluation including slit-lamp and fundus examinations, and ancillary testing (Table 3-1). If the patient is a good candidate for surgery, the appropriate refractive surgery procedures, benefits, and risks need to be discussed, and informed consent must be obtained.

Because accurate testing results are critical to the success of refractive surgery, the refractive surgeon must closely supervise office staff who are performing the various tests in the preoperative evaluation (eg, corneal topography or pachymetry). Likewise, the surgeon should make sure the instruments used in the evaluation are properly calibrated, as miscalibrated instruments can result in faulty data and poor surgical results.

Patient Expectations

One of the most important aspects of the entire evaluation is assessing the patient's expectations. The surgeon should explore expectations relating to both the refractive result (eg, uncorrected visual acuity) and the emotional result (eg, improved self-esteem). Patients need to understand that they should not expect refractive surgery to improve their best-corrected visual acuity. In addition, refractive surgery will not prevent possible future ocular problems such as cataract, glaucoma, or retinal detachment. If the patient has obviously unrealistic desires, such as a guarantee of 20/20 uncorrected visual acuity, or perfect uncorrected reading *and* distance vision even though he or she is presbyopic,

Table 3-1 Important Parts of the Preoperative Refractive Surgery Examination

PATIENT EXPECTATIONS
Assessment of specific patient expectations
Discussion of uncorrected distance versus reading vision
HISTORY
Social history, including visual requirements of profession and hobbies
Medical history, including systemic medications and diseases such as diabetes and rheumatologic diseases
Ocular history, including history of contact lens wear
OCULAR EXAMINATION
Uncorrected near and distance vision
Manifest refraction (pushing plus)
Monovision demonstration, if indicated
Pupillary evaluation
Motility
Slit-lamp examination, including IOP measurement
Corneal topography
Wavefront analysis, if indicated
Pachymetry
Cycloplegic refraction (refining sphere, not cylinder)
Dilated fundus examination
Discussion of findings
INFORMED CONSENT
Discussion of medical and surgical alternatives and risks
Answering of patient questions
Having patient read and sign informed consent, before dilation and before day of procedure

the patient may need to be told that refractive surgery cannot currently fulfill his or her needs. The refractive surgeon should exclude patients with unrealistic expectations.

Social History

The social history and medical history can identify the visual requirements of the patient's profession. Certain jobs require that best vision be at a specific distance. For example, a preacher may desire that best uncorrected vision be at arm's length, so that reading can be done at the pulpit without glasses. Soldiers, fire fighters, or police may have restrictions on the type of refractive surgery they can have. The type of sports and recreational activities a patient prefers may help select the best refractive procedure or determine whether that patient is even a good candidate for refractive surgery. For example, a surface laser procedure may be preferable to a lamellar procedure for a patient who wrestles, boxes, or rides horses and is at high risk of ocular trauma. A highly myopic stamp collector or jeweler, who is used to examining objects without glasses a few inches from the eyes, may not be happy with postoperative emmetropia.

Medical History

The medical history should include systemic conditions, prior surgeries, and current and prior medications. Certain systemic conditions, such as connective tissue disorders, can lead to poor healing after refractive surgery. An immunocompromised state, for example from cancer or HIV/AIDS, may increase the risk of infection after refractive surgery. Medications that affect healing or the ability to fight infection, such as systemic corticosteroids or chemotherapeutic agents, should be specifically noted. The use of corticosteroids, and some diseases such as diabetes, increase the risk of cataract development, which could compromise the long-term postoperative visual outcome. Certain medications may increase the risk of poor results with PRK and LASIK, for example, isotretinoin (Accutane) and amiodarone (Cordarone), due to potentially increased risk of poor corneal healing. In addition, caution needs to be taken with patients using sumatriptan (Imitrex) who are undergoing PRK and LASIK, and with patients using hormone replacement therapy or antihistamines who are undergoing PRK, due to possible increased risk of delayed epithelial healing.

Caution should be taken in performing any excimer laser surgery in patients with cardiac pacemakers and implanted defibrillators, due to the unknown effects of the laser's electromagnetic emissions. Refractive surgery is also generally contraindicated in pregnant and nursing women, due to possible changes in refraction and corneal hydration status. Many surgeons recommend waiting at least 3 months after delivery and cessation of nursing before performing refractive surgery.

Pertinent Ocular History

The ocular history should focus on previous and current eye problems such as dry eye symptoms, blepharitis, recurrent erosions, and retinal tears or detachments. Ocular medications should be noted. A history of previous methods of optical correction, such as glasses and contact lenses, should be taken. The stability of the current refraction is very important. Have the glasses or the contact lens prescription changed significantly in the past few years? A significant change is generally thought to be greater than 0.5 D in either sphere or cylinder over the past year. A contact lens history should be taken. Important information includes the type of lens (eg, soft, rigid gas-permeable, PMMA); the wearing schedule (eg, daily wear disposable, daily wear frequent replacement, overnight wear indicating number of nights worn in a row); the type of cleaning, disinfection, and enzyming; and how old the lenses are. Occasionally, a patient may have been happy with contact lens wear and only needs a change in lens material or wearing schedule to eliminate the recent onset of discomfort symptoms.

Because contact lens wear can change the shape of the cornea (corneal warpage), discontinuing contact lens wear is recommended prior to the refractive surgery evaluation and also prior to the surgery. The exact amount of time the patient should be out of contact lenses has not been established. Current clinical practice typically involves discontinuing soft contact lenses for at least 3 days to 2 weeks and rigid contact lenses for at least 2 to 3 weeks. Patients with irregular or unstable corneas should discontinue their contact lenses longer and then be re-refracted every few weeks until the refraction is stable before being considered for refractive surgery. Some surgeons will change patients from rigid lenses to soft lenses for a period of time to aid stabilization of the corneal curvature in those patients who wear gas-permeable lenses but find glasses a significant hardship.

Patient Age, Presbyopia, and Monovision

The age of the patient is very important in predicting postoperative patient satisfaction. The loss of near vision with aging should be discussed with all patients. Prior to age 40 years, emmetropic patients generally do not require reading adds to see a near target. After this age patients need to understand that if they are made emmetropic with refractive surgery, they will require reading glasses for near vision. This point cannot be overemphasized for myopes who are approaching age 40. These patients can read well with and without their glasses. Some may even read well with their contact lenses. If they are emmetropic after surgery, many of these patients will not read well without reading glasses. The patient needs to understand this phenomenon and must be willing to accept this result, prior to undergoing any refractive surgery that aims for emmetropia. A trial with contact lenses will approximate the patient's reading ability after surgery.

A discussion of monovision (one eye corrected for distance and the other eye for near) often fits well in the evaluation at this point. The alternative of monovision correction should be discussed with all patients in the prepresbyopic and presbyopic age groups. Generally the dominant eye is corrected for distance and the nondominant eye is corrected to approximately −1.50 to −1.75 D. Such a refraction allows good uncorrected distance and near vision without intolerable anisometropia for most patients. Some surgeons prefer a "mini-monovision" procedure, where the near-vision eye is corrected to approximately −0.75 D, allowing some near vision with better distance vision and less anisometropia. The exact amount of monovision depends on the desires of the patient. Higher amounts of monovision (up to −2.50 D) can be used successfully in selected patients who desire excellent postoperative near vision. While improving the near vision, loss of depth perception and anisometropia may be unwanted side effects from the higher add in some patients.

Many patients have successfully used monovision in contact lenses and want it after refractive surgery. Others have never tried it but would like to, and still others have no interest. If a patient has not used monovision before but is interested, the attempted result should be demonstrated to them in glasses at near and distance. It is often best to try it in contact lenses prior to refractive surgery to make sure the patient is happy with the refractive goal. Although typically the nondominant eye is corrected for near, some patients prefer the dominant eye corrected for near. There are several methods to test ocular dominance. One of the simplest is to have the patient point to a distant object, such as a small letter on the eye chart, and then close each eye to determine which eye he or she was using to point, which is the dominant eye, or to have a patient make an "okay sign" with one hand and look at the examiner through the opening.

Examination

Uncorrected Visual Acuity and Manifest and Cycloplegic Refraction Acuity

The refractive elements of the preoperative examination are critically important because they directly determine the amount of surgery that is performed. Uncorrected visual acuity at distance and near should be measured. The current glasses prescription and vision with those glasses should also be measured. The manifest refraction should then be performed. The sharpest visual acuity with the least amount of minus ("pushing plus") should be the final endpoint. The Duochrome test should not be used as the final endpoint because it tends to overminus patients. Document the best visual acuity obtainable, even if it is better than 20/20. After the patient's eyes are dilated, a cycloplegic refraction is also necessary. Appropriate cycloplegic drops and enough waiting time between the drops and the cycloplegic refraction are required. Tropicamide 1% or cyclopentolate 1% is generally used. Waiting at least 30 or 60 minutes, respectively, for full cycloplegia is recommended. The cycloplegic refraction should refine the sphere and not the cylinder from the manifest refraction. For eyes with greater than 5 D of refractive error, a vertex distance measurement should be performed to obtain the most accurate refraction. When there is a large difference between the manifest and cycloplegic refractions (eg, >0.75 D), a postcycloplegic refraction should be performed to recheck the manifest refraction. In myopes, this is often caused by an overminused manifest refraction. In hyperopes, there may be significant latent hyperopia, and in such cases the surgeon and patient need to decide on exactly how much hyperopia to treat. If there is significant latent hyperopia, a pushed plus spectacle or contact lens correction can be worn for several weeks preoperatively to lessen the postoperative adjustment of treating the true refraction.

Pupillary Examination

After the manifest refraction (but before placing dilating drops) the external and anterior segment examinations are performed. Specific attention should be given to the pupillary examination, evaluating the pupil size in bright room light and dim illumination and looking for an afferent pupillary defect. There are a variety of techniques to measure pupil size in dim illumination, including a near card with pupil sizes on the edge (with the patient fixating at distance), a light amplification pupillometer (eg, Colvard pupillometer), or an infrared pupillometer. The actual amount of light entering the eye during the dim light measurement should closely approximate normal nighttime activities, such as night driving, and not necessarily complete darkness.

It is important to try to standardize pupil size measurements as much as possible. Large pupil size may be one of the risk factors for postoperative glare and halo symptoms after refractive surgery. Another risk factor for postoperative glare includes a higher degree of myopia or astigmatism. As a general rule, pupil size greater than the effective optical zone (usually 6 to 8 mm) increases the risk of glare, but large pupil size is certainly not the only determinant of glare. When asked, patients often have glare under dim light conditions even before refractive surgery. It is important to make patients aware of their glare and halo symptoms preoperatively, as this may minimize postoperative complaints.

Measuring the low-light pupil diameter preoperatively and using the measurement to direct surgery remains controversial. Conventional wisdom suggests that the optical zone should be larger than the pupil diameter to minimize visual disturbances such as glare and haloes. However, it is not clear that pupil size can be used to predict which patients are more likely to have symptoms. It is possible that the size of the effective optical zone, which is related to the ablation profile and the level of refractive error, is more important in minimizing visual side effects than the low-light pupil diameter.

Ocular Motility, Confrontation Fields, and Ocular Anatomy

Ocular motility should also be evaluated. Patients with an asymptomatic tropia or phoria may develop symptoms after refractive surgery if the change in refraction causes the motility status to break down. If there is a history of strabismus (see Chapter 10) or there is a concern regarding ocular alignment postoperatively, a trial with contact lenses before surgery should be considered. An orthoptic evaluation can be obtained preoperatively if strabismus is an issue. Confrontation fields should be performed in all patients.

The general anatomy of the orbits should also be assessed. Patients with small palpebral fissures and/or large brows may not be ideal candidates for LASIK because there may be inadequate exposure and difficulty in achieving suction with the microkeratome.

Intraocular Pressure

The IOP should be checked after performing the manifest refraction and corneal topography measurements. Patients with glaucoma (see Chapter 10) should be aware that certain refractive surgery procedures elevate the IOP dramatically during the procedure, potentially aggravating optic nerve damage. Also, topical corticosteroids are used after most refractive surgery procedures and may be used for months after PRK or LASEK. Long-term topical corticosteroids may cause marked elevation of IOP in corticosteroid responders. Laser refractive surgery procedures such as PRK and LASIK thin the cornea and typically cause a falsely low measurement of IOP postoperatively. Patients and surgeons need to be aware of this issue, especially if the patient has glaucoma or is a glaucoma suspect.

Slit-Lamp Examination

A complete slit-lamp examination of the eyelids and anterior segment should be performed. The eyelids should be checked for significant blepharitis and meibomitis. The tear lake should be assessed for aqueous tear deficiency. The conjunctiva should be examined, looking specifically for conjunctival scarring which may cause problems with microkeratome suction. The cornea should be evaluated for surface abnormalities such as decreased tear break-up time (Fig 3-1) and punctate epithelial erosions (Fig 3-2). Significant blepharitis (Fig 3-3), meibomitis, and dry eye syndrome should be addressed prior to refractive surgery, as they are associated with increased postoperative discomfort and decreased vision. A careful examination for epithelial basement membrane dystrophy (Fig 3-4) is required, because its presence increases the risk of flap complications during LASIK. Patients with epithelial basement membrane dystrophy are not good candidates for LASIK; they may be better candidates for PRK. Signs of keratoconus, such as corneal thinning and steepening, may also be found. Keratoconus is typically an absolute contraindication to refractive surgery (but see Other Potential Uses for Intrastromal Corneal Ring Segments in Chapter 5). The endothelium should be examined carefully, looking for signs of cornea guttata and Fuchs and other dystrophies. Corneal edema is generally considered a contraindication to refractive surgery.

The anterior chamber, iris, and crystalline lens should be examined. A shallow anterior chamber depth may be a contraindication for insertion of certain phakic IOLs (see Chapter 8). Careful undilated and dilated evaluation of the crystalline lens for clarity is

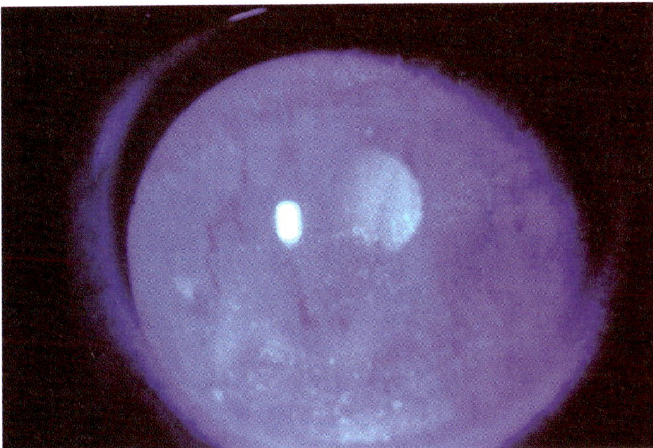

Figure 3-1 Decreased tear break-up time. After instillation of fluorescein dye, the patient keeps the eye open and the tear film is examined with cobalt blue light. Breaks, or dry spots, in the tear film can be seen in this patient. Punctate epithelial erosions are also present. *(Photograph courtesy of Christopher J. Rapuano, MD.)*

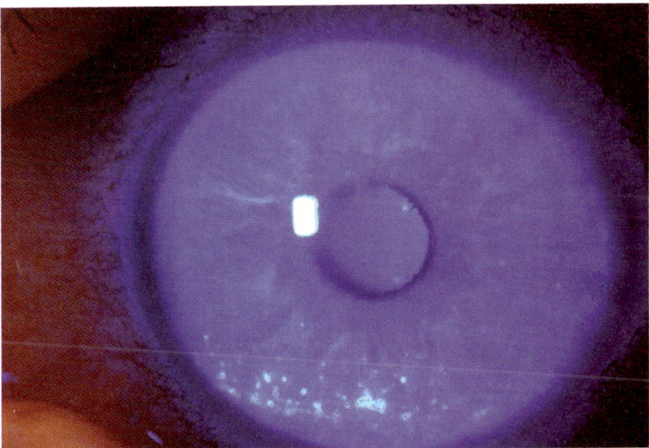

Figure 3-2 Punctate epithelial erosions. Inferior punctate fluorescein staining is noted in this patient with moderately dry eyes. *(Photograph courtesy of Christopher J. Rapuano, MD.)*

essential, especially in patients over age 50. Patients with mild lens changes that are visually insignificant should be informed of these findings and of the fact that the changes may become more significant in the future, independent of refractive surgery. In patients with moderate lens opacities, cataract extraction may be the best form of refractive surgery. Patients should be informed that if they do not undergo refractive surgery at this time, significant refractive error could be addressed at the time of future cataract surgery. Some surgeons give patients a record of their preoperative refractions and keratometry measurements along with the amount of laser ablation performed and the postoperative refraction. This information should help improve the accuracy of the IOL calculation should cataract surgery be required at some future date.

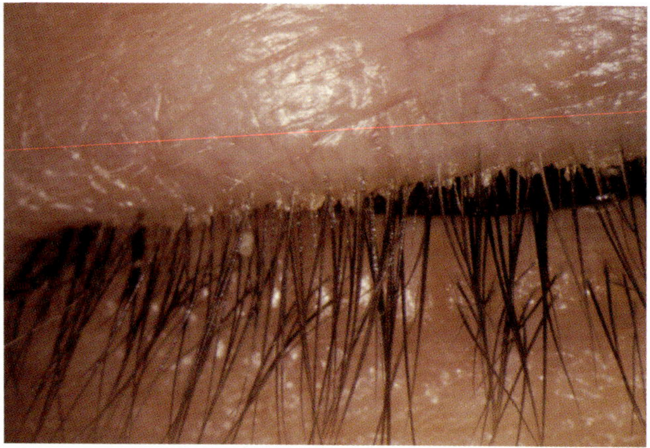

Figure 3-3 Blepharitis. Moderate crusting at the base of the lashes is found in this patient with seborrheic blepharitis. *(Photograph courtesy of Christopher J. Rapuano, MD.)*

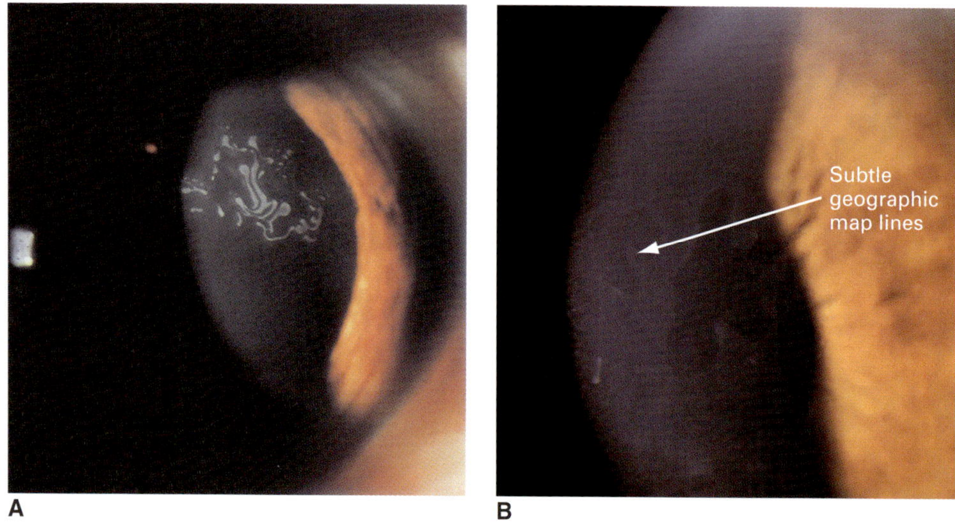

Figure 3-4 Epithelial basement membrane dystrophy. Epithelial map changes can be obvious **(A)** or subtle **(B).** Arrow shows geographic map lines. *(A courtesy of Vincent P. deLuise, MD; B courtesy of Christopher J. Rapuano, MD.)*

Dilated Fundus Examination

A dilated fundus examination is also important prior to refractive surgery to be certain the posterior segment is normal. Special attention should be given to the optic nerve (glaucoma, optic nerve drusen) and peripheral retina (retinal breaks, detachment). Patients and surgeons should realize that highly myopic eyes (see Chapter 10) are at increased risk for retinal detachment, even after the refractive error has been corrected.

Ancillary Tests

Corneal Topography

An evaluation of corneal curvature is necessary. While manual keratometry readings can be quite informative, they have largely been replaced by computerized videokeratographic analyses. There are several different methods with which to analyze the corneal curvature, including Placido disk systems and scanning-slit-beam methods. (See also the extensive discussion of corneal topography in Chapter 1.) These techniques image the cornea and provide color maps representing corneal power and/or elevation. This analysis gives a "simulated keratometry" reading and an overall evaluation of the corneal curvature. Eyes with visually significant irregular astigmatism are generally not good candidates for corneal refractive surgery. The curvature analysis should reveal a spherical cornea or regular astigmatism. Early keratoconus, pellucid marginal degeneration (Fig 3-5), or contact lens warpage should be considered as causes in eyes with visually significant irregular astigmatism. Irregular astigmatism secondary to contact lens warpage usually reverses over time, although it may take months; serial corneal topography should be performed to document the disappearance of visually significant irregular astigmatism prior to any refractive surgery.

Unusually steep or unusually flat corneas can increase the risk of poor flap creation with the microkeratome. Flat corneas (flatter than 40 D) increase the risk of small flaps and free caps and steep corneas (steeper than 48 D) increase the risk of buttonhole flaps. Femtosecond laser (eg, IntraLase) flap creation theoretically may avoid these risks. Excessive corneal flattening and steepening after refractive surgery may increase the risk of poor quality of vision. Patients with corneas flatter than approximately 34 D or steeper than approximately 50 D postoperatively may be at risk for this complication. Postoperative keratometry for myopes is estimated by subtracting approximately 80% of the refractive correction from the average preoperative keratometry reading. For example, if the preoperative keratometry reading is 42 D and 5 D of myopia is being corrected, an estimated postoperative keratometry reading would be 42 D – (0.8 × 5 D) = 38 D. Postoperative keratometry for hyperopes is estimated by adding 100% of the refractive correction to the average preoperative keratometry reading. For example, if the preoperative keratometry reading is 42 D and 3 D of hyperopia is being corrected, the estimated postoperative keratometry reading would be 42 D + (1 × 3 D) = 45 D.

When keratometric or corneal topographic measurements reveal an amount or an axis of astigmatism significantly different from the refraction, the refraction should be rechecked for accuracy. Lenticular astigmatism or posterior corneal curvature may account for the difference between refractive and keratometric/topographic astigmatism. Most surgeons decide to treat the amount and axis of the refractive astigmatism, with the understanding that after cataract surgery, some astigmatism may reappear (after the astigmatism contributed by the natural lens has been eliminated).

Pachymetry

A measurement of corneal thickness should be done to determine whether the cornea is of adequate thickness for keratorefractive surgery. This procedure is usually performed

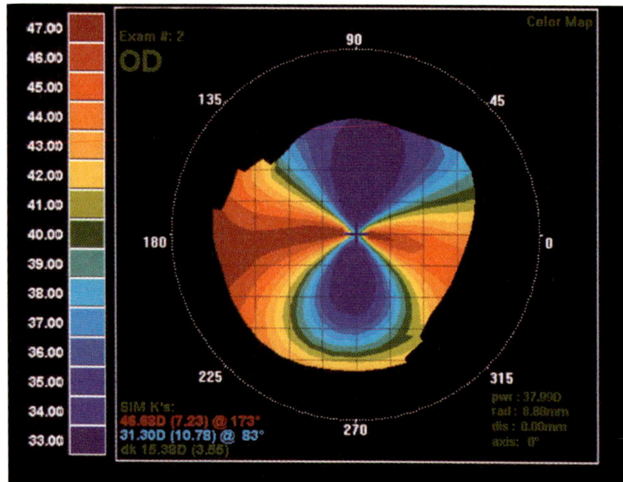

Figure 3-5 A corneal topographic map of the typical irregular against-the-rule astigmatism that is seen in eyes with pellucid marginal degeneration. Note that the steepening nasally and temporally connects inferiorly. *(Photograph courtesy of Christopher J. Rapuano, MD.)*

with ultrasound pachymetry; however, certain corneal topography systems (eg, scanning-slit-beam, such as Orbscan) can also be used. This latter system can provide a map representing the relative thickness of the cornea at various locations. The accuracy of the pachymetry measurements of scanning-slit-beam systems decreases markedly after keratorefractive surgery is performed. Because the thinnest part of the cornea is typically located centrally, a central measurement should always be performed. Unusually thin corneas may reveal early keratoconus. Some surgeons also check the midperipheral corneal thickness for inferior thinning, which may suggest early keratoconus. Unusually thick corneas may suggest mild Fuchs dystrophy. The thickness of the cornea is an important factor in determining whether the patient is a candidate for refractive surgery and which procedure may be best. In a study of 896 eyes undergoing LASIK, the mean central corneal thickness was 550 μm ± 33 μm, with a range of 472 to 651 μm. It is unclear whether an unusually thin cornea (beyond perhaps 2 standard deviations) suggests inherent instability that would not be ideal for any refractive surgery. Consequently, even if there is adequate stromal tissue for an excimer ablation, most refractive surgeons will not consider LASIK below a certain lower limit of corneal thickness. If LASIK is performed and results in a relatively thin residual stromal bed, for example around 250 μm, future enhancement surgery that further thins the stromal bed may not be possible. If there is a question of endothelial integrity causing an abnormally thick cornea, specular microscopy may be helpful to assess the health of the endothelium.

Price FW Jr, Koller DL, Price MO. Central corneal pachymetry in patients undergoing laser in situ keratomileusis. *Ophthalmology.* 1999;106:2216–2220.

Wavefront Analysis

Wavefront analysis is a relatively new technique that can provide an objective refraction measurement (see also discussion of this topic in Chapter 1 and Chapter 6). Certain excimer lasers can use this wavefront analysis information directly to perform the ablation, a procedure called wavefront-guided or "custom" ablation. Some surgeons are using wavefront analysis to document levels of preoperative higher-order aberrations. Refraction data from the wavefront analysis unit can also be used to refine the manifest refraction.

Calculation of Residual Stromal Bed Thickness After LASIK

A lamellar laser refractive procedure such as LASIK involves creation of a corneal flap, ablation of the stromal bed, and replacement of the flap. The strength and integrity of the cornea postoperatively depends on the thickness of the residual stromal bed. Stromal bed thickness is calculated by taking the preoperative central corneal thickness and subtracting the flap thickness and the calculated laser ablation depth for the particular refraction. For example, if the central corneal thickness is 550 μm, the flap thickness is estimated to be 160 μm, and the ablation depth for the patient's refraction is 50 μm, the residual stromal bed thickness would be 550 μm – (160 μm + 50 μm) = 340 μm. When calculating residual bed thickness, the amount of actual tissue removal should be based on the actual intended refractive correction, not on the nomogram-adjusted number entered into the laser computer. For example, if a −10 D myope is being fully corrected, the amount of tissue removal for −10 D is 128 μm for a 6.5 mm ablation zone for the VISX laser. Even if the surgeon usually takes off 15% of the refraction and enters that number into the laser computer, approximately 128 μm of tissue will be removed, not 85% of 128 μm.

Exactly how thick the residual stromal bed needs to be is unclear. However, most surgeons believe that it should be at least 250 μm thick, and many surgeons believe it should be even thicker, in the 275 to 300 μm range. Others want the residual bed thickness to be greater than 50% of the original corneal thickness. If the calculation reveals a residual stromal bed thickness that is thinner than desired, LASIK may not be the best surgical option. In these cases, a surface laser procedure such as PRK or epithelial-sparing PRK (LASEK) may be a better option because no stromal flap is required.

Discussion of Findings and Informed Consent

Once the evaluation is complete, the surgeon must analyze all the information and discuss the findings with the patient. If the patient is a candidate for refractive surgery, the risks and benefits of the various medical and surgical alternatives are discussed (Table 3-2). Important aspects of this discussion are the expected uncorrected visual acuity results for their refractive error (including the need for distance and/or reading glasses, the chance of needing an enhancement, and whether maximal surgery is being performed initially), the risk of decreased best-corrected visual acuity or severe visual loss, the side effects of glare/haloes or dry eyes, the change in "quality" of vision, and the need to revise a corneal flap (for flap displacement, significant striae, or epithelial ingrowth). The

Table 3-2 Summary of the Most Common Refractive Surgery Procedures

Procedure	Typical Spherical Range	Typical Cylinder Range	Limitations
LASIK	−10.0 to +4.0 D	Up to 4.0 D	Thin corneas (thin residual stromal bed); epithelial basement membrane dystrophy; small palpebral fissures; microkeratome flap complications with flat and steep corneas; preoperative severe dry eye syndrome; significant glaucoma; certain medications; wavefront-guided ablations may have more restricted FDA-approved treatment parameters
PRK/LASEK	−8.0 to +4.0 D	Up to 4.0 D	Postoperative haze at high end of treatment range; preoperative dry eye syndrome; certain medications
Intrastromal corneal ring segments	−0.75 to −3.0 D	None	Does not correct cylinder; glare symptoms; white opacities at edge of ring segments
Holmium laser thermokeratoplasty	+0.75 to +2.5 D	None	Does not correct cylinder; regression of effect
Conductive keratoplasty	+0.75 to +3.0 D	None	Does not correct cylinder; possible regression of effect
Phakic intraocular lenses	−5.0 to −20.0 D	None	FDA approved for myopia; long-term complications such as glaucoma, iritis, cataract, pupil distortion, corneal edema

patient should understand that the laser ablation might need to be aborted if there is an incomplete, decentered, or buttonholed flap. The pros and cons of surgery on one eye versus both eyes on the same day should also be discussed, allowing patients to decide which is best for them. While the risk of bilateral infection may be higher with bilateral surgery, serial unilateral surgery may result in temporary anisometropia and is more inconvenient. Of course, nonsurgical alternatives, such as glasses, contact lenses, and orthokeratology (see Chapter 5), should also be explained.

If the patient is considering refractive surgery, he or she should be given the informed consent document either prior to dilation or to take home and review once dilation has worn off. The patient should be given an opportunity to discuss any questions related to the informed consent form with the surgeon preoperatively. This discussion and the signing of the consent form should take place well before the surgery and never when the patient is dilated and/or sedated. See Appendixes 3-1 and 3-2 for sample informed consent forms.

APPENDIX 3-1: Model Informed Consent Form-A *(Courtesy of Ophthalmic Mutual Insurance Company, www.OMIC.com)*

INFORMED CONSENT FOR LASER IN SITU KERATOMILEUSIS (LASIK)

Introduction

This information is being provided to you so that you can make an informed decision about the use of a device known as a microkeratome, combined with the use of a device known as an excimer laser, to perform LASIK. LASIK is one of a number of alternatives for correcting nearsightedness, farsightedness and astigmatism. In LASIK, the microkeratome is used to shave the cornea to create a flap. The flap then is opened like the page of a book to expose tissue just below the cornea's surface. Next, the excimer laser is used to remove ultra-thin layers from the cornea to reshape it to reduce nearsightedness. Finally, the flap is returned to its original position, without sutures.

LASIK is an elective procedure: There is no emergency condition or other reason that requires or demands that you have it performed. You could continue wearing contact lenses or glasses and have adequate visual acuity. This procedure, like all surgery, presents some risks, many of which are listed below. You should also understand that there may be other risks not known to your doctor, which may become known later. Despite the best of care, complications and side effects may occur; should this happen in your case, the result might be affected even to the extent of making your vision worse.

Alternatives to Lasik

If you decide not to have LASIK, there are other methods of correcting your nearsightedness, farsightedness or astigmatism. These alternatives include, among others, eyeglasses, contact lenses and other refractive surgical procedures.

Patient Consent

In giving my permission for LASIK, I understand the following: The long-term risks and effects of LASIK are unknown. I have received no guarantee as to the success of my particular case. I understand that the following risks are associated with the procedure:

Vision Threatening Complications

1. I understand that the microkeratome or the excimer laser could malfunction, requiring the procedure to be stopped before completion. Depending on the type of malfunction, this may or may not be accompanied by visual loss.
2. I understand that, in using the microkeratome, instead of making a flap, an entire portion of the central cornea could be cut off, and very rarely could be lost. If preserved, I understand that my doctor would put this tissue back on the eye after the laser treatment, using sutures, according to the ALK procedure method. It is also possible that the flap incision could result in an incomplete flap, or a flap

Patient Initials: ______

that is too thin. If this happens, it is likely that the laser part of the procedure will have to be postponed until the cornea has a chance to heal sufficiently to try to create the flap again.

3. I understand that irregular healing of the flap could result in a distorted cornea. This would mean that glasses or contact lenses may not correct my vision to the level possible before undergoing LASIK. If this distortion in vision is severe, a partial or complete corneal transplant might be necessary to repair the cornea.
4. I understand that it is possible a perforation of the cornea could occur, causing devastating complications, including loss of some or all of my vision. This could also be caused by an internal or external eye infection that could not be controlled with antibiotics or other means.
5. I understand that mild or severe infection is possible. Mild infection can usually be treated with antibiotics and usually does not lead to permanent visual loss. Severe infection, even if successfully treated with antibiotics, could lead to permanent scarring and loss of vision that may require corrective laser surgery or, if very severe, corneal transplantation or even loss of the eye.
6. I understand that other very rare complications threatening vision include, but are not limited to, corneal swelling, corneal thinning (ectasia), appearance of "floaters" and retinal detachment, hemorrhage, venous and arterial blockage, cataract formation, total blindness, and even loss of my eye.

Non–Vision Threatening Side Effects

1. I understand that there may be increased sensitivity to light, glare, and fluctuations in the sharpness of vision. I understand these conditions usually occur during the normal stabilization period of from 1 to 3 months, but they may also be permanent.
2. I understand that there is an increased risk of eye irritation related to drying of the corneal surface following the LASIK procedure. These symptoms may be temporary or, on rare occasions, permanent, and may require frequent application of artificial tears and/or closure of the tear duct openings in the eyelid.
3. I understand that an overcorrection or undercorrection could occur, causing me to become farsighted or nearsighted or increase my astigmatism and that this could be either permanent or treatable. I understand an overcorrection or undercorrection is more likely in people over the age of 40 years and may require the use of glasses for reading or for distance vision some or all of the time.
4. I understand that at night there may be a "starbursting" or halo effect around lights. I understand that this condition usually diminishes with time, but could be permanent. I understand that my vision may not seem as sharp at night as during the day and that I may need to wear glasses at night. I understand that I should not drive until my vision is adequate both during the day and at night.
5. I understand that I may not get a full correction from my LASIK procedure and this may require future enhancement procedures, such as more laser treatment or the use of glasses or contact lenses.

Patient Initials: ______

6. I understand that there may be a "balance" problem between my two eyes after LASIK has been performed on one eye, but not the other. This phenomenon is called anisometropia. I understand this would cause eyestrain and make judging distance or depth perception more difficult. I understand that my first eye may take longer to heal than is usual, prolonging the time I could experience anisometropia.
7. I understand that, after LASIK, the eye may be more fragile to trauma from impact. Evidence has shown that, as with any scar, the corneal incision will not be as strong as the cornea originally was at that site. I understand that the treated eye, therefore, is somewhat more vulnerable to all varieties of injuries, at least for the first year following LASIK. I understand it would be advisable for me to wear protective eyewear when engaging in sports or other activities in which the possibility of a ball, projectile, elbow, fist, or other traumatizing object contacting the eye may be high.
8. I understand that there is a natural tendency of the eyelids to droop with age and that eye surgery may hasten this process.
9. I understand that there may be pain or a foreign body sensation, particularly during the first 48 hours after surgery.
10. I understand that temporary glasses either for distance or reading may be necessary while healing occurs and that more than one pair of glasses may be needed.
11. I understand that the long-term effects of LASIK are unknown and that unforeseen complications or side effects could possibly occur.
12. I understand that visual acuity I initially gain from LASIK could regress, and that my vision may go partially back to a level that may require glasses or contact lens use to see clearly.
13. I understand that the correction that I can expect to gain from LASIK may not be perfect. I understand that it is not realistic to expect that this procedure will result in perfect vision, at all times, under all circumstances, for the rest of my life. I understand I may need glasses to refine my vision for some purposes requiring fine detailed vision after some point in my life, and that this might occur soon after surgery or years later.
14. I understand that I may be given medication in conjunction with the procedure and that my eye may be patched afterward. I therefore understand that I must not drive the day of surgery and not until I am certain that my vision is adequate for driving.
15. I understand that if I currently need reading glasses, I will still likely need reading glasses after this treatment. It is possible that dependence on reading glasses may increase or that reading glasses may be required at an earlier age if I have this surgery.
16. Even 90% clarity of vision is still slightly blurry. Enhancement surgeries can be performed when vision is stable UNLESS it is unwise or unsafe. If the enhancement is performed within the first 6 months following surgery, there generally is no need to make another cut with the microkeratome. The original flap can usually be lifted with specialized techniques. After 6 months of healing, a new

Patient Initials: ______

LASIK incision **may be** required, incurring greater risk. In order to perform an enhancement surgery, there must be adequate tissue remaining. If there is inadequate tissue, it may not be possible to perform an enhancement. An assessment and consultation will be held with the surgeon at which time the benefits and risks of an enhancement surgery will be discussed.

17. I understand that, as with all types of surgery, there is a possibility of complications due to anesthesia, drug reactions, or other factors that may involve other parts of my body. I understand that, since it is impossible to state every complication that may occur as a result of any surgery, the list of complications in this form may not be complete.

For Presbyopic Patients (those requiring a separate prescription for reading)
The option of monovision has been discussed with my ophthalmologist.

Patient's Statement of Acceptance and Understanding

The details of the procedure known as LASIK have been presented to me in detail in this document and explained to me by my ophthalmologist. My ophthalmologist has answered all my questions to my satisfaction. I therefore consent to LASIK surgery.

I give permission for my ophthalmologist to record on video or photographic equipment my procedure, for purposes of education, research, or training of other health care professionals. I also give my permission for my ophthalmologist to use data about my procedure and subsequent treatment to further understand LASIK. I understand that my name will remain confidential, unless I give subsequent written permission for it to be disclosed outside my ophthalmologist's office or the center where my LASIK procedure will be performed.

______________________________ _______________
Patient signature Date

______________________________ _______________
Witness Date

I have been offered a copy of this consent form (please initial). ______

APPENDIX 3-2: Model Informed Consent Form-B *(Courtesy of Ophthalmic Mutual Insurance Company, www.OMIC.com)*

Addendum: Consent for Bilateral Simultaneous LASIK

LASIK has become a common procedure for many refractive surgery patients. While many patients choose to have both eyes treated at the same surgical setting, there may be risks associated with simultaneous treatment that are not present when the eyes are treated on different days. **If you elect to have surgery performed on both eyes at the same time, you should understand both the possible advantages and disadvantages of your decision.**

Safety: The risks of infection, severe inflammation, delayed clouding of the cornea, corneal scarring and internal bleeding or retinal damage are very rare but potentially devastating. If these complications occur in one eye, they may also occur in the other. Should any of these complications happen, you could experience significant loss of vision or even temporary or permanent legal blindness. By choosing to have LASIK performed on separate days, you avoid the risk of having one or more of these complications in both eyes at the same time.

Accuracy: If there is an over-correction or under-correction in one eye, chances are it may happen in both eyes. If a retreatment is required in one eye, it is quite possible that your fellow eye may also require a retreatment. By having surgery on separate days, the doctor can monitor the healing process and visual recovery in the first eye and may be able to make appropriate modifications to the treatment plan for the second eye. In some patients, this might improve the accuracy of the result in the second eye. By correcting both eyes simultaneously, there is no opportunity to learn from the healing patterns of the first eye before treating the second eye.

Visual Recovery: Most LASIK patients experience rapid visual recovery, but some may experience symptoms such as blurred vision, night glare or ghost images that can result in prolonged recovery of normal vision. Blurred vision may rarely continue for several weeks, which could make driving difficult or dangerous and could interfere with your ability to work if it occurs in both eyes. There is no way of predicting how long your eyes will take to heal. If the eyes are operated separately, you can generally function with the fellow eye while the first eye fully recovers. However, there may be a period of imbalance in vision between your two eyes, producing a form of double vision. If you are able to wear a contact lens in your unoperated eye, the corrective lens could minimize this imbalance. The balance in vision between your two eyes will usually be restored more rapidly if they are operated on the same day.

The healing corneal flap is most susceptible to trauma during the first several weeks after surgery. Should both flaps become accidentally displaced, significant visual loss in both eyes may result.

Patient Initials: ______

Satisfaction: Both eyes tend to experience similar side effects. If you experience undesirable side effects such as glare, ghost images, increased light sensitivity, or corneal haze in one eye, you will likely experience them in both eyes. These side effects may cause a decrease in vision or other negative effects, and some patients have elected to not have their second eye treated. By having each eye treated on separate dates, you will have the opportunity to determine whether the LASIK procedure has produced satisfactory visual results without loss of vision or other uncommon undesirable side effects. If you are over age 40, you will also have an opportunity to experience the change in your close vision that results from the correction of your nearsightedness or farsightedness. This could influence your decision on whether or not to fully correct your other eye to maintain some degree of close vision without the need for glasses (monovision).

Convenience: It may be inconvenient for you to have each eye treated at separate visits because it would necessitate two periods of recovery from the laser surgery and might require additional time away from work.

Cost: Professional and facility fees may be greater if the eyes are operated on different days, and the additional time off work that may also be needed can be costly.

____

Initial

Consent Statement: I have read and understand the above risks and benefits of bilateral simultaneous LASIK, and I understand that this summary does not include every possible risk, benefit and complication that can result from bilateral simultaneous LASIK. My doctor has answered all of my questions about the LASIK procedure. I wish to have both of my eyes treated during the same treatment session if my doctor determines that the treatment in the first eye appeared to be technically satisfactory.

The reason(s) I wish to have both eyes treated at the same time are:

Greater convenience

Possible faster recovery

Less time away from work

Contact lens intolerance and/or difficulty wearing contacts

Elimination of possible vision imbalance between treated and untreated eyes

Other: ____

__________________________ ______________

Patient signature Date

__________________________ ______________

Witness Date

I have been offered a copy of this consent form (please initial). ________

PART II

Specific Procedures in Refractive Surgery

CHAPTER 4

Incisional Corneal Surgery

Since its inception in the late 1890s incisional corneal surgery has had periods of adoption, refinement, and abandonment. Incisional surgery for myopia and hyperopia has been all but replaced by excimer laser procedures, but astigmatic keratotomy still has a role in the treatment of astigmatism after cataract surgery (limbal relaxing incisions) and after penetrating keratoplasty (arcuate keratotomy).

Incisional Procedure for Myopia (Radial Keratotomy)

History of Radial Keratotomy (RK)

The first organized examination of incisional keratotomy has been attributed to a Dutch ophthalmologist, Lans, in the 1890s. Lans examined astigmatic changes induced in rabbits after partial-thickness corneal incisions and thermal cautery.

An ophthalmologist in Japan, Sato, made significant contributions to incisional refractive surgery in the 1930s and 1940s even though his long-term results in humans were poor. He observed central corneal flattening and improvement in vision after the healing of spontaneous ruptures of Descemet's membrane (hydrops) in advanced keratoconus patients, and he developed a technique to induce artificial ruptures of Descemet's membrane. Using a specially developed knife, he performed posterior keratotomy on keratoconus patients by making a series of incisions through the endothelium, Descemet's membrane, and the posterior stroma with good initial results. Short-term follow-up of eyes with myopia of −2.50 to −15.00 D that were undergoing anterior and posterior keratotomy demonstrated a reduction of myopia by an average of 3.00 D. However, 75% of patients developed corneal edema an average of 20 years after the operation (Fig 4-1). We now understand that the age-related loss of corneal endothelium, superimposed on the immediate surgically induced cell loss, resulted in the delayed corneal decompensation.

Russian researchers investigated keratotomy techniques in the 1960s and 1970s. Fyodorov is credited with laying the foundation of modern radial and astigmatic keratotomy. He established that the diameter of the central clear zone was inversely related to the amount of refractive correction: smaller central clear zones yield greater myopic corrections. He also developed the forerunners of modern keratotomy instrumentation, including a micrometer blade handle with footplate, gauge blocks for calibrating blade depth, and corneal marking devices.

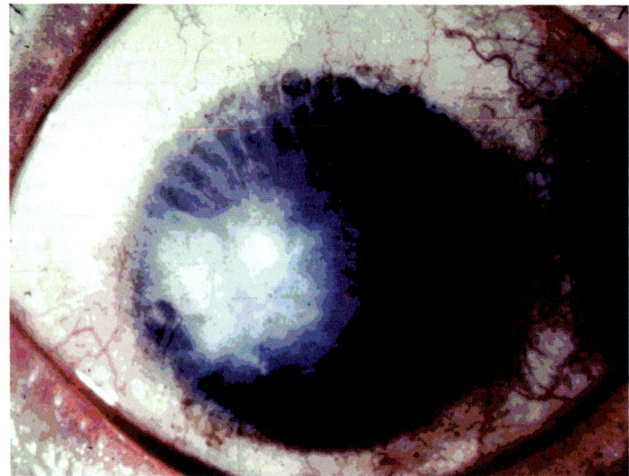

Figure 4-1 Corneal edema that occurred years after a Sato posterior keratotomy. Multiple peripheral keratotomy incisions are visible. *(Photograph courtesy of Steven C. Schallhorn, MD.)*

Radial Keratotomy in the United States

Following its introduction into the United States, radial keratotomy was modified and advanced as researchers and clinicians sought to improve its safety and predictability. These advances included the use of better equipment (diamond blades, ultrasonic pachymetry, etc), more accurate nomograms (incorporating variables such as patient age and IOP), and technique modification (reduced number of incisions and mini–radial keratotomy with shorter incisions). Salz and colleagues found that 80% to 90% of corneal flattening could be produced with the first 8 incisions, and as a result, the generally accepted number of radial incisions was gradually reduced from 16 to 8 or 4.

In order to evaluate the safety and efficacy of RK, the Prospective Evaluation of Radial Keratotomy (PERK) study was undertaken in 1982 and 1983 for patients with myopia from −2.00 to −8.75 D (mean, −3.875 D). The sole surgical variable was the diameter of the central clear zone (either 3.0, 3.5, or 4.0 mm) based on the level of preoperative myopia. Eight radial incisions were used for all patients; repeat surgery, if necessary, added an additional 8 incisions. Ten years after the procedure, 53% of patients had achieved 20/20 or better uncorrected visual acuity and 85% were 20/40 or better. Of the patients who had bilateral surgery, only 30% reported the use of spectacles or contact lenses for distance refractive correction at 10 years. Complications related to the procedure included a loss of best-corrected visual acuity (3%), delayed bacterial keratitis, corneal scarring, irregular astigmatism, and epithelial erosions.

The most important finding in the 10-year PERK study was the continuing long-term instability of the procedure. A hyperopic shift of 1.0 D or greater was found in 43% of eyes between 6 months and 10 years postoperatively. More worrisome was the fact that there was no evidence that the amount of hyperopic shift decreased between 5 and 10 years after RK. There was an association between the length of the incision and the hyperopic shift. Two techniques were developed in response to the hyperopic shift after RK, intentional undercorrection and use of shorter incisions (mini-RK).

Waring GO III, Lynn MJ, McDonnell PJ, and the PERK Study Group. Results of the Prospective Evaluation of Radial Keratotomy (PERK) study 10 years after surgery. *Arch Ophthalmol.* 1994;112:1298–1308.

Patient Selection

RK was used most commonly to treat patients with −1.00 to −4.00 D of myopia. Serious complications resulted from more aggressive treatment with optical zones smaller than 3.0 mm or more than 8 incisions. RK surgery differs from PRK and LASIK in that it does not involve removal of tissue from the central cornea. Disadvantages of RK are the limited range of refractive error that can be treated, the potential for long-term hyperopic drift, its detrimental effect on ocular integrity, the risk of intraoperative perforation, and the risk of infectious keratitis or endophthalmitis. Further, RK may not be appropriate for individuals who spend time at high altitude because of possible abrupt hyperopic refractive shifts.

Surgical Technique

Radial corneal incisions sever collagen fibrils in the corneal stroma. This produces a wound gape that increases the radius of curvature in the central cornea, flattening it and decreasing its refractive power, thereby decreasing myopia (Fig 4-2).

The design of the diamond-blade micrometer knife (angle and sharpness of cutting edge, width of blade, and footplate design) influences both the depth and contour of incisions. The length of the knife blade is set based on the corneal thickness, which is usually measured with an ultrasonic pachymeter.

A vertical blade pushed from the periphery toward the center of the cornea (centripetal or Russian technique) will cut deeper than an angled blade pulled from the center to the periphery (centrifugal or American technique). The latter method minimizes the risk of an inadvertent cut into the visual axis. The use of a combination (bidirectional) blade combines the effectiveness of the centripetal blade with the safety of the centrifugal blade.

Outcomes

Surgical and patient variables affecting outcome

Surgical variables include the following:

- *Centering.* Corneal surgical procedures are preferably centered on the entrance pupil of the eye.
- *Optical zone diameter.* Smaller optical zones produce more flattening and a greater reduction of myopic power.
- *Depth of incisions.* The ideal depth of radial incisions is 85% to 95% of the corneal thickness. The deeper the incisions, the more the flattening, but deeper incisions may reduce the stability of the refractive outcome.

The primary patient variable is the age of the patient. The older the patient, the greater the effect achieved with the same surgical technique. The increase is approximately 0.50 to 1.00 D per decade.

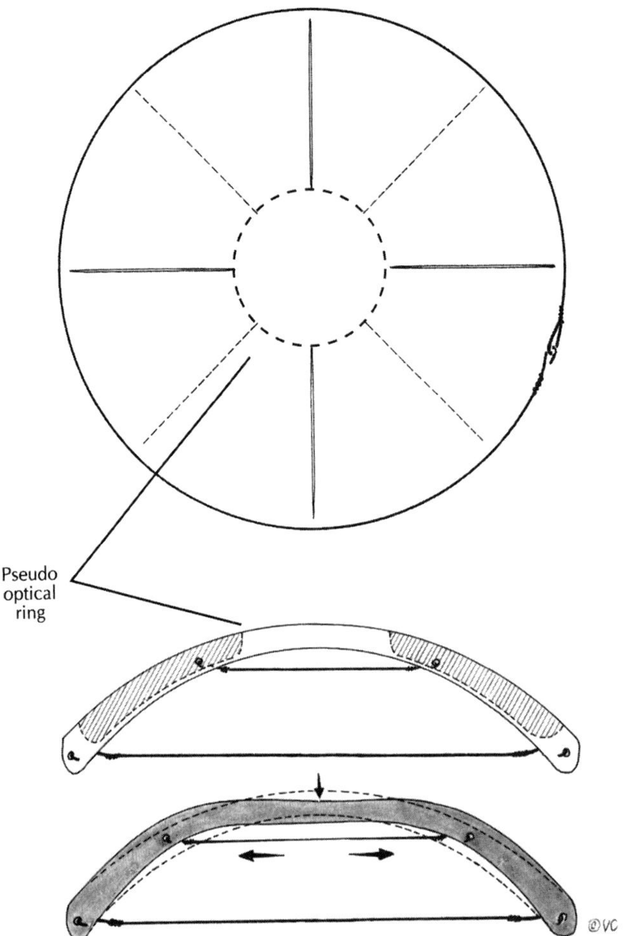

Figure 4-2 Effect of radial incisions. Flattening is induced in the optical zone central to incision-induced ectasia in the peripheral support zone. *(Reprinted with permission from Troutman RC, Buzard KA.* Corneal Astigmatism: Etiology, Prevention, and Management. *St. Louis: Mosby-Year Book; 1992.)*

Several nomograms have been generated to determine the optimal size of the optical zone and number of incisions, based on the patient's age and degree of myopia. These nomograms generally try to leave the patient slightly myopic (undercorrection), which is recognized to be preferable to overcorrection. Overcorrection is difficult to treat, while undercorrection can be treated by lengthening, deepening, or increasing the number of incisions.

Efficacy and predictability

The ideal result after surgery is mild residual myopia, on the order of −0.50 D, because residual myopia delays the onset of symptomatic presbyopia and offsets the continued tendency toward hyperopia that occurs in some RK patients.

The percentage of eyes with final spherical equivalent refractive error within ±1.00 D ranged from 54% to 96% in various studies. Series that included reoperations for undercorrection generally showed a higher percentage of emmetropic eyes. Among 310 patients with bilateral radial keratotomy in the PERK study, 70% reported not wearing spectacles or contact lenses for distance vision at 10 years.

Postoperative refraction, visual acuity, and corneal topography

RK changes not only the curvature of the central cornea but also its overall topography, creating a multifocal cornea. The result is a decrease in the direct correlation among refraction, central keratometry, and uncorrected visual acuity, presumably because the new corneal topography creates a more complex optical system consisting of central flattening and peripheral steepening. Thus, keratometric readings that sample only two points approximately 3.0 mm apart may show amounts of astigmatism different from those detected by refraction. Similarly, uncorrected visual acuity may vary, particularly depending on pupil diameter: the smaller the pupil, the less the multifocal effect of postoperative changes in the cornea.

Stability of refraction

Almost all eyes show a decrease in myopia immediately following radial keratotomy. Some regression occurs with healing, but most eyes are generally stable by 3 months after surgery. However, two phenomena of postoperative refractive instability—diurnal fluctuation of vision and a continued effect of surgery—may persist for several years.

Diurnal fluctuation of vision can occur because the cornea is flatter upon awakening and gradually steepens during the patient's waking hours. In a subset of the PERK study at 10 years, the mean change in the spherical equivalent of refraction between the morning (waking) and evening examinations was an increase of 0.31 ± 0.58 D in minus power in first eyes.

The continued effect of surgery is one of the major unknowns about RK. The refractive error in 43% of eyes in the PERK study changed in the hyperopic direction by 1.00 D or more between 6 months and 10 years postoperatively. The hyperopic shift was statistically associated with the diameter of the central clear zone.

Complications

Probably the best measure of the safety of RK is the rate of loss of best spectacle-corrected visual acuity; 1% to 3% of eyes lose two or more Snellen lines. Mild to moderate irregular astigmatism can cause visual distortion and glare, especially in patients who have more than 8 incisions, incisions extending inside a 3.0 mm central clear zone, intersecting radial and transverse incisions (Fig 4-3A and B), and hypertrophic scarring.

Many patients report seeing a starburst pattern around lights at night after RK. This presumably results from light scattering off the radial incisions and/or scars. While most patients find the starburst effect comparable to looking through dirty spectacles or contact lenses, some patients cannot drive at night because of this complication. Other side effects that do not reduce best-corrected visual acuity include postoperative pain, undercorrection and overcorrection, increased astigmatism, epithelial plugs (see Figure 4-3), vascularization of stromal scars, and nonprogressive endothelial disruption beneath the incisions.

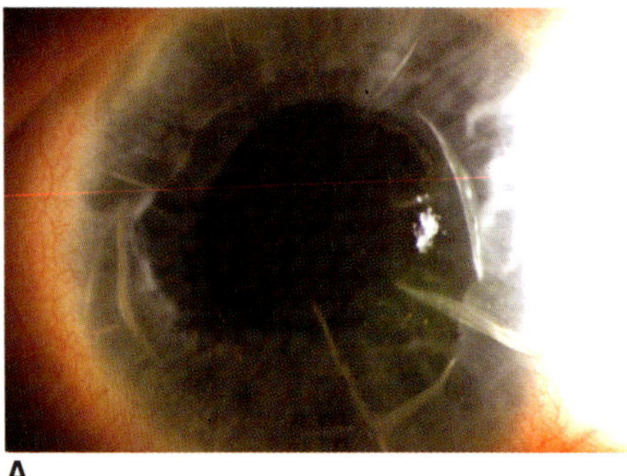
A

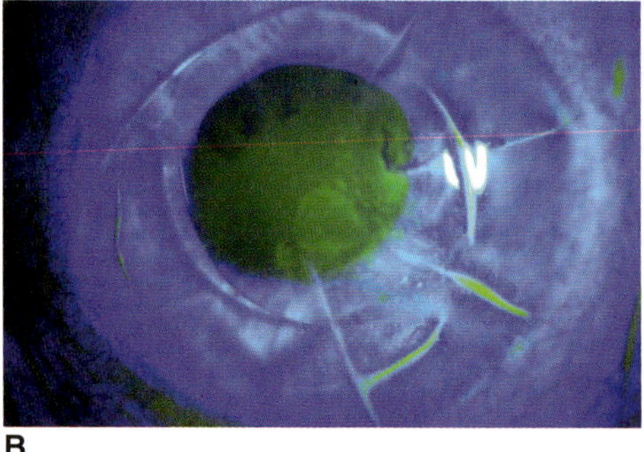
B

Figure 4-3 **A,** Crossed RK and arcuate keratotomy incisions with epithelial plugs in a patient who had intraoperative corneal perforation. **B,** Fluorescein staining demonstrates gaping of the incisions, causing persistent ocular irritation. *(Photographs courtesy of Jayne S. Weiss, MD.)*

Potentially blinding complications occur rarely after RK. These include:

- Perforation of the cornea, which can lead to endophthalmitis, epithelial ingrowth, and traumatic cataract.
- Traumatic rupture of the globe occurring through a keratotomy incision (Fig 4-4). This complication has been reported as long as 13 years after RK.
- Bacterial keratitis, which can occur immediately after surgery or up to 1 to 3 years later, presumably because the epithelium of the incision scars heals slowly and is constantly turning over, creating a site for bacterial adherence. Early-onset corneal ulcers are usually paracentral and deep, whereas late-onset ulcers are usually peripheral and superficial.

Ocular Surgery After Radial Keratotomy

Prior to the advent of excimer laser surgery, unacceptable residual myopia after RK was treated by opening the incisions with a blunt instrument and deepening or extending them to a smaller clear zone, or by making additional incisions between the initial ones.

A major finding in the 10-year PERK study was the continuing long-term instability of the procedure. A hyperopic shift of 1.0 D or greater was found in 43% of eyes between 6 months and 12 years postoperatively. More worrisome, there was no evidence that the amount of hyperopic shift was slowing between 5 and 10 years. It remains unknown if or when the refractive errors of this population will stabilize. There was an association between the length of the incision, as determined by the corneal diameter and the central clear zone diameter, and the amount of hyperopic shift. This association supports the theory that the more the cornea is weakened, the greater the long-term refractive instability. It is likely that all forms of refractive surgery that act by weakening the cornea will be susceptible to some degree of instability. Accordingly, surgical procedures that act by weakening the cornea may not be advisable in patients with progressive hyperopia after RK. LASIK and PRK have been shown to be effective in correcting residual myopia after RK, but these procedures are less effective in correcting progressive hyperopia after RK. Because unpublished reports suggest that corneal scarring may increase if PRK is per-

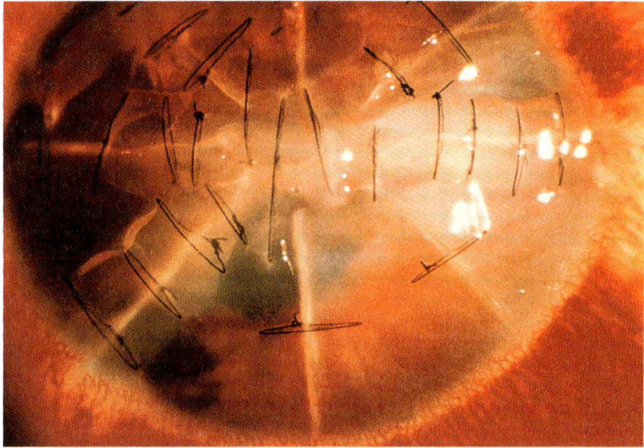

Figure 4-4 Traumatic rupture of an 8-incision RK, showing communication between two horizontal RK incisions. Interrupted 10–0 nylon sutures were used to close the incision. *(Reprinted with permission from* External Disease and Cornea: A Multimedia Collection. *San Francisco: American Academy of Ophthalmology; 2000.)*

formed after RK, LASIK may be preferable for treatment of undercorrected RK. While central keratometric measurement may be very flat after RK, the surgeon should realize that the peripheral cornea remains steeper. Consequently, many corneas that have had prior RK can have uncomplicated LASIK flaps despite keratometric measurements that are very flat (<40 D).

In patients with endothelial dystrophy, corneal infection, irregular astigmatism, severe visual fluctuations, and starburst effects, penetrating keratoplasty may be needed to restore visual functioning. Penetrating keratoplasty should be avoided if the patient's visual problems are correctable with glasses or contact lenses. If penetrating keratoplasty is deemed to be necessary, the RK incisions may need to be sutured before trephination to allow adequate suturing of the donor corneal graft to the recipient bed.

Linebarger EJ, Hardten DR, Lindstrom RL. Laser assisted in situ keratomileusis for correction of secondary hyperopia after radial keratotomy. *Int Ophthalmol Clin.* 2000;40:125–132.

Salamon SA, Hjortdal JO, Ehlers N. Refractive results of radial keratotomy: a ten-year retrospective study. *Acta Ophthalmol Scand.* 2000;78:566–568.

Cataract extraction with IOL implantation may lead to unintentional hyperopia following RK. In addition, IOL power calculation may be problematic and may result in undercorrection and hyperopia. Calculation of implant power for cataract surgery after RK is done using a third-generation formula (eg, Haigis, Hoffer Q, Holladay 2, or SRK/T) rather than a regression formula (eg, SRK I or SRK II) and then choosing the highest resulting IOL power. Keratometric power is determined in one of three ways: direct measurement using computerized videography; knowledge of pre-RK keratometry minus the refractive change; or adjustment of the base curve of a plano contact lens by the overrefraction (see Chapter 11).

Seitz B, Langenbucher A. Intraocular lens calculations status after corneal refractive surgery. *Curr Opin Ophthalmol.* 2000;11:35–46.

Waring GO III. Radial keratotomy for myopia. In: *Focal Points: Clinical Modules for Ophthalmologists.* San Francisco: American Academy of Ophthalmology; 1992: vol 10, no 5.

Incisional Procedure for Hyperopia (Hexagonal Keratotomy)

Hexagonal keratotomy is an example of a procedure that generated considerable interest when it was introduced but that was abandoned when subsequent studies uncovered significant safety concerns. It involved making a series of paracentral incisions in a hexagonal pattern, resulting in steepening of the central cornea and correction of hyperopia. This presumably occurred because the central cornea mechanically "decouples" from the rest of the cornea and bulges forward. We now know that procedures that induce corneal ectasia can lead to significant visual problems including glare, photophobia, polyopia, fluctuating vision, and irregular astigmatism.

Basuk WL, Zisman M, Waring GO III, et al. Complications of hexagonal keratotomy. *Am J Ophthalmol.* 1994;117:37–49.

Incisional Correction of Astigmatism

Several techniques of incisional surgery have been used to correct astigmatism including transverse keratotomy, arcuate keratotomy (AK), and limbal relaxing incisions (LRIs). Transverse keratotomy was frequently used in combination with RK to correct myopic astigmatism, but it is seldom used today. AK was also employed for the correction of naturally occurring astigmatism, but it is now used primarily for the correction of postkeratoplasty astigmatism (Fig 4-5). LRIs are used in the management of astigmatism during or after phacoemulsification and IOL implantation.

Transverse Keratotomy

Transverse keratotomy is a surgical procedure in which diametrically opposite linear (transverse) incisions are placed in the steep corneal meridian, resulting in flattening of the cornea along this meridian. A substantial amount of concomitant steepening of the orthogonal meridian, known as *coupling* (Fig 4-6), often occurs after a transverse keratotomy incision. This is in contrast to a radial incision, which does not induce corneal steepening in the orthogonal meridian. (In addition to flattening the incision meridian, a radial incision results in overall corneal flattening and hyperopic shift instead of coupling.)

When the coupling ratio (the amount of flattening in the incision meridian divided by the induced steepening in the opposite meridian) is 1, the spherical equivalent is unchanged. The type of incision (arcuate versus tangential) and the length and number of parallel incisions can influence the coupling ratio. Short, straight, and tangential incisions induce less steepening in the opposite meridian than do arcuate or longer incisions.

For transverse keratotomy, the instruments used are similar to those used for RK, but the diamond blade designs are different. Thin trapezoid-shaped blades and front-

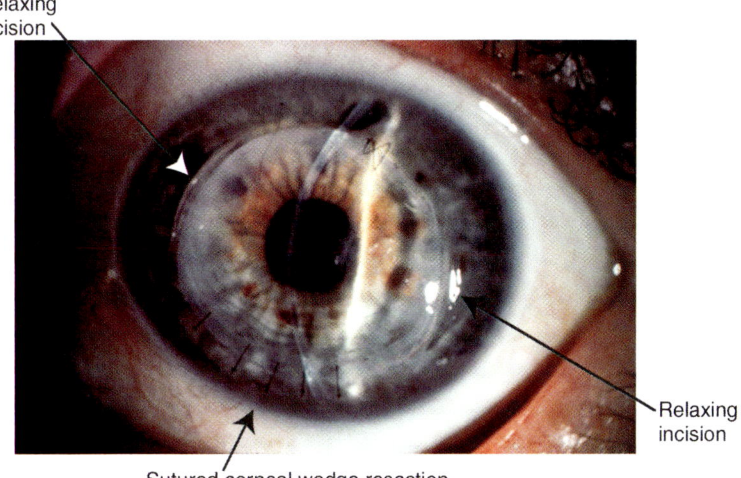

Figure 4-5 Corneal wedge resection (to steepen flat meridian) and relaxing incisions (to flatten steep meridian) to correct astigmatism after penetrating keratoplasty. *(Photograph courtesy of Jayne S. Weiss, MD.)*

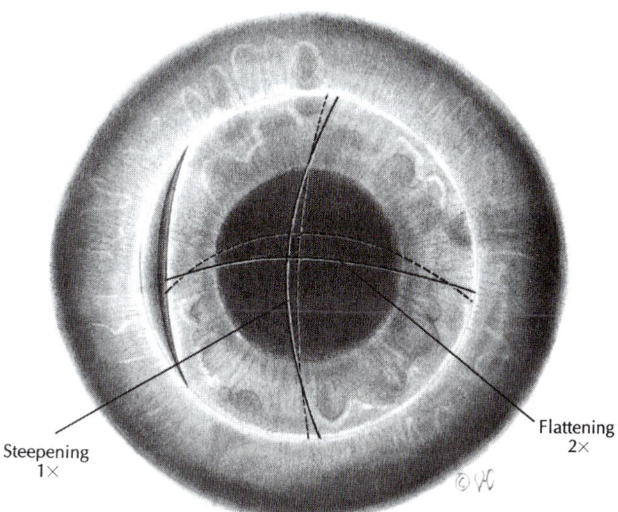

Figure 4-6 Coupling. A relaxing incision in a graft scar (pseudo-optical ring) across the steeper corneal meridian flattens the incisional meridian, inducing steepening of the meridian at 90° in a 2:1 ratio. *(Reprinted with permission from Troutman RC, Buzard KA.* Corneal Astigmatism: Etiology, Prevention, and Management. *St. Louis: Mosby-Year Book; 1992.)*

cutting diamond blades are used, which allow better visibility and maneuverability. The principles of astigmatic correction are similar to those discussed below for AK and for LRIs. The primary indication for transverse keratotomy was to treat simple myopic astigmatism and compound myopic astigmatism. At the time of writing, however, this technique has essentially been replaced by LASIK and PRK.

Arcuate Keratotomy and Limbal Relaxing Incisions

AK is an incisional surgical procedure in which arcuate incisions of approximately 95% depth are made in the corneal midperipheral zone centered on the steep corneal meridian(s). LRIs are incisions set at approximately 600 µm depth and placed in the peripheral cornea just anterior to the limbus. AK differs from LRIs by its midperipheral location and its greater relative depth. Due to the concomitant steepening of the orthogonal meridian (coupling), AK and LRIs correct astigmatism without inducing a substantial hyperopic change of the spherical equivalent of the preoperative refraction. Increased effect in LRIs is achieved primarily by increasing the length of the incision. For astigmatic keratotomy, cylindrical correction can be increased by increasing the length or depth of the incision, using multiple incisions, or reducing the distance between the AK incisions.

Instrumentation

The instruments used in AK and LRIs are similar to those used for transverse keratotomy. Front-cutting diamond blades are more often used in AK, and back-cutting diamond blades are more often used in LRI surgery. A mechanized trephine, the Hanna arcuate trephine, has been shown to make smooth curvilinear AK incisions of specified optical zone and arc length. This has led to the development of other mechanized systems aimed at achieving smooth AK and LRI incisions.

Surgical Techniques

With any system, accurate assessment of the steep meridian (plus cylinder axis for AK, and steep meridian on topography or keratometry for LRIs) is essential. The axis should be identified preoperatively and verified intraoperatively. AK incisions may be used in pairs along the steep meridian, no closer than 3.5 mm from the center of the pupil because of induced glare and aberrations. LRIs are placed during or after cataract surgery in the peripheral cornea. They result in lower amounts of astigmatic correction than AK, but they have the advantage of minimizing optical aberration in astigmatic patients undergoing cataract surgery. AK incisions used to correct post–penetrating keratoplasty astigmatism are usually made in the graft. When AK incisions are made in the graft–host junction or in the host, the effect of the incisions is reduced.

Outcomes

Although AK incisions are primarily used to correct post–penetrating keratoplasty astigmatism and LRIs are primarily used during or after cataract surgery, these procedures have been employed for the correction of naturally occurring astigmatism, a condition that is currently corrected primarily using PRK, LASEK, or LASIK. The outcome of AK and LRIs depends on several variables, including patient age; the distance separating the incision pairs; and the length, depth, and number of incisions.

Few large prospective trials exist. The ARC-T trial of AK, which used a 7.0 mm optical zone and varying arc lengths, showed a reduction in astigmatism of 1.6 ± 1.1 D in patients with preoperative naturally occurring astigmatism of 2.8 ± 1.2 D. Other studies have shown a final uncorrected visual acuity of 20/40 in 65% to 80% eyes. Overcorrections have been reported in 4% to 20% of patients.

Studies of LRIs are limited, but these incisions are used with seemingly good results in astigmatic patients undergoing cataract surgery. One study showed an absolute change in refractive astigmatism of 1.72 ± 0.81 D after LRIs in patients with mixed astigmatism. Astigmatism was decreased by 0.91 D, or 44%, in another series of LRIs in 22 eyes of 13 patients. Incisions in the horizontal meridian have been reported to cause approximately twice as much astigmatic correction as vertical incisions (Table 4-1).

Anecdotal evidence suggests that AK incisions show progressive flattening over time secondary to corneal thinning and (notable) gaping of the edges of incisions, especially with arc lengths of 90° or greater. In contrast, LRIs show evidence of stability by day 4, especially when the incisions are <45°.

Complications

Corneal topography after AK and LRIs shows flattening of the incision meridian coupled with steepening of the orthogonal meridian, although irregular astigmatism occurs often postoperatively. Off-axis astigmatic keratotomy can lead to undercorrection or worsening of preexisting astigmatism. To avoid creating an isolated block or edge of cornea that swells and cannot be epithelialized, arcuate incisions and LRIs should not intersect other incisions (see Figure 4-3). Corneal perforation has been reported.

Ocular Surgery After Arcuate Keratotomy and Limbal Relaxing Incisions

AK can be combined with or done after cataract, RK, PRK, or LASIK surgery. Penetrating keratoplasty can be done after extensive AK, but the wounds may have to be sutured before trephination as discussed above for RK. As noted above, the use of LRIs is usually reserved for the correction of preexisting astigmatism in patients undergoing cataract surgery. A prerequisite for this approach is the use of astigmatically neutral, small-incision, clear corneal phacoemulsification with self-sealing peripheral corneal incisions.

Table 4-1 Current Nomogram for Peripheral Corneal Relaxing Incisions to Correct Keratometric Astigmatism During Cataract Surgery

Preoperative Astigmatism (D)	Age (Years)	Number	Length (Degrees)
With-the-rule			
0.75–1.00	<65	2	45
	≥65	1	45
1.01–1.50	<65	2	60
	≥65	2	45 (or 1 × 60)
>1.50	<65	2	80
	≥65	2	60
Against-the-rule/oblique*			
1.00–1.25†	–	1	35
1.26–2.00	–	1	45
>2.00	–	2	45

* Combined with temporal corneal incision.
† Especially if cataract incision is not directly centered on the steep meridian.

(From Wang L, Misra M, Koch DD. Peripheral corneal relaxing incisions combined with cataract surgery. *J Cataract Refract Surg.* 2003;29:712–722.)

Bayramlar HH, Daglioglu MC, Borazan M. Limbal relaxing incisions for primary mixed astigmatism and mixed astigmatism after cataract surgery. *J Cataract Refract Surg.* 2003;29:723–728.

Budak K, Yilmaz G, Aslan BS, et al. Limbal relaxing incisions in congenital astigmatism: 6-month follow-up. *J Cataract Refract Surg.* 2001;27:715–719.

Faktorovich EG, Maloney RK, Price FW Jr. Effect of astigmatic keratotomy on spherical equivalent: results of the Astigmatism Reduction Clinical Trial. *Am J Ophthalmol.* 1999;127:260–269.

Gills JP, Gayton JL. Reducing pre-existing astigmatism. In: Gills JP, Fenzl R, Martin RG, eds. *Cataract Surgery: The State of the Art.* Thorofare, NJ: Slack, Inc; 1998:53–66.

Müller-Jensen K, Fischer P, Siepe U. Limbal relaxing incisions to correct astigmatism in clear corneal cataract surgery. *J Refract Surg.* 1999;15:586–589.

Price FW Jr, Grene RB, Marks RG,et al and the ARC-T Study Group. Astigmatism Reduction Clinical Trial: a multicenter prospective evaluation of the predictability of arcuate keratotomy. *Arch Ophthalmol.* 1995;113:277–282.

CHAPTER 5

Onlays and Inlays

Refractive errors can be corrected by placing preformed tissue or synthetic material onto or into the cornea. This alters the optical power of the cornea by changing the shape of the anterior corneal surface or by creating a lens with a higher index of refraction than the corneal stroma. Tissue addition procedures, such as epikeratoplasty, have fallen out of favor because of the difficulty of obtaining donor tissue as well as the poor predictability of the refractive and visual results. Synthetic material holds greater promise because it can be shaped to greater precision than tissue and can also be mass produced. Because of problems with re-epithelialization, synthetic material generally has to be placed in the corneal stroma. This requires a partial or complete lamellar dissection with specialized instruments. Early work using lenticules of glass and plastic resulted in necrosis of the overlying stroma because these substances are impermeable to water and nutrients. Current techniques use lenticule inlays made of more permeable substances such as hydrogel. Another type of inlay indirectly alters the shape of the cornea using ring segments of polymethylmethacrylate (Intacs). Because the ring segments are narrow, the overlying stroma can receive nutrients from surrounding tissue.

Keratophakia

In keratophakia, a plus-power lens is placed intrastromally to increase the curvature of the anterior cornea for the correction of hyperopia. After a central lamellar keratectomy with a microkeratome, the lenticule is placed onto the host bed and the anterior lamellar cap is sutured in place. The lens can be prepared either from donor cornea (homoplastic) or synthetic material (alloplastic). The homoplastic implant is prepared from a donor cornea by a lamellar keratectomy after removal of the epithelium and Bowman's layer. The tissue (fresh or frozen) is then shaped into a lens with an automated lathe. The lens of tissue can be preserved either fresh in refrigerated tissue culture medium, frozen at subzero temperatures, or freeze dried.

Homoplastic Corneal Inlays

Keratophakia has been used to correct aphakia and hyperopia of up to 20 D, but there have been few published studies on this procedure. Troutman and colleagues reported on 32 eyes treated with homoplastic keratophakia, 29 of which also underwent cataract extraction. Even when the surgeons were more experienced in their second series, predictability was still low: 25% of patients were more than 3 D from the intended correction.

Complications included irregular lamellar resection, wound dehiscence, and postoperative corneal edema. Although the procedure was originally intended to be used in conjunction with cataract extraction for the correction of aphakia, the complexity of the procedure and the unpredictable refractive results could not compete with aphakic contact lenses or the improved technology of IOL implantation in the early 1980s. Homoplastic keratophakia thus quickly became a secondary procedure for use in the contact lens–intolerant aphakic patient for whom intraocular surgery was contraindicated, and the procedure fell further out of favor when prelathed lenticules became available for epikeratoplasty in the 1980s.

Alloplastic Corneal Inlays

Synthetic corneal inlays change the refractive power of the eye either by mechanically altering the curvature of the cornea or by acting as an intrastromal lens that has an index of refraction greater than that of the corneal stroma. They are placed under a stromal flap or in a pocket over the pupillary aperture as an alloplastic form of keratophakia. Synthetic inlays offer several potential advantages, such as the ability to be mass produced in a wide range of sizes and powers that can be measured and verified. Also, synthetic material may have optical properties superior to tissue lenses, which are difficult to accurately lathe. Unlike synthetic material, tissue lenticules can become distorted upon insertion and may undergo remodeling, which can prolong postoperative visual recovery and can lead to refractive instability.

A variety of materials have been tried for the inlays. Beginning in 1949, Barraquer experimented with flint glass and Plexiglas intracorneal lenses (6 mm diameter) in rabbits and cats, but he abandoned their use because of anterior corneal stromal necrosis and eventual implant extrusion. Polysulfone is an impermeable material with excellent optical qualities and a high index of refraction (1.633). Because it can serve as an intrastromal lens, no change in anterior corneal curvature is required, as in hydrogel implants. A technically easier stromal pocket dissection can be used for insertion rather than a complete lamellar keratectomy. Experiments in the early 1980s had disappointing results because of corneal opacities, nonhealing epithelial erosions, and diurnal fluctuations in vision. This led to the incorporation of microperforations into the inlay for the transfer of fluid and nutrients to the anterior cornea. Although fenestrated polysulfone (35 μm fenestrations) showed increased safety in cat corneas, it proved to be optically unsatisfactory. Smaller fenestrations (10 μm) may preserve the optical properties of implanted polysulfone and still provide adequate nourishment to the anterior cornea. Smaller-diameter, high index of refraction implants are also being investigated as a technique for correcting presbyopia.

Knowles and many other subsequent investigators have demonstrated the importance of fluid and nutrient permeability of the implant to the nourishment of the overlying anterior stroma. For this reason, most succeeding studies used water-permeable hydrogel implants. Hydrogel lenses have an index of refraction similar to that of the corneal stroma, so they have little intrinsic optical power when implanted. To be effective, they must change the curvature of the anterior cornea.

The PermaVision lens (Anamed) is undergoing clinical trials in the United States (Fig 5-1). It is composed of a hydrogel material called Nutrapore with a 78% water

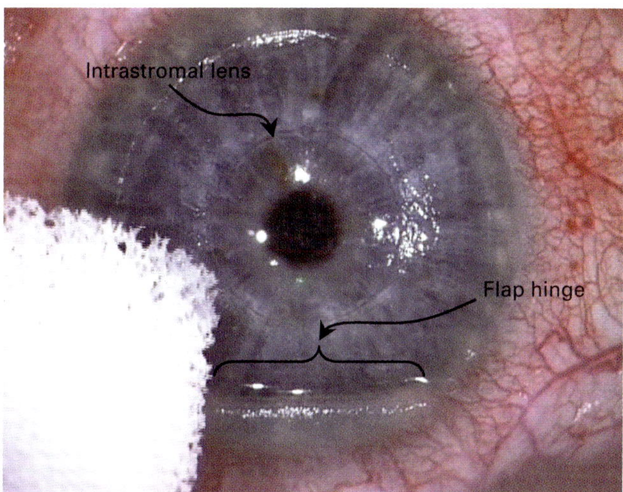

Figure 5-1 After the corneal flap is made, the PermaVision lens is placed in the central stromal bed to change the anterior corneal curvature and refraction. *(Courtesy of Anamed, Inc.)*

content. Studies have demonstrated that the lens is well tolerated in an animal model. The lens is 5.0 to 5.5 mm wide with a 30 to 60 μm central thickness. The PermaVision lens has the same index of refraction as the stroma and acts by changing the shape of the anterior cornea. The surgeon uses a microkeratome to create the corneal flap. The flap is reflected, the appropriate power lens implant is centered over the pupil on the stromal bed, and then the flap is put back in place. A convex lens steepens the central cornea to correct hyperopia and a concave lens flattens the central cornea to correct myopia. One of the advantages of the inlay is that the refractive result is potentially reversible and adjustable by removing the lens or replacing it with another of a different power.

Barraquer JI. Modification of refraction by means of intracorneal inclusions. *Int Ophthalmol Clin.* 1966;6:53–78.

Ismail MM. Correction of hyperopia with intracorneal implants. *J Cataract Refract Surg.* 2002;28:527–530.

Jankov M, Mrochen MC, Bueeler M, et al. Experimental results of preparing laser-shaped stromal implants for laser-assisted intrastromal keratophakia in extremely complicated laser in situ keratomileusis cases. *J Refract Surg.* 2002;18:S639–S643.

Knowles WF. Effect of intralamellar plastic membranes on corneal physiology. *Am J Ophthalmol.* 1961;51:1146–1156.

Troutman RC. Indications, techniques, and complications of keratophakia. *Int Ophthalmol Clin.* 1983;23:11–23.

Epikeratoplasty

Background

To eliminate the complexity of the lamellar dissection and intraoperative lathing of early keratomileusis procedures, in which a corneal cap was dissected from the eye, shaped on a cryolathe, and then repositioned with sutures, Kaufman and Werblin developed epikeratoplasty (also called epikeratophakia) in the early 1980s. Epikeratoplasty involves suturing a preformed lenticule of human donor corneal tissue directly onto Bowman's layer of the host cornea (Fig 5-2). Because no viable cells exist in the donor tissue, classic graft rejection does not occur. Epikeratoplasty was originally intended as a "living contact lens" for aphakic patients who were unable to wear contact lenses. By eliminating the central lamellar dissection, it was hoped that the procedure would be safer, easier to perform, and that the "living lens" could be removed, allowing reversibility of the refractive result. Epikeratoplasty was later expanded to include the treatment of hyperopia and myopia.

Patient Selection

In 1988, the FDA made the following recommendations for indications for epikeratoplasty:

- A visually disabled monocular aphake for whom secondary IOL insertion is contraindicated
- An aphakic child who is contact lens intolerant and who is unable to use spectacles for visual correction
- A visually disabled patient with keratoconus who is contact lens intolerant, in whom keratoplasty is contraindicated or associated with a high risk for failure
- A patch graft used for tectonic purposes

In light of the disappointing results of the myopia trials, no application for myopic epikeratoplasty was submitted to the FDA for review. The FDA also had concerns that the refractive power of the lenticule could not be reproducibly measured after creation. The manufacturer of the commercially prepared lenticules ceased production, and only those few centers with corneal lathe equipment have been able to continue performing this procedure.

Instrumentation

The primary requirement for epikeratoplasty is the lenticule. This is donor corneal tissue that is cut to size, frozen, and lathed to a predetermined shape. The curvature of the anterior surface produced by the lenticule provides the refractive correction. This can theoretically change the refractive status of the cornea by up to 37 D. Plus (convex) lenses are used for aphakia and hyperopia, minus (concave) lenses for myopia, and plano lenses for keratoconus.

In the most refined technique, donor lenticules are made 1.5 mm larger than the recipient. A typical lenticule would be 8.5 mm in diameter with a 7.0 mm prepared host bed. Storage of the lathed lenticule changed from lyophilization to a "moist pack" in an effort to promote more rapid epithelialization and clearing of the cornea.

Technique

To prepare the host cornea, the epithelium is removed followed by an annular keratectomy with resection of a 0.5 to 1.0 mm wedge of Bowman's layer and anterior stroma from the inner aspect of a partial-thickness 7 to 8 mm trephine. A partial lamellar dissection peripheral to the trephine allows the wing of the lenticule to be tucked under the host tissue. This preparation helps to scar the lenticule to the host cornea and permits repopulation of the donor with host keratocytes. Interrupted and/or running 10–0 nylon sutures are used to secure the tissue and are removed 6 to 12 weeks later (Fig 5-3A and B).

Outcomes

Studies were conducted initially on nonhuman primates and were later expanded to include human adults. Four large nationwide studies (on adult and pediatric aphakia, keratoconus, and myopia) with a collective total of 1389 cases were conducted after commercially prepared tissue became available in 1984.

The refractive results of myopic epikeratoplasty were disappointing. The mean spherical equivalent refractive error decreased from −12.52 to −1.38 D postoperatively. However, the postoperative standard deviation was 3.64 D, indicating considerable variability in refractive outcome. Overall, 33% of patients attained 20/40 or better uncorrected

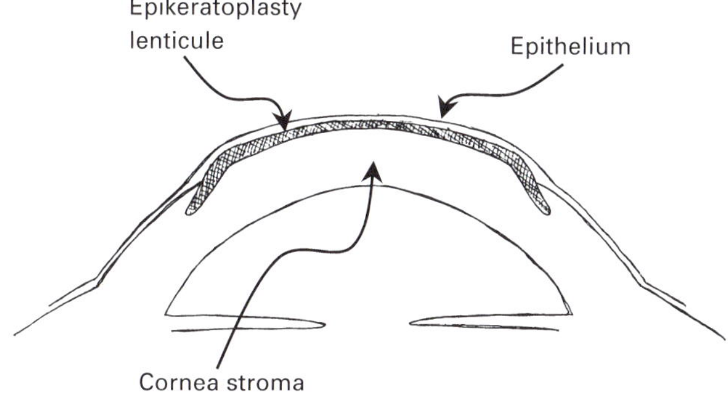

Figure 5-2 The lenticule in epikeratoplasty is sutured onto the cornea after removal of the epithelium. The edge of the lenticule is placed into a shallow lamellar dissection.

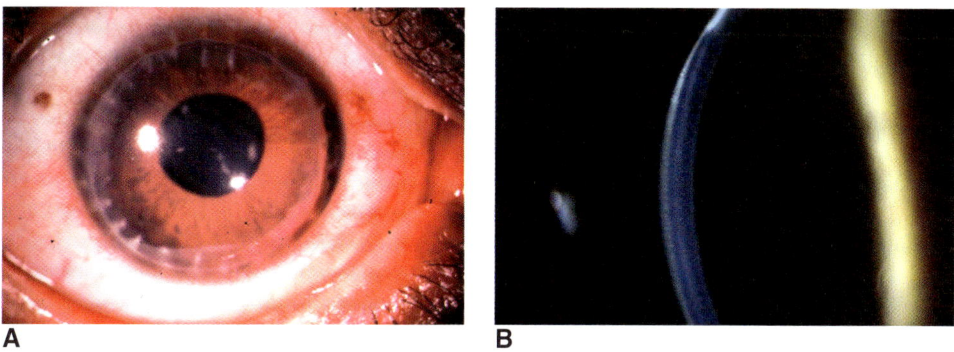

Figure 5-3 **A,** Epikeratoplasty after suture removal. **B,** A slit-lamp cross section shows the interface between the lenticule and the host cornea. *(A courtesy of Jayne S. Weiss, MD; B courtesy of Steven C. Schallhorn, MD.)*

vision, and only 35% were corrected to within 10% of emmetropia (based on their preoperative myopia). A total of 15% of patients lost 2 or more lines of best-corrected visual acuity and the mean astigmatism increased from 1.4 ± 0.8 D to 2.6 ± 2.1 D. Early and late regression of refractive effect were also noted.

The results for aphakic epikeratoplasty were also disappointing. In the nationwide aphakia study, the mean spherical-equivalent refractive error decreased from +11.5 ± 1.92 D to +0.90 ± 2.83 D postoperatively. Again the high postoperative standard deviation (2.83 D) indicated considerable variability in refractive outcome, especially when compared with the standard deviation for IOL implantation, which is generally 1.0 D. Visual recovery time was also substantially longer after epikeratoplasty than after IOL implantation. Still, the procedure did offer an alternative method to correct anisometropia in the unilaterally aphakic, contact lens–intolerant patient in whom intraocular surgery was contraindicated.

For keratoconus, epikeratoplasty was envisioned to provide tectonic support where severe corneal distortion and steepness made it impossible to fit contact lenses. Epikeratoplasty could then restore vision by allowing the resumption of contact lens use, while avoiding the risks of penetrating keratoplasty. The nationwide study of epikeratoplasty for keratoconus resulted in improvement in uncorrected vision in 98% (80/82) of patients. There was a higher proportion of patients who achieved 20/40 or better best-corrected visual acuity (78% post-epikeratoplasty compared with 69% before surgery). Astigmatism was slightly reduced from an average of 5.97 D before the procedure to 4.65 D afterward. When compared with penetrating keratoplasty, both procedures were shown to have similar results in obtaining 20/40 or better best-corrected visual acuity. However, penetrating keratoplasty resulted in a significantly higher proportion of eyes with 20/20 best-corrected visual acuity (73% after penetrating keratoplasty vs 24% after epikeratoplasty).

Complications

Delayed re-epithelialization over the lenticule was a major complication that was never fully solved. Bandage contact lenses, patching, temporary tarsorrhaphies, and changes in lathing and preservation techniques of the lenticule were tried. The incidence of nonhealing defects in the large nationwide series was 2.5% to 3.5%. The mean time to re-epithelialization was 7.1 days in adult aphakia cases, but it could take weeks to months before the epithelium had a normal histologic appearance and barrier function. The consequences of failure to re-epithelialize were severe and included necrosis, infection, and melting of the graft. The overall graft removal rate in the four nationwide studies was 7.7%, with the most common reason being a persistent epithelial defect. Other complications and causes for lenticule removal included graft haze/scar, infection, stromal infiltrates, melt, dehiscence, refractive error, irregular astigmatism, epithelial ingrowth and interface cysts, and severe glare symptoms. After lenticule removal, 14% of patients who had undergone epikeratoplasty for myopia had a reduction of best-corrected visual acuity. Central scarring of the host after donor removal was also reported, which cast doubt on the reversibility of the procedure.

Alloplastic Corneal Onlays

Laser-adjustable synthetic epikeratoplasty has been proposed as an adjustable and reversible refractive procedure. It is similar to standard epikeratoplasty except that a synthetic lenticule is used. This eliminates many of the disadvantages of human tissue, such as the difficulty of lathing, the production of consistent and measurable lenticules, distortion upon suturing, and postoperative remodeling that causes changes in refraction. If further refractive correction is required after placing the synthetic lenticule, a laser is used to remodel the anterior surface. The properties of the synthetic material are the key to the success of this technique. It must have satisfactory optical quality and biocompatibility without in vivo degradation. It must also be able to promote stable epithelial attachments. Laser-adjustable synthetic epikeratoplasty has not progressed beyond the experimental stage in search of the ideal synthetic material.

American Academy of Ophthalmology. Epikeratoplasty: Ophthalmic Procedure Assessment. *Ophthalmology*. 1996;103:983–991.

Kaufman HE. The correction of aphakia. *Am J Ophthalmol.* 1980;89:1–10.

Intrastromal Corneal Ring Segments

Background

Intrastromal corneal ring segments (Intacs, Addition Technology) can treat low amounts of myopia by displacing the lamellar bundles and shortening the corneal arc length. These circular rings of polymethylmethacrylate (PMMA) are placed in the midperipheral corneal stroma in a lamellar channel (Figs 5-4, 5-5). The thicker the segment, the greater the flattening of the cornea and the greater the reduction in myopia.

There are several potential advantages of ring segments over other forms of refractive surgery. The ring segments can be explanted, making the refractive result of the procedure potentially reversible, and the ring segments can be replaced with ring segments of different thickness to titrate the refractive result. Unlike PRK or LASIK, the central clear zone of the cornea is not directly treated. The normal cornea is generally prolate, or steeper centrally than peripherally: the central cornea profile after placement of ring segments has been shown to maintain an aspheric, prolate shape because the ring segments flatten the peripheral cornea more than the central cornea. It has been suggested that a prolate cornea may minimize visual disturbances, such as glare and halo symptoms. Conventional myopic excimer laser procedures flatten the central cornea more than the peripheral cornea, which typically produces an oblate (flattened) central corneal shape.

There are several disadvantages of intrastromal ring segments. Specialized equipment and training is required to create the lamellar channels and to insert the ring segments. The procedure generally takes longer to perform than LASIK. Patients can experience ocular discomfort after surgery and some complain of visual disturbances such as glare. Only low levels of myopia can be treated. Ring segments cannot correct astigmatism or hyperopia. Even in the low myopia range, ring segments have declined in popularity and have not captured a significant portion of the refractive surgery market; LASIK remains much more popular.

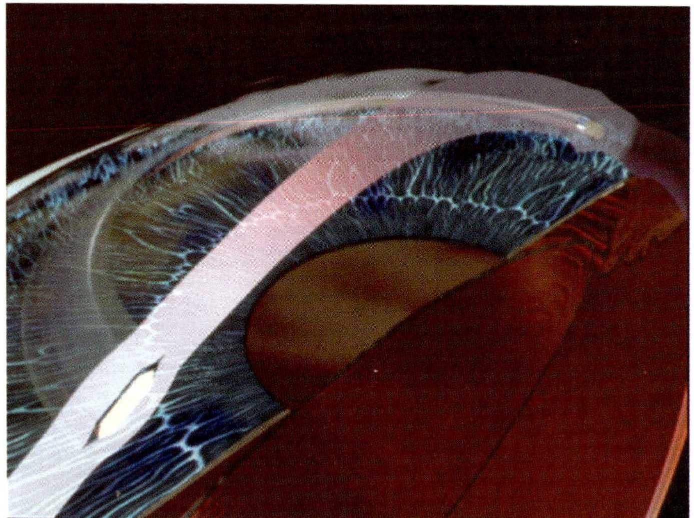

Figure 5-4 Cross section of the cornea with an intrastromal corneal ring segment. The ring segment displaces the lamellar bundles, which shortens the corneal arc length and reduces the myopia. *(Courtesy of Addition Technology.)*

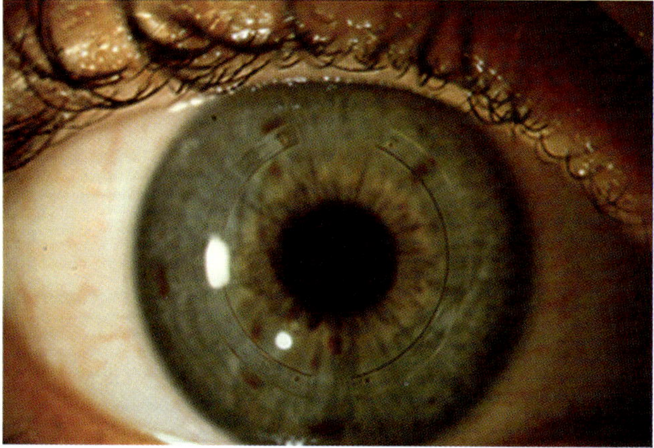

Figure 5-5 Ring segments implanted in an eye to treat low myopia. Note the vertical placement of the ring segments with a clear central zone. *(Photograph courtesy of Steven C. Schallhorn, MD.)*

Patient Selection

Intacs are approved by the FDA for low levels of myopia (−1.00 to −3.00 D spherical equivalent) but cannot correct astigmatism. Additional selection criteria are for patients

- With an age of 21 years or older
- With documented stability of refraction as demonstrated by a change of less than or equal to 0.50 D for at least 12 months prior to the preoperative examination
- With 1.0 D of astigmatism or less

Intacs are typically contraindicated

- In patients with collagen vascular, autoimmune, or immunodeficiency diseases
- In pregnant or nursing women
- In the presence of ocular conditions (such as keratoconus, recurrent corneal erosion syndrome, or corneal dystrophy) that may predispose the patient to future complications

Intacs are not recommended

- In patients with a low-light pupil diameter of 7.0 mm or larger because of the predisposition to low-light visual symptoms (the ring segments are placed at approximately 7.5 mm diameter around the visual axis)
- In patients with systemic diseases likely to affect wound healing, such as insulin-dependent diabetes or severe atopic disease
- In patients with a history of ophthalmic herpes simplex or herpes zoster
- In eyes with a central corneal thickness of less than 480 µm or a peripheral thickness of less than 570 µm
- In eyes with a corneal keratometry steeper than 46 D or flatter than 40 D

Intacs recently received a Humanitarian Device Exemption (HDE) from the FDA for use in reducing or eliminating myopia and astigmatism in certain patients with keratoconus, specifically those who are no longer able to achieve adequate vision with their contact lenses or spectacles. The intent is to restore functional vision and defer the need for a corneal transplant. Selection criteria for patients include

- experience with a progressive deterioration in vision, such that the patient can no longer achieve adequate functional vision on a daily basis with contact lenses or spectacles
- age 21 years or older
- clear central corneas
- a corneal thickness of 450 µm or greater at the proposed incision site
- corneal transplantation is the only remaining option for improving functional vision

Instrumentation

The Intacs ring segments consist of two arc-shaped segments made of PMMA. Initially a 330° segment was used but this was difficult to insert. The procedure was changed to the insertion of two segments of 150° of arc. They have a fixed outer diameter of 8.10 mm and are available in five thicknesses: 0.250, 0.275, 0.300, 0.325, and 0.350 mm. Two additional segments, 0.400 and 0.450 mm, are available outside of the United States. The amount of correction achieved is related to the thickness of the ring segments; the thicker ring segments are used for higher amounts of correction (Table 5-1).

A special set of surgical instruments has been developed for placement of the ring segments. This set includes an incision and placement marker, glide tip, ring forceps,

Table 5-1 Ring Segment Thickness and Predicted Correction for Intrastromal Corneal Ring Segments (Intacs)

Ring Segment Thickness	Predicted Correction	Recommended Prescribing Range
0.250 mm	−1.30 D	−1.00 to −1.63 D
0.275 mm	−1.65 D	−1.625 to −1.75 D
0.300 mm	−2.00 D	−1.75 to −2.25 D
0.325 mm	−2.35 D	−2.25 to −2.50 D
0.350 mm	−2.70 D	−2.375 to −3.00 D

NOTE: There is overlap in the prescribing ranges. For instance, the predicted correction for the 0.275 mm ring segments is −1.65 D and for the 0.300 mm ring segments is −2.00 D. To treat −1.75 D, the 0.275 mm ring segments would have a nominal postoperative refraction of −0.10 D and the 0.300 mm ring segments would have a nominal postoperative refraction of +0.25 D. So the choice of ring size would depend on whether the target was slightly myopic or slightly hyperopic.

stromal spreader, vacuum centering guide with vacuum system, and clockwise and counterclockwise dissectors. Other necessary equipment is an ultrasonic pachymeter and a guarded diamond knife.

Technique

The ring segment procedure involves the creation of a lamellar channel at approximately ⅔ stromal depth followed by the insertion of the ring segments (see Figure 5-4). The procedure usually takes 15 to 30 minutes per eye to complete.

The eye is prepped with a topical anesthetic and an iodine solution, after which an eyelid speculum is inserted. The geometric center of the cornea is marked with a blunt hook using light pressure. Using the center of the cornea as a reference, the incision and placement device marks the radial incision superiorly at an optical zone of 7.5 mm and also indicates the ring segments' final positions. An ultrasound pachymeter is used to measure the thickness of the cornea over the radial incision mark. A diamond knife is set to 68% of the stromal depth and is then used to create a 1.0 mm radial incision at the 12 o'clock position. A lamellar channel is started with the stromal spreader tool. The vacuum centering guide is placed over the eye using the central corneal mark. Vacuum is applied and confirmed. The clockwise glide tip is placed into the lamellar channel and the clockwise dissector is engaged into the centering guide and the tip is placed under the glide. While vacuum is maintained to stabilize the eye, the dissector is rotated clockwise to create the left-hand side of the intrastromal tunnel (Fig 5-6). This is followed by the counterclockwise dissection for the right-hand tunnel. The suction device is removed. A ring segment forceps is used to insert one ring segment and to rotate it into position, followed by the other ring segment. One or two 10–0 nylon sutures are used to close the radial incision.

Outcomes

The FDA clinical trials provided the most complete outcome analysis of Intacs. A total of 452 patients enrolled in these trials. The patients received either the 0.250, 0.300, or 0.350 mm ring segments to correct an average preoperative mean spherical equivalent

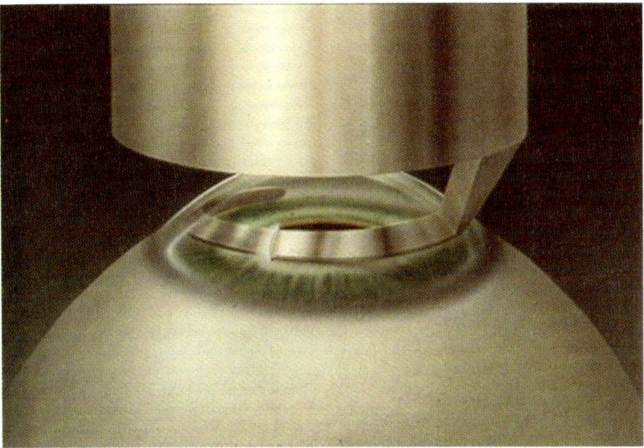

Figure 5-6 The Intacs dissector tool is being rotated to create the intrastromal tunnel. The suction ring and centering guide are not shown. *(Courtesy of Addition Technology.)*

of −2.24 D, with a range of −0.75 to −4.125 D. At 12 months postoperatively, 97% of eyes had 20/40 or better uncorrected vision and 74% had achieved 20/20 or better. In addition, 69% and 92% of eyes were within ±0.50 and 1.0 D of emmetropia, respectively. These clinical outcomes were similar to early PRK and LASIK results, although excimer laser studies generally had a broader range of preoperative myopia.

Patients who receive the 0.350 mm ring segment are more likely to have a worse outcome, both in terms of refractive accuracy and postoperative uncorrected visual acuity. The larger ring segment is also associated with a higher rate of removal due to patient dissatisfaction. In clinical trials, the 0.350 mm ring segments were removed at a rate of 13.3% versus a removal rate of 3.4% and 6.4% for the 0.250 and 0.300 mm ring segments, respectively.

A unique advantage of Intacs is that the ring segments can be removed or exchanged, making the refractive result potentially reversible. The removal or exchange rate has been reported to vary between 3% and 15%. The most common reason for a ring segment exchange is residual myopia. Ring segment removal is most often performed for disabling visual symptoms such as glare, double vision, or photophobia. There are few complications associated with ring segment removal. In one series of 684 eyes that received Intacs, 46 underwent removal (6.7%). Most patients returned to their original preoperative myopia by 3 months postremoval (73% returned to within 0.50 D of preoperative mean spherical equivalent). No patient had a loss of best-corrected visual acuity of more than 2 lines. However, up to 15% of patients have reported new or worsening symptoms after removal.

Intacs and Keratoconus

Other than penetrating keratoplasty, very few surgical options are available for keratoconus. Excimer laser procedures, which correct ametropia by removing tissue, are considered an absolute contraindication in treating keratoconus. Intacs have been used to correct patients with mild keratoconus with promising results. In one study of 26 keratoconus patients, a horizontal orientation for the ring segments was used with a thick ring (0.45 mm, not currently available in the United States) in the inferior cornea and a thinner one (0.25 mm) in the superior cornea. In another study of 50 patients (74 eyes), the orientation of the ring segments was adjusted according to the refractive cylinder. Based on the level of myopia, either the 0.30-mm or the 0.35-mm ring (the largest currently available in the United States) was placed inferiorly, and the 0.25-mm ring was placed superiorly. Patients had mild to severe keratoconus with or without scarring. A superficial channel with Bowman's layer perforation on one eye was the only operative complication. A total of six rings were explanted for segment migration and externalization (1 ring) and foreign-body sensation (5 rings).

The visual improvement was significant. With an average follow-up of 9 months, the mean UCVA improved from approximately 20/200 (1.05 logMAR) to 20/80 (0.61 logMAR) ($P < .01$). The mean BCVA also improved from approximately 20/50 (0.41 logMAR) to 20/32 (0.24 logMAR) ($P < .01$). Most patients still required optical correction to achieve their best-corrected vision. Eyes with corneal scarring had a similar improvement in UCVA and BCVA. There was a reduction in the inferior steepening on topography. The dioptric power of the inferior cornea relative to the superior (I-S value) was reduced from a preoperative mean of 25.62 D to 6.60 D postoperatively. It was due to these favorable results that the FDA granted a Humanitarian Device Exemption for the treatment of keratoconus in those patients not able to achieve adequate vision with either glasses or contact lenses.

Complications

The loss of best-corrected visual acuity (≥2 lines of vision) after Intacs is approximately 1% at 1 year postoperatively. Adverse events (defined as events that if left untreated could be serious or result in permanent sequelae) occur in approximately 1% of patients. Reported adverse events include

- Anterior chamber perforation
- Microbial keratitis (Fig 5-7A)
- Implant expulsion (Fig 5-7B)
- Shallow ring segment placement

Ocular complications (defined as clinically significant events that will not result in permanent sequelae) have been reported in 11% of patients at 12 months postoperatively. These include

- Reduced corneal sensitivity (5.5%)
- Induced astigmatism between 1.0 and 2.0 D (3.7%)
- Deep neovascularization at the incision site (1.2%)
- Persistent epithelial defect (0.2%)
- Iritis/uveitis (0.2%)

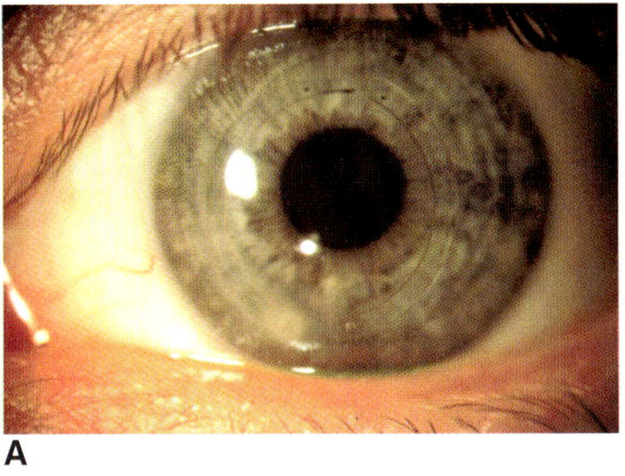
A

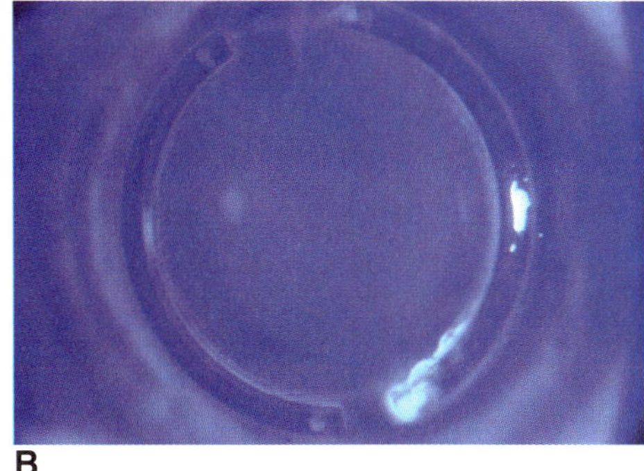
B

Figure 5-7 Complications of Intacs. **A,** Inferior infiltrate. **B,** Inferior ring segment expulsion. *(Courtesy of Addition Technology.)*

Visual symptoms rated as always present and severe in nature have been reported in approximately 14% of patients and include

- Difficulty with night vision (4.8%)
- Blurry vision (2.9%)
- Diplopia (1.6%)
- Glare (1.3%)
- Haloes (1.3%)
- Fluctuating distance vision (1.0%)
- Fluctuating near vision (0.3%)
- Photophobia (0.3%)

Fine white deposits occur frequently within the lamellar ring channels after Intacs placement (Fig 5-8). The incidence and density of the deposits increase with the ring segment thickness and the duration of implantation. Deposits do not seem to alter the optical performance of the ring segments or to result in corneal thinning or necrosis, although some patients are bothered by their appearance.

Other Potential Uses for Intrastromal Corneal Ring Segments

Applications of corneal ring segments that are currently under investigation (ie, that are not FDA-approved, and hence are off label) include use before or after LASIK and ectasia after LASIK. If these prove effective, there may be a resurgence of interest in ring segment technology.

Before or after LASIK

Corneal ring segments have been used to correct residual myopia following LASIK with good initial results. This procedure may be useful in patients whose stromal bed would not support repeat excimer laser ablation. Additional intraoperative pachymetry has been recommended to make sure there is adequate tissue for ring segment insertion.

Conversely, LASIK has been performed after ring segment removal with good success. The flap is created in a plane superficial to the previous ring segment channel.

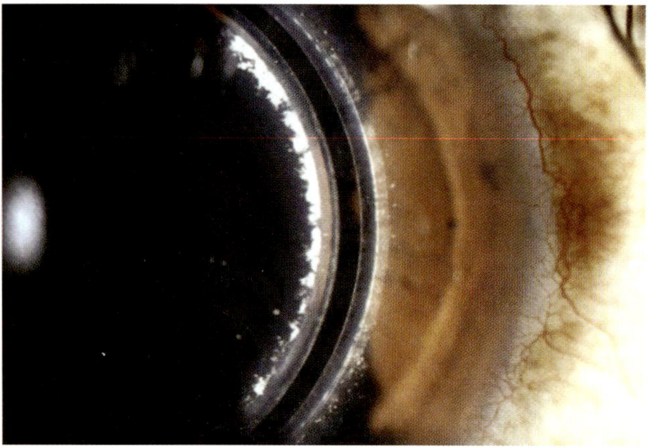

Figure 5-8 Grade 4 deposits around ring segments. The deposits can be graded on a 0 (none) to 4 (confluent) scale. These channel deposits are typically not seen until weeks or months after surgery. Although the corneal opacities may cause cosmetic complaints, they usually do not cause other ocular problems. *(Courtesy of Addition Technology.)*

With ectasia after LASIK

Ring segments have also been used for the postoperative management of corneal ectasia after LASIK. As in the treatment of keratoconus, few surgical options are available to treat corneal ectasia. Use of the excimer laser to remove additional tissue is considered a contraindication. A lamellar graft or penetrating keratoplasty can have significant morbidity, such as irregular astigmatism, delayed visual recovery, and tissue rejection. In limited early trials using Intacs to treat post-LASIK ectasia, myopia was reduced and uncorrected visual acuity was improved. However, the long-term effect of such an approach for the management of post-LASIK ectasia is unknown.

Boxer Wachler BS, Christie JP, Chandra NS, et al. Intacs for keratoconus. *Ophthalmology.* 2003;110:1031–1040.

Holmes-Higgin DK, Burris TE. Corneal surface topography and associated visual performance with Intacs for myopia: phase III clinical trial results. The Intacs Study Group. *Ophthalmology.* 2000;107:2061–2071.

Kymionis GD, Siganos CS, Kounis G, et al. Management of post-LASIK corneal ectasia with Intacs inserts: one-year results. *Arch Ophthalmol.* 2003;121:322–326.

Rapuano CJ, Sugar A, Kolch DD, et al. Intrastromal corneal ring segments for low myopia. *Ophthalmology.* 2001;108:1922–1928.

Siganos CS, Kymionis GD, Kartakis N, et al. Management of keratoconus with Intacs. *Am J Ophthalmol.* 2003;135:64–70.

U.S. Food and Drug Administration. *KeraVision Intacs. Part 2. Summary of Safety and Effectiveness Data.* P980031. April 30, 1999 (http://www.fda.gov/cdrh/pdf/p980031.html).

Orthokeratology

Orthokeratology, or corneal refractive therapy, refers to the overnight use of gas-permeable contact lenses to temporarily reduce myopia. The goal of this nonsurgical method of temporary myopia reduction is to achieve functional uncorrected visual acuity during the day. The contact lens is fitted at a flatter base curve than the corneal curvature. Temporary corneal flattening results from redistribution of corneal tissue (mostly the epithelium). A mean of 1 D temporary reduction of myopia was reported 20 years ago by Polse and colleagues in a National Eye Institute orthokeratology clinical trial.

More recently, the FDA approved a rigid contact lens (Paragon CRT) for overnight orthokeratology and temporary reduction of naturally occurring myopia of from −0.50 to −6.00 D of sphere with up to 1.75 D of astigmatism. The contact lens used in this clinical trial had three zones. The center zone had an apical radius greater than the underlying corneal apical radius; the secondary midperipheral zone returned the contact lens to the proximity of the cornea; and the third zone was tangent to the cornea in the peripheral area. Special training was mandated for dispensing practitioners because of the unique challenges associated with fitting these contact lenses. The contact lenses were inserted every night before the patient went to sleep and were removed on awakening. Vision was optimal for 8 hours after removal. The refractive error increased to baseline after an undetermined period of time.

A total of 408 eyes were studied; 34.6% of patients discontinued contact lens use. The contact lenses did not affect the magnitude of pretreatment astigmatism. The mean reduction of myopia was 2.59 D. In the study, 89% of all eyes were within 1 D of emmetropia and 50% were within 0.5 D. At 9 months, uncorrected visual acuity of 20/20 was achieved in 58.4% of patients and uncorrected visual acuity of 20/40 was achieved in 89.8%. The study found that 90% of patients with 1 to 2 D of myopia achieved 20/40 uncorrected visual acuity while 76% of patients with more than 4 D achieved 20/40 uncorrected visual acuity. At 9 months, 68% of patients had no change in best-corrected visual acuity, 13% had a 1-line increase in best-corrected visual acuity, 1.6% had more than a 2-line increase in best-corrected visual acuity, and 4% had a loss of 2 lines of more of best-corrected visual acuity. Safety and efficacy in patients under 18 years of age was not determined.

In this study, 75% of patients complained of some degree of discomfort but this decreased to 20% by 9 months. There was one case of corneal abrasion and 18 cases of corneal edema. Corneal edema was reported more frequently in patients fitted at higher altitudes. No cases of corneal ulceration were reported. Because the effect of the contact lens is temporary, the patient may notice blurring of vision during regression of effect. During this time, the gas-permeable contact lenses can be reinserted to achieve the best-corrected visual acuity.

Orthokeratology is most appropriate for highly motivated low myopes who do not want refractive surgery but who want to be free of contact lenses and spectacles during the day. The contact lens does not treat astigmatism or hyperopia. Prospective patients should be informed that in clinical trials, approximately one third of patients discontinued contact lens use and most patients (75%) experienced discomfort at some point during contact lens wear.

Polse KA, Brand RJ, Vastine DW, et al. Corneal change accompanying orthokeratology. Plastic or elastic? Results of a randomized controlled clinical trial. *Arch Ophthalmol.* 1983; 101:1873–1878.

Conclusion

Corneal inlay and onlay procedures to correct ametropia have been performed for many years. Many procedures, such as epikeratoplasty, have been abandoned because of poor predictability or safety concerns. Intrastromal corneal ring segments are being implanted in a small percentage of patients with low spherical myopia, but the popularity of the procedure is declining. There may be a resurgence with the recent approval to use them to treat keratoconus. Other possible uses under investigation are in the treatment of residual myopia after LASIK and LASIK-induced ectasia. Alloplastic keratophakia inlays remain investigational but are promising.

CHAPTER 6

Photoablation

The 193 nm argon-fluoride excimer laser decreases refractive error by ablating the anterior corneal stroma to a new radius of curvature. There are three major refractive surgical techniques that employ excimer laser ablation. While the epithelium is debrided in photorefractive keratectomy (PRK), it is preserved as an epithelial flap in the PRK variant, laser subepithelial keratomileusis (LASEK). The excimer laser ablation is performed under a lamellar flap formed with a microkeratome or scanning pulsed laser in laser in situ keratomileusis (LASIK).

Background

Trokel and Srinivasan demonstrated a new form of laser–tissue interaction, *photoablation,* in 1983. Srinivasan, an IBM engineer, was studying the far-UV (193 nm) argon-fluoride excimer laser for photoetching of computer chips (the term *excimer* is a contraction of "excited dimer," referring to the unstable molecular combination of argon and fluorine, created transiently by a high-voltage electrical charge and emitting a UV photon when the molecule reverts to separate atoms). Trokel, an ophthalmologist, not only showed that the excimer laser could remove corneal tissue precisely, with minimal adjacent corneal damage, but also recognized the potential for refractive and therapeutic corneal surgery.

Photoablation occurs because the cornea has an extremely high absorption coefficient at 193 nm. A single 193 nm photon has sufficient energy to directly break carbon-carbon and carbon-nitrogen bonds that form the peptide backbone of the corneal collagen molecules. Excimer laser radiation ruptures the collagen polymer into small fragments, expelling a discrete volume of corneal tissue from the surface with each pulse of the laser (Fig 6-1). Because the laser removes tissue rather than incises it, the excimer laser is a poor replacement for a cutting scalpel.

Photorefractive keratectomy, the sculpting of the de-epithelialized corneal surface to alter refractive power, underwent extensive preclinical investigation before it was applied to sighted human eyes. Results of early animal studies provided evidence for normal wound healing in laser-ablated corneas. McDonald and co-workers treated the first sighted human eye in 1988.

The popularity of PRK faded rapidly when LASIK began to be performed frequently in the late 1990s because of LASIK's faster visual recovery and decreased postoperative discomfort. LASIK represents the combination of two refractive technologies: excimer

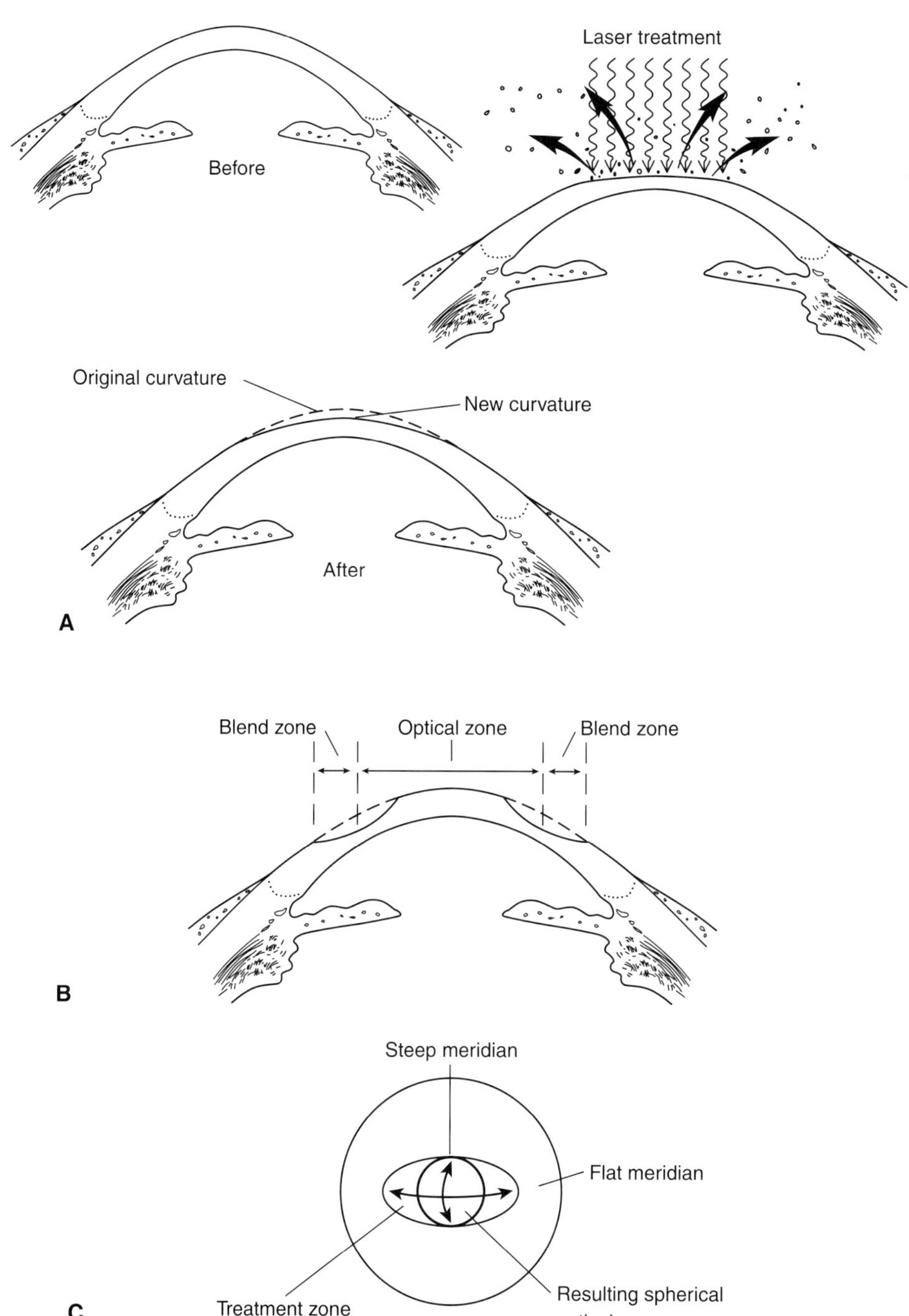

Figure 6-1 Schematic representation of corneal recontouring by the excimer laser. **A,** Correction of myopia by flattening the central cornea. **B,** Correction of hyperopia by relative steepening of the central corneal optical zone and blending the periphery. **C,** Correction of astigmatism by differential tissue removal 90° apart. Note that in correction of myopic astigmatism, the steeper meridian with more tissue removal corresponds to the smaller dimension of the ellipse. **D,** In LASIK, a flap is reflected back, the excimer laser ablation is performed on the exposed stromal bed, and then the flap is replaced. The altered corneal contour of the bed causes the same alteration in the anterior surface of the flap. *(Continues)*

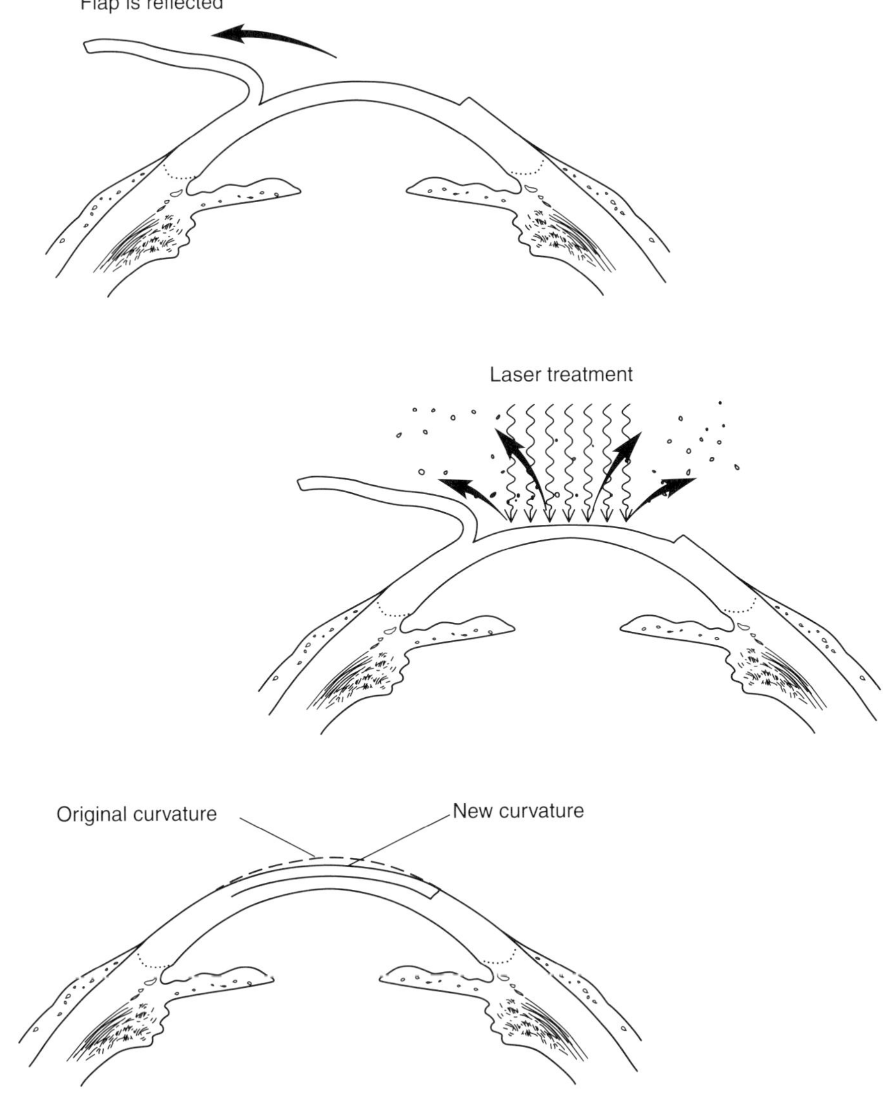

Figure 6-1 *(Continued) (Illustration by Jeanne Koelling.)*

laser stromal ablation and the placement of the ablation beneath a stromal flap made by a microkeratome. The microkeratome evolved from the original type designed by Barraquer to perform his frozen-tissue keratomileusis procedures; it was modified in the subsequent evolution of automated lamellar keratomileusis (ALK) by Ruiz, who used a second pass of the microkeratome to remove a refractive-shifting wedge of tissue. While more LASIK procedures continue to be performed than PRK, PRK is an attractive alternative in specific indications, such as very low refractive corrections, epithelial basement membrane disease (often called map-dot-fingerprint dystrophy), thin corneas, and for treatment of some LASIK flap complications such as buttonholed flaps. In addition, with the advent of wavefront-guided laser ablation, the popularity of PRK may increase. The LASIK flap is associated with a greater increase in postoperative higher-order optical aberrations than PRK, so it is possible that the postoperative quality of vision may be higher with wavefront-guided PRK than with LASIK.

Srinivasan R. Ablation of polymers and biological tissue by ultraviolet lasers. *Science.* 1983;234:559–565.

Trokel SL, Srinivasan R, Braren B. Excimer laser surgery of the cornea. *Am J Ophthalmol.* 1983;96:710–715.

Photorefractive Keratectomy (PRK) and Laser Subepithelial Keratomileusis (LASEK)

Patient Selection

The preoperative evaluation of patients considering refractive surgery is presented in detail in Chapter 3. This section reviews only the aspects of the preoperative evaluation that are specific to PRK and its variant, LASEK.

A history of connective tissue diseases such as rheumatoid arthritis, systemic lupus erythematosus, or Sjögren syndrome is considered a contraindication to PRK because of less predictable corneal wound healing with the potential for corneal melting. Although keloid scar formation is a commonly listed contraindication to PRK, one study found that African Americans with a history of keloid formation did well after PRK. Prior herpes simplex keratitis is another commonly listed contraindication to PRK, but systemic antiviral prophylaxis preoperatively and for several months after surgery may make PRK safer for these patients. Diabetes needs to be well controlled preoperatively due to instability of the refractive error and potential poor wound healing with fluctuating blood sugar levels (see Chapter 10). Extreme caution should be exercised if PRK or any refractive surgery is considered for a normal eye when the fellow eye is highly amblyopic. The refractive procedure puts the patient's better eye at risk, and this patient should be wearing protective spectacles rather than undergoing surgery to reduce spectacle use (see Chapter 10).

The orbital anatomy must be carefully inspected. A high brow, deep-set globe, or narrow palpebral fissure each increases the difficulty of performing a successful microkeratome flap and may lead a surgeon to consider surface ablation over LASIK.

Measurement of the low-light scotopic pupil size is important in the preoperative assessment. Although conventional wisdom previously suggested that the optical zone should be larger than the pupil diameter to minimize visual disturbances such as glare and haloes, more recent findings have demonstrated that this belief may be too simplistic. In fact, some patients with large pupils have no night vision complaints. Higher-order optical aberrations increase in the corneal periphery and the interaction with pupil size probably explains complaints of poor night vision.

Patients with epithelial basement membrane dystrophy are better candidates for PRK than LASIK because PRK may be therapeutic, enhancing epithelial adhesion, while the microkeratome friction in LASIK may cause a frank epithelial defect.

In addition, the surgeon must evaluate any clinically significant disparity between the manifest and cycloplegic refractions. Most patients will have a cycloplegic refraction between 0.25 and 1.0 D shifted in the hyperopic direction. Some or all of this disparity can be attributed to the optics of the peripheral cornea and a small posterior shift of the crystalline lens with cycloplegia. Refractive surgeons have their own preferences on whether to program the laser using manifest or cycloplegic refraction, based on their individual nomogram and technique. Many surgeons will plan their laser input based on the manifest refraction, especially in younger patients, if the manifest refraction has been performed with a careful defogging technique. A disparity between the manifest and cycloplegic refractions of more than 1.0 D of sphere warrants reevaluation, often including a postcycloplegic manifest refraction "pushing plus" to overcome accommodative spasm. Accommodative spasm is common in both myopes who have become "overminused" in their contact lenses or spectacles (extra minus causes a slight minification of the image, which causes a perception of higher contrast) and in hyperopes who have a lifelong habit of accommodation to improve distance vision. In middle-aged patients, a cycloplegic refraction is still mandatory, because surprising amounts of accommodative spasm may remain. Some refractive surgeons use the cycloplegic refraction to plan the laser input in these patients. Tropicamide 1% is usually strong enough to relax accommodation in patients over age 40, but Cyclogyl 1% (cyclopentolate) may be advisable in younger patients, especially hyperopes.

Several clinical tests are helpful in resolving disparities between the manifest and cycloplegic refractions. In addition to a "defogging" technique that "pushes plus," a time-honored technique is the duochrome chart, where one half of the chart is green and the other half is red. Because of chromatic aberration, the longer red wavelengths are focused slightly behind the shorter green wavelengths. An overminused refraction will cause the focal point to be behind the retina. Red wavelengths will be further retrofocused and therefore letters on the red half of the chart appear more blurred than letters on the green half of the chart. Other helpful clinical strategies include placing a 4 mm aperture in the trial frame during the cycloplegic refraction to restrict vision to the more central cornea, and comparing the refraction to the readings from an autorefractor with a defogging device system.

Ambrosio R Jr, Klyce SD, Wilson SE. Corneal topographic and pachymetric screening of keratorefractive patients. *J Refract Surg.* 2003;19:24–29.

Cua IY, Pepose JS. Late corneal scarring after photorefractive keratectomy concurrent with development of systemic lupus erythematosus. *J Refract Surg.* 2002;18:750–752.

Surgical Technique

Calibration of the excimer laser

The laser should be checked for an adequate homogeneous beam profile, alignment, and power output daily and in between patients, according to the instructions of the manufacturer.

Preoperative planning and laser programming

Often the manifest and cycloplegic refractions differ, or the amount and axis of astigmatism observed on topographic and refractive examination differs. Consequently, it may be unclear what refraction to enter into the laser. The surgeon's decision about whether to use the manifest or the cycloplegic refraction is based on his or her individual nomogram and technique. The manifest refraction is more accurate that the cycloplegic refraction in determining cylinder axis and amount. If the refractive cylinder is confirmed to differ from the topographic cylinder, lenticular astigmatism or posterior corneal curvature is assumed to be the cause. In this case, the laser is still programmed with the axis and amount of cylinder noted on refraction. The surgeon should take particular care to check the consistency of the axis on the refraction and topography with the value programmed into the laser, because this is a common source of error, particularly when there is a conversion between plus and minus cylinder formats.

In many laser models, the surgeon also must enter the size of the optical zone and whether or not a blend of the ablation zone should be performed. If there is sufficient corneal tissue, an ablation zone larger than the scotopic pupil size is usually selected. A "blend zone" is an area of peripheral asphericity designed to reduce the possible undesirable effects of an abrupt transition from the optical zone to the untreated cornea (see Figure 1-1B). A common approach to the creation of a blend zone would be to have, for example, a −6 D correction consist of a −5 D correction at a 6 mm optical zone and a −1 D correction at an 8 mm optical zone. The larger the treatment area, the deeper the ablation. The surgeon must calculate whether an adequate stromal bed will remain. Although this is rarely an issue for surface ablation, there may be inadequate tissue for LASIK in thinner corneas and higher dioptric treatments, which would be an indication to select surface ablation.

Preoperative preparation of the patient

Some surgeons use topical antibiotic prophylaxis preoperatively. The skin is prepped with povidone-iodine (Betadine) or alcohol wipes before or after entering the laser suite, and 5% povidone-iodine solution is sometimes applied as drops to the ocular surface for further antisepsis. There is no consensus about the utility of these measures. Prior to having the laser treatment performed, the patient should be instructed regarding the sounds and smell of the laser. Anxious patients may receive an oral sedative such as diazepam and the operative eye (in unilateral treatments) should be indicated with an adhesive label on the forehead.

If a large amount of astigmatism is being treated, some surgeons elect to mark the cornea at the horizontal or vertical axis to ensure accurate alignment of the patient under the laser. A 15° offset in the axis of treatment can decrease the effective cylinder change by 50% and can result in a significant axis shift.

After placing the patient under the laser, a sterile drape may be placed over the skin and eyelashes according to the surgeon's preference. Topical tetracaine and/or proparacaine anesthetic drops are placed in the eye. An eyelid speculum is placed in the operative eye and a patch is placed over the fellow eye to avoid cross-fixation. A gauze pad may be taped over the temple between the operative eye and the ear to absorb any excess eye drops. The patient is asked to fixate on the laser centration light while the surgeon focuses and centers the laser. For most patients, line-of-sight fixation by the patient during PRK produces more accurate centration than globe immobilization by the surgeon.

Epithelial debridement techniques for PRK

The epithelium can be removed by a sharp blade or a blunt spatula, by a rotating corneal brush, by application of diluted absolute alcohol (typically around 20% concentration) to the corneal surface to loosen the epithelium, or by transepithelial ablation by the excimer laser itself (Fig 6-2). With transepithelial ablation, the peripheral margin of the de-epithelialization is defined by the laser itself. For other epithelial debridement techniques, the surgeon defines the outer limit of de-epithelialization with an optical zone marker and then debrides the periphery first, followed by the center. An ophthalmic surgical cellulose sponge lightly moistened with an artificial tear lubricant such as carboxymethylcellulose 0.5% can be uniformly brushed over the surface of the cornea to remove any residual epithelium and to provide a smooth surface. The epithelium should be removed efficiently and consistently in order to prevent hydration changes in the stroma, because the rate of excimer laser ablation may be increased by excessive corneal

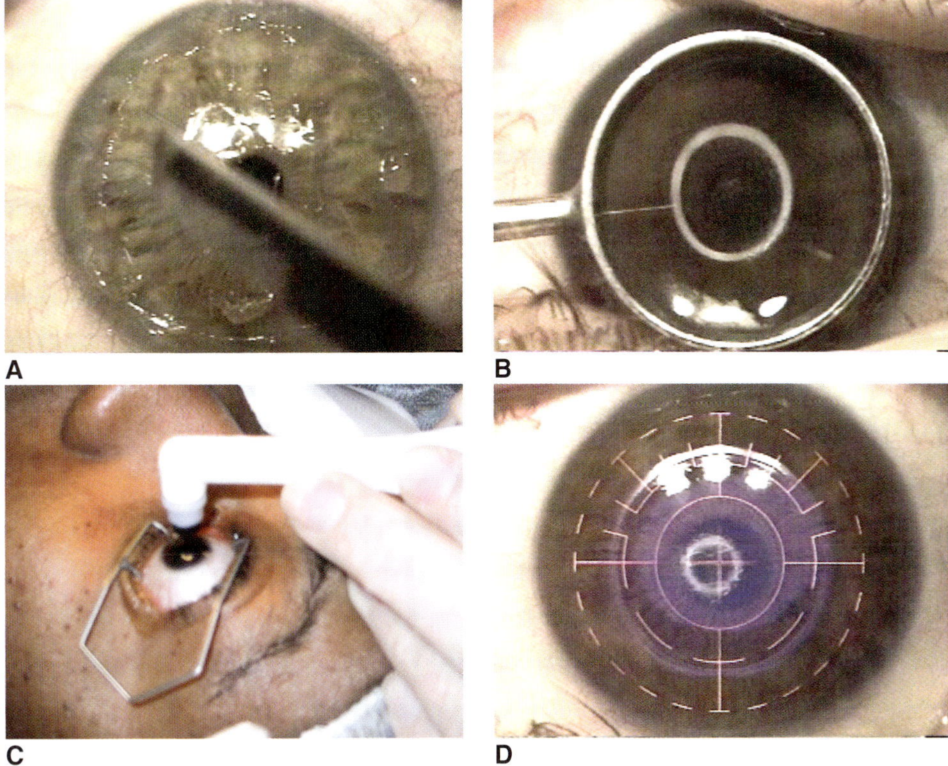

Figure 6-2 Techniques for de-epithelialization for PRK. **A,** Scraping with a blade; **B,** 20% dilution of absolute ethanol in an optical zone marker well; **C,** a rotary brush debridement; **D,** "laser scrape," where a broad-beam laser exposes the entire treatment zone to ablation pulses that remove most of the epithelium that is fluorescing brightly, after which the basal epithelial layer is removed by scraping with a blade. *(A, B, and D courtesy of Roger F. Steinert, MD; C courtesy of Steven C. Schallhorn, MD.)*

stromal dehydration, resulting in an overcorrection. The optical zone must be free of epithelial cells, debris, and excess fluid before ablation.

Epithelial preservation techniques for LASEK

In the LASEK variant of PRK, the goal is the preservation of the patient's epithelium. Instead of debriding and discarding the epithelium, or ablating the epithelium with the excimer laser, the surgeon folds back an intact sheet of epithelium (Fig 6-3). Placing a radial mark of gentian violet ink can aid in later realignment of the epithelial flap. A solution of approximately 20% diluted absolute alcohol is then applied for between 20 to 30 seconds. An 8.0 to 9.0 mm diameter optical zone marker pressed onto the corneal surface will restrict the alcohol to the area to be de-epithelialized. After the desired exposure time, the alcohol is removed from the "well" of the optical zone marker by absorption into a microsurgical spear sponge. After full absorption of the alcohol and removal of the optical zone marker, the ocular surface is immediately copiously irrigated

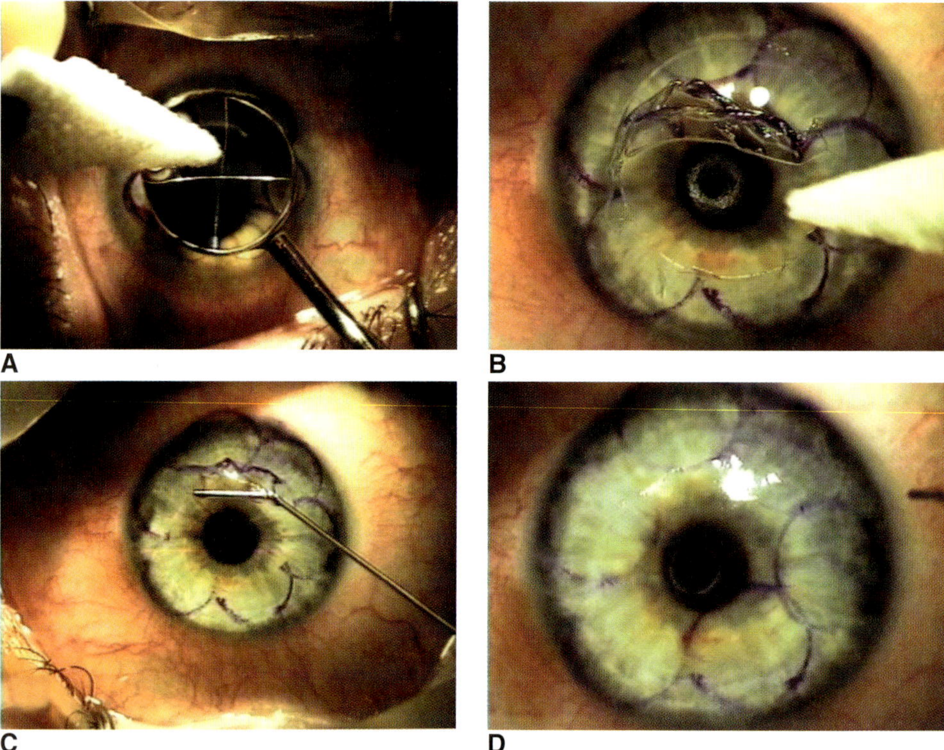

Figure 6-3 LASEK technique. **A,** 18% ethanol is released into the marker well. Care is taken to avoid spillage by using a dry sponge to absorb the overflowing ethanol. **B,** A dry, nonfragmenting sponge is used to peel the epithelial flap. **C,** After laser ablation is applied to the exposed Bowman's layer and stroma, a 30-gauge Rycroft irrigating cannula is used to hydrate and reposition the epithelial flap. **D,** The flap edges are aligned, and no epithelial defects are noted after flap repositioning and during the 5-minute waiting period. A bandage soft contact lens is applied at the end of the procedure. *(Reprinted with permission from Azar DT, Ang RT. Laser subepithelial keratomileusis: evolution of alcohol-assisted flap surface ablation.* Int Ophthalmol Clin. *2002;42:89–97.)*

with balanced salt solution to minimize toxicity to the limbal germinal epithelium. The surgeon then uses an instrument, often with a hoe or spatula configuration, to carefully separate a flap of full-thickness epithelium from the underlying Bowman's layer. The epithelium is delicately folded back on itself until all of the epithelium has been removed except for a small "hinge," typically located superiorly.

Although the goal of LASEK is to reduce postoperative pain, to speed the recovery of visual acuity, and to decrease postoperative haze formation, controlled studies have not supported these claims. With LASEK, vision may be slighter better on the first postoperative day compared with PRK, but some reports show more discomfort and a delay in recovery of vision with LASEK compared with PRK after the first day.

Development of a variant of the microkeratome used in LASIK (modified with a dull blade and a thin applanation plate to mechanically remove an epithelial flap without the use of toxic agents such as the alcohol used in LASEK) may improve the results of LASEK. The goal is to create an epithelial flap that will remain viable and successfully readhere postoperatively.

Ambrosio R, Wilson S. LASIK vs LASEK vs PRK: advantages and indications. *Sem Ophthalmol.* 2003;18:2–10.

The Laser Treatment

Centration and ablation

The laser is centered and focused according to the manufacturer's recommendations. In general, improved centration occurs when the aiming beams or reticule are centered on the entrance pupil instead of on the corneal apical light reflex. The patient is instructed to maintain good fixation during the stromal ablation. Small microsaccades should not adversely affect the outcome of the procedure. If the patient begins to lose fixation, however, the surgeon should immediately stop the treatment until adequate refixation is achieved. If the laser includes a tracking mechanism, it is still important for the surgeon to monitor for excessive eye roll, which can result in decentration despite the tracking device.

Although the excimer laser beam at 193 nm is invisible to the human eye, a faint fluorescence of deep blue light is sometimes visible during stromal ablation (Fig 6-4). The sound of the laser firing is the main feedback signal to the surgeon, along with an alteration in the light reflex as the stromal ablation progresses.

In order to attempt to decrease the chance of postoperative corneal haze after enhancement of a prior PRK scar or after PRK is applied to a LASIK flap, a soaked pledget or "corneal light shield" of mitomycin (usually 0.02% or 0.2 mg/mL mitomycin) can be placed on the ablated surface for 30 seconds to 2 minutes at the end of the laser exposure. The cornea is then irrigated with balanced salt solution to remove the excess mitomycin. In order to avoid damage to limbal stem cells, care should be taken to avoid exposure of the limbus or conjunctiva to the mitomycin. Animal studies have shown a reduced keratocyte population and less haze in eyes that had mitomycin, but vision-threatening complications of mitomycin have been reported in other settings, including glaucoma and corneal perforation. The search continues for the ideal topical wound-healing modulator that has high specificity for inhibiting collagen synthesis without toxic side effects.

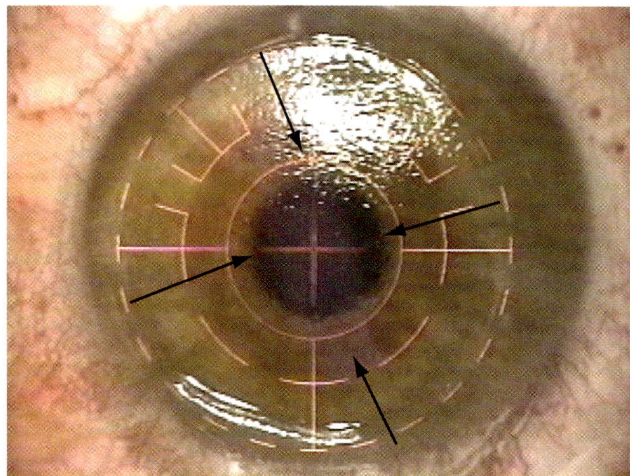

Figure 6-4 Excimer laser ablation of the stromal bed. Note the faint blue fluorescence of the stromal bed from the laser pulse *(arrows)*. The rectangular shape of the exposure by this broad-beam laser indicates that the laser is correcting the cylindrical portion of the treatment. (Photograph is enhanced to visualize fluorescence; the surgeon usually sees minimal or no fluorescence through the operating microscope.) *(Photograph courtesy of Roger F. Steinert, MD.)*

Carones F, Vigo L, Scandola E, et al. Evaluation of the prophylactic use of mitomycin-C to inhibit haze formation after photorefractive keratectomy. *J Cataract Refract Surg.* 2002;28:2088–2095.

Chen CC, Chang JH, Lee JB, et al. Human corneal epithelial cell viability and morphology after dilute alcohol exposure. *Invest Ophthalmol Vis Sci.* 2002;43:2593–2602.

Gabler B, Winkler von Mohrenfels C, Dreiss AK, et al. Vitality of epithelial cells after alcohol exposure during laser-assisted subepithelial flap preparation. *J Cataract Refract Surg.* 2002;28:1841–1846.

Majmudar PA, Forstot SL, Dennis RF, et al. Topical mitomycin-C for subepithelial fibrosis after refractive corneal surgery. *Ophthalmology.* 2000;107:89–94.

Immediate postablation measures

After the procedure is completed, drops of antibiotic, corticosteroid, and sometimes a nonsteroidal anti-inflammatory drug (NSAID) are placed in the eye, followed by a bandage soft contact lens. If the LASEK variant has been performed, the surgeon carefully floats and repositions the epithelial sheet back into position with balanced salt solution prior to applying the medications and the bandage soft contact lens. Some surgeons also apply chilled balanced salt solution before and/or after the PRK procedure in the belief that cooling reduces pain and haze formation, although the advantage of this practice has not been substantiated in a controlled study. If the patient cannot tolerate a bandage soft contact lens, a pressure patch may be used.

Operative day postablation treatment

During the first 24 hours, patients experience a variable amount of pain, from minimal to severe, which may need to be relieved by an oral narcotic pain medication in many patients. Some studies have shown that topical NSAID drops reduce postoperative pain, although they may also slow the rate of re-epithelialization and promote sterile infiltrates (see Figure 6-8). Corneal melting has been described after diclofenac therapy. Studies have also demonstrated a reduction in pain with the use of topical anesthetic drops. The patient must be carefully warned not to overuse topical anesthetic drops because they may cause severe corneal complications when used excessively over a prolonged period. However, topical nonpreserved tetracaine used ad libitum (generally every 1 to 4 hours if needed) in conjunction with a bandage soft contact lens for 1 or 2 days after PRK does not seem to delay re-epithelialization or cause keratopathy.

Subsequent postoperative care

The patient should be followed closely until the epithelium is completely healed, which usually occurs within 72 hours. As long as the bandage soft contact lens is in place, patients are treated with topical broad-spectrum antibiotics and corticosteroids, usually 4 times daily. At this point, the bandage soft contact lens, antibiotic drops, and NSAID drops (if used) may be discontinued. If used at all, topical anesthetic drops are confiscated from the patient to prevent prolonged use.

The administration of topical corticosteroids to modulate postoperative wound healing, to reduce anterior stromal haze, and to decrease regression of the refractive effect remains controversial. While some studies have demonstrated that corticosteroids have no significant long-term effect on corneal haze or visual outcome after PRK, other studies have shown that corticosteroids are effective in limiting haze and myopic regression after PRK, particularly after higher myopic corrections. Some surgeons who advocate topical corticosteroids after the removal of the bandage soft contact lens restrict them to patients with higher levels of myopia (eg, greater than −4 or −5 D). When used after bandage soft contact lens removal, corticosteroid drops are typically tapered over a 3- to 4-month period, depending on the patient's corneal haze and refractive outcome. For example, the corticosteroids may be used 4 times daily for the first month, 3 times daily for the second month, 2 times daily for the third month, and once a day for the fourth month. Patients undergoing hyperopic PRK should be informed about the longer epithelial healing time because of the larger ablation zone as well as the temporary reduction in best-corrected visual acuity in the first week to month, which usually improves with time.

Corbett MC, O'Brart DP, Marshall J. Do topical corticosteroids have a role following excimer laser photorefractive keratectomy? *J Refract Surg.* 1995;11:380–387.

Kapadia MS, Meisler DM, Wilson SE. Epithelial removal with the excimer laser (laser-scrape) in photorefractive keratectomy retreatment. *Ophthalmology.* 1999;106:29–34.

Verma S, Marshall J. Control of pain after photorefractive keratectomy. *J Refract Surg.* 1996;12:358–364.

Outcomes

Evolving technology

As the early broad-beam excimer laser systems improved and as surgeon experience increased, PRK results improved markedly. The ablation zone diameter enlarged because small ablation zones, originally selected to limit depth of tissue removal, produced more haze and regression as well as subjective glare and haloes. The larger treatment diameters used today, including optical zones and aspheric peripheral blend zones, improve both optical quality and refractive stability in both myopic and hyperopic treatments. Central island elevations have become less common with improvements in beam quality and with the development of scanning excimer lasers.

Tracking devices

Scanning laser technology necessitated the development of tracking technology because of the longer ablation times associated with the smaller scanning lasers. Subsequently, all manufacturers introduced trackers because of the potential for improved centration.

Two types of tracker technology are commonly employed. In so-called closed-loop trackers, high-speed oscillating infrared beams scan across the edge of a fixed dilated pupil. These beams detect the abrupt change in reflected light at the edge of the pupil. This signal then directs rapidly responding mirrors to create a space-stabilized image, and the laser treatment is located on the cornea based on that image.

The second type of tracker, a so-called open-loop system, uses video technology to monitor the location of an infrared image of the pupil and to shift the laser beam accordingly.

Myopic spherical PRK

The first excimer lasers that were approved by the FDA for myopic PRK were manufactured by Summit and VISX. Clinical trials of conventional (non–wavefront driven) excimer laser treatments limited to low myopia (generally < -6.0 D) reveal that 56% to 71% of eyes achieved uncorrected visual acuity (UCVA) of at least 20/20, 88% to 97% achieved UCVA of at least 20/40, and 82% to 94% were within 1.0 D of emmetropia. In the original Summit study, 6.8% had a loss of 2 or more lines of best-corrected visual acuity (BCVA). More recent clinical trials, however, have reported a 0% loss of BCVA postoperatively. FDA clinical trials of patients with moderate myopia (-6.0 to -10.0 D) report that 32% to 49% of eyes achieved UCVA of at least 20/20, 67% to 86% achieved at least 20/40 UCVA, 53% to 77% were within 1.0 D of emmetropia, and up to 6.7% lost more than 2 lines of BCVA. In other published studies, of patients with high myopia (> -10.0 D), 26% to 42% achieved at least 20/40 UCVA, 28% to 48% were within 1.0 D of emmetropia, and 7.7% to 22% lost at least 2 lines of BCVA.

Greater amounts of attempted correction are associated with decreased predictability, increased severity of haze and loss of BCVA, increased regression, and decreased likelihood of obtaining 20/40 or better UCVA. Consequently, many surgeons limit their treatment to a maximum of -10.0 D of myopia. However, pharmacological mediators of wound healing, including but not limited to intraoperative topical mitomycin, may decrease the postoperative haze in higher myopes who are undergoing excimer laser ablation.

Toric PRK

Astigmatism is corrected with the excimer laser by performing an elliptical ablation to flatten the steeper meridian of the cornea to match the flatter meridian (see Figure 6-1C). Because the treatment zone becomes elliptical, the effective optical zone of the ablation is smaller than the treated area. The results of photoastigmatic keratectomy (often termed PARK in the earlier literature) are difficult to interpret because the various studies use different techniques, nomograms, and variables to measure efficacy. In addition, a thorough evaluation of astigmatism requires vector analysis, which is not performed in many of the studies.

FDA clinical trials of photoastigmatic keratectomy reveal that 45% to 64% of eyes achieved postoperative UCVA of 20/20 or better, 83% to 93% achieved UCVA of 20/40, 80% to 92% were within 1.0 D of emmetropia, and 1.6% to 8.5% lost 2 or more lines of BCVA. Initial clinical trials of toric PRK showed that it was not as predictable as spherical PRK and that it tended to undercorrect the cylinder, probably because of conservative nomograms. By allowing more direct recontouring of the toric corneal surface into a sphere, in conjunction with simultaneous correction of hyperopia or myopia, the newer scanning lasers usually remove less tissue than the earlier broad-beam lasers.

Hyperopic PRK

In contrast to myopic PRK in which the central cornea is flattened, in hyperopic PRK more tissue is removed from the midperiphery than the central cornea, resulting in an effective steepening (see Figure 6-1B). A sharp transition between treated and untreated cornea in the periphery can cause significant haze and regression. For this reason, additional pulses are applied to blend the maximally ablated midperipheral area with the untreated peripheral cornea. Hyperopic PRK therefore requires a large ablation area in order to maintain an adequate size of central hyperopic treatment.

Initial studies using hyperopic treatment zones of 4.0 mm combined with a total blended area out to 7.0 mm revealed unacceptable regression of effect. In addition, a significant number of eyes lost BCVA, largely secondary to mild decentration combined with the small optical zones.

Later studies were performed using larger hyperopic treatment zones with transition zones out to 9.0 to 9.5 mm. FDA clinical trials of hyperopic PRK up to +6.0 D reveal postoperative UCVA of 20/20 or better in 46% to 53% of eyes, postoperative UCVA of 20/40 or better in 92% to 96%, 84% to 91% within 1.0 D of emmetropia, and loss of greater than 2 lines of BCVA in 1%. The period from surgery to postoperative stabilization for the same quantity of correction is longer for hyperopic than myopic corrections. Treatment of higher degrees of hyperopia results in poorer predictability and stability.

Hyperopic astigmatic PRK

The VISX FDA clinical trial of hyperopic astigmatic PRK up to +6.0 D sphere and +4.0 D cylinder reported an approximate postoperative UCVA of 20/20 or better in 50% of eyes, UCVA of 20/40 or better in 97%, and 87% within ±1.0 D of emmetropia, with loss of more than 2 lines of BCVA in 1.5%.

Mixed astigmatic PRK

No excimer lasers have been approved by the FDA nor have major studies been published for mixed astigmatic PRK.

Enhancements

After the stabilization of the UCVA and refraction, typically around 3 to 6 months after the PRK, the patient and surgeon assess their satisfaction with the result of the PRK. If the patient is dissatisfied with the UCVA and the surgeon agrees it is prudent, reoperation or enhancement can be performed to treat the residual refractive error. The surgeon should avoid performing an enhancement for a patient with unrealistic expectations. The patient who wants enhancement to improve the UCVA of 20/20 in his "bad eye" to UCVA of "20/15" that his "good eye" has achieved should instead be re-educated about the realistic results. The goal of refractive surgery is improvement in UCVA, not perfect vision. When enhancement of myopic PRK is contemplated, the surgeon must be aware that the epithelium is often thickened (hyperplastic) centrally as a reaction to the flattened corneal profile created by the myopic ablation. Initial undercorrection of the laser ablation must be differentiated from regression of the initial ablation. Regression may be due to stromal collagen healing, epithelial hyperplasia, or a combination. A PRK enhancement may result in overcorrection if the regression due to epithelial hyperplasia is included in the enhancement and an equal amount of epithelial hyperplasia does not recur.

Hersh PS, Stulting RD, Steinert RF, et al. Results of phase III excimer laser photorefractive keratectomy for myopia. *Ophthalmology.* 1997;104:1535–1553.

Litwak S, Zadok D, Garcia-de Quevedo V, et al. Laser-assisted subepithelial keratectomy versus photorefractive keratectomy for the correction of myopia: a prospective comparative study. *J Cataract Refract Surg.* 2002;28:1330–1333.

McDonald MB, Deitz MR, Frantz JM, et al. Photorefractive keratectomy for low-to-moderate myopia and astigmatism with a small-beam, tracker-directed excimer laser. *Ophthalmology.* 2000;107:814–816.

Steinert RF, Hersh PS. Spherical and aspherical photorefractive keratectomy and laser in-situ keratomileusis for moderate to high myopia: two prospective, randomized clinical trials. Summit Technology PRK-LASIK Study Group. *Trans Am Ophthalmol Soc.* 1998;96: 197–221.

Complications

Overcorrection

Overcorrection of more than +1.0 D at 1 year occurs in less than 5% of myopes. Myopic or hyperopic PRK typically undergoes regression for at least 3 to 6 months. Refractive stability must be achieved before deciding whether the overcorrection requires retreatment. For example, with myopic corrections, a 1-month low hyperopic response (planned overcorrection) is followed by regression of 0.5 to 1.0 D toward myopia over the next few months.

An overcorrection may occur if substantial stromal dehydration develops prior to commencing the laser treatment, because more stromal tissue will be ablated per pulse. Overcorrection tends to occur more often in older individuals because they do not have as strong a wound-healing response. Studies reveal that older patients (ages 35 to 54) with moderate to high myopia have a greater response to the same amount of dioptric correction than younger patients do. There are various modalities available to attempt to treat small amounts of overcorrection. Myopic regression can be induced by the abrupt discontinuation of corticosteroids. The administration of topical NSAIDs (usually 4 times a day) in conjunction with a bandage soft contact lens over several months may decrease small amounts of overcorrection (see Chapter 11).

Undercorrection

Undercorrection occurs much more frequently at higher degrees of myopia and hyperopia because of decreased predictability resulting from the greater frequency and severity of regression. Regression is markedly increased with optical zones of less than 6.0 mm diameter. Patients with regression after treatment of their first eye have an increased likelihood of regression in their second eye. Sometimes the regression may be reversed with aggressive topical corticosteroids. The patient may undergo a retreatment after the refraction has remained stable for at least 3 months. A patient with significant corneal haze and regression is at higher risk after retreatment for further regression and recurrence of visually significant corneal haze and loss of BCVA. Topical mitomycin, administered at the time of retreatment, can be used to modulate the response. It is recommended that the surgeon wait at least 12 months for the haze to improve naturally before repeating PRK.

Central islands

A central island is disclosed by computerized videokeratography as an area of central corneal elevation surrounded by an area of flattening corresponding to the myopic treatment zone in the paracentral region (Fig 6-5). A central island is defined at a minimum as an elevation of at least 1 D with a diameter of more than 1 mm as compared with the paracentral flattened area. Islands generally occurred with the older broad-beam laser systems rather than the more recent scanning delivery systems. They have been reported more frequently in ablations larger than 5.0 mm in diameter and with greater attempted corrections. Central topographic islands may be associated with decreased visual acuity, monocular diplopia and multiplopia, ghost images, and decreased contrast sensitivity.

There have been several theories proposed to explain the etiology of central islands. The plume theory states that a plume of gaseous and particulate debris is emitted from the corneal surface whenever the energy delivered by the laser strikes the cornea. Another theory suggests that poor homogeneity leads to less laser energy being delivered to the central cornea, which would explain why central islands are more frequently seen with broad-beam lasers. Another potential cause of central island formation is uneven corneal surface hydration. One proposed mechanism of differential corneal hydration is the "shock wave" theory, which postulates that during the ablation, as laser energy strikes

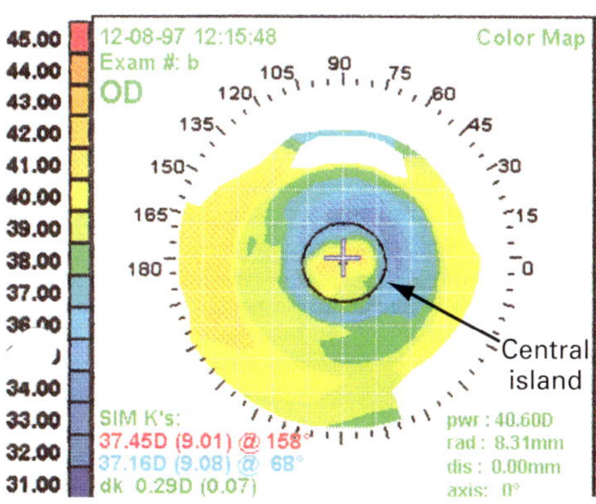

Figure 6-5 Corneal topography of a myopic ablation *(blue)* with a central island *(yellow)* in the visual axis. *(Topography scan courtesy of Roger F. Steinert, MD.)*

the cornea, the laser pressure wave may force water from the underlying stroma to the center of the cornea. This fluid then acts as a masking agent, reducing the central corneal ablation rate.

Applying extra laser pulses to the central cornea, usually calculated as a fixed percentage of the total number of treatment pulses, reduces the incidence of central islands in broad-beam lasers. In addition, multizone and multipass techniques have been proposed to result in a smoother ablation. If the islands do not resolve spontaneously by 6 to 12 months, they may be re-treated directly with the excimer laser. With the majority of laser ablations performed today with scanning rather than broad-beam excimer lasers, central islands have become an infrequent occurrence.

Optical aberrations

Some patients report optical aberrations after PRK, including glare, ghost images, and haloes. These symptoms are most prevalent after treatment with smaller ablation zones and after higher attempted correction. These complaints seem to be exacerbated at night and are most prevalent in young, myopic patients with large pupillary diameters, due to an optical zone that is smaller than the entrance pupil under conditions of dim illumination. Wavefront mapping may reveal higher-order aberrations associated with these subjective complaints. In general, a larger, more uniform, and well-centered optical zone will provide a better quality of vision, especially at night.

Night vision complaints are often caused by spherical aberration, although other higher-order aberrations will also contribute to distortions. The cornea and lens have spherical aberration. In addition, excimer laser ablation increases spherical aberration in the midperipheral cornea. Larger pupil size correlates with frequency of complaints about aberrations because spherical aberration increases when the midperipheral corneal optics contribute to the light energy passing to the retina. Customized wavefront-guided corneal treatment patterns are designed to reduce both existing aberrations and the creation of new or worsening of preexisting aberrations, with the goal of achieving better quality of vision after laser ablation.

Decentered ablation

Accurate centration during the PRK procedure is important to optimize the visual potential. Centration is even more critical for hyperopic than myopic treatments. A decentered stromal ablation may occur if the patient's eye slowly begins to drift and loses fixation or if the surgeon initially improperly positions the patient's head (Fig 6-6). In

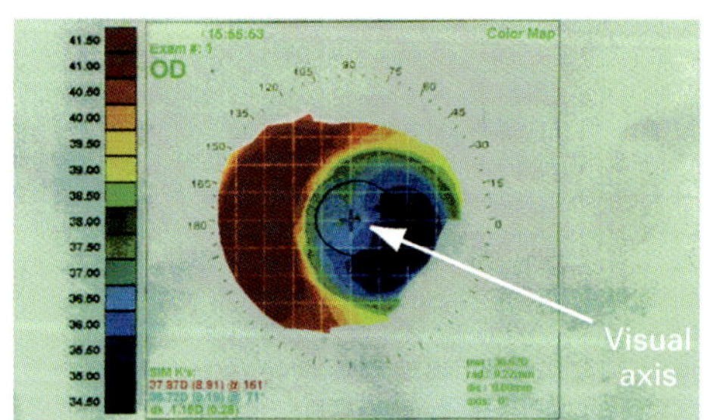

Figure 6-6 Corneal topography of a decentered ablation. *(Topography scan courtesy of Roger F. Steinert, MD.)*

addition, centering the ablation on a pharmacologically miotic pupil may be inaccurate due to the nasal and sometimes superior shift of the pupil that frequently occurs with miosis. Decentration incidence increases with surgeon inexperience and with higher refractive correction, probably because of the associated longer ablation time with increased duration of fixation. Larger decentrations may cause complaints of glare, haloes, and decreased visual acuity. The patient may experience more symptoms if the decentration is more than 1.0 mm but may not necessarily have any symptoms if it is less than 0.5 mm. Patients with larger pupils may experience symptoms with smaller amounts of decentration, because the edge of the decentered ablation will more easily be perceived within the patient's visual axis. Decentrations may be prevented by proper stabilization of the patient's head and by alertness of the surgeon in stopping the ablation if the patient begins to lose fixation.

Corneal haze

Wound-healing patterns after PRK can be separated into three groups:

- Normal healers, who have trace to 1+ haze and a refraction of 0 to +1.0 D at 1 month
- Inadequate healers, who have no haze and a refraction >+1.0 D beyond the target correction at 1 month
- Aggressive healers, who have 1+ or greater haze that increases in months 2 and 3 accompanied by regression of the correction

Subepithelial corneal haze typically appears several weeks after PRK, peaks in intensity at 1 to 2 months, and gradually disappears during the following 6 to 12 months (Fig 6-7). Late-onset corneal haze has been described that occurs several months or even 1 year or more postoperatively after a prior period of a relatively clear cornea. Histologic studies in animals with corneal haze after PRK demonstrate abnormal glycosaminoglycans and/or nonlamellar collagen deposited in the anterior stroma as a consequence of epithelial–stromal wound healing. Most histologic studies from animals and humans

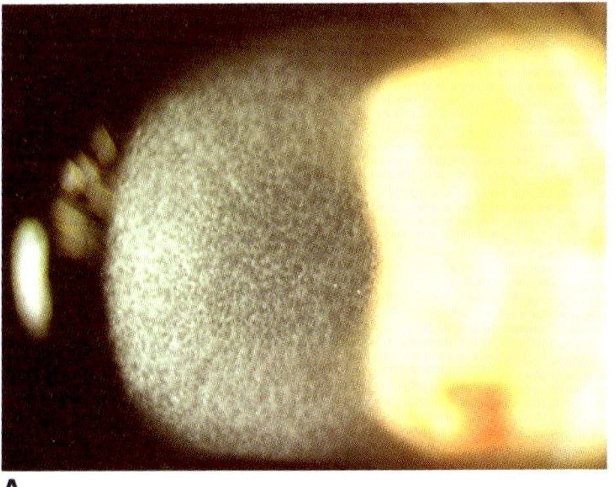

A

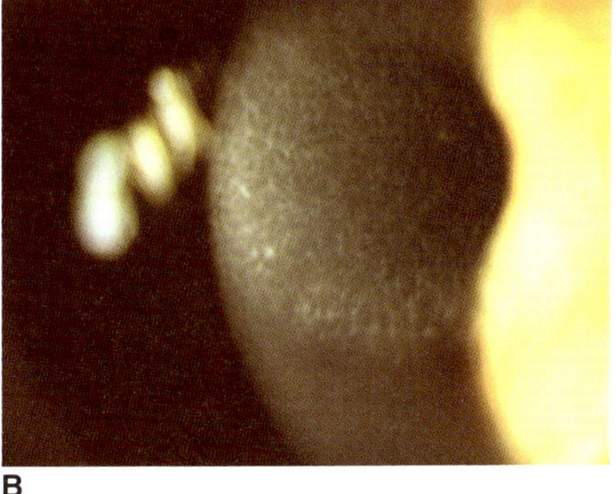

B

Figure 6-7 PRK haze. **A,** Severe haze 5 months after PRK. The reticular pattern is characteristic of PRK-induced haze. **B,** Haze has improved to moderate level by 13 months postoperatively. *(Photographs courtesy of Roger F. Steinert, MD.)*

show an increase in the number and activity of stromal keratocytes, which suggests that increased keratocyte activity may be the source for the extracellular deposits.

Persistent severe haze is usually associated with greater amounts of correction or smaller ablation diameters. Animal studies have demonstrated that UV-B exposure after PRK prolongs the stromal healing process with increase in subepithelial haze. Clinical cases of haze after high UV exposure (such as high altitude) corroborate these studies.

If clinically unacceptable haze persists, a superficial keratectomy or phototherapeutic keratectomy may be performed. In addition, topical mitomycin (0.02%) may be used to prevent recurrence of subepithelial fibrosis after debridement or phototherapeutic keratectomy. Because haze is known to resolve spontaneously with normal wound remodeling, reablation should be delayed for at least 6 months. The clinician should be aware that in the presence of haze, refraction is often inaccurate, with an overestimation of the amount of myopia.

Epithelial defect

Usually, the epithelial defect created during PRK heals within 3 to 4 days with the aid of a bandage soft contact lens or pressure patching. A frequent cause of delayed re-epithelialization is keratoconjunctivitis sicca, which may be treated with increased lubrication and/or temporary punctal occlusion. Patients with undiagnosed autoimmune connective tissue disease or diabetes mellitus may also have poor epithelial healing. The importance of closely monitoring patients until re-epithelialization occurs cannot be overemphasized.

Infiltrates

The use of therapeutic contact lenses to aid in epithelial healing is associated with sterile infiltrates, especially in patients using topical NSAIDs for longer than 24 hours without concomitant topical corticosteroids. The infiltrates, which have been reported in approximately 1 in 300 cases, are usually sterile and secondary to an immune reaction (Fig 6-8). The incidence of infectious keratitis has been reported as 0.2%; all infiltrates must be suspected to be infectious and managed appropriately.

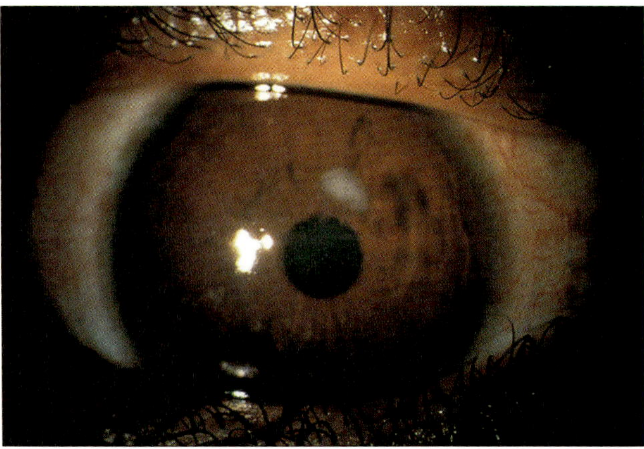

Figure 6-8 Stromal infiltrates seen with a bandage soft contact lens after PRK. *(Photograph courtesy of Jayne S. Weiss, MD.)*

Corticosteroid-induced complications

The incidence of increased IOP after PRK has been reported to range from 11% to 25%. Occasionally, the IOP may be quite high. In one study, 2% of patients had IOP greater than 40 mm Hg. The majority of cases of elevated IOP are associated with prolonged topical corticosteroid therapy. Corticosteroid-induced glaucoma occurs in 1.5% to 3.0% of patients using fluorometholone but in up to 25% of patients using dexamethasone or stronger corticosteroids. The increase in IOP is usually controlled with topical IOP-lowering medications and typically normalizes after the corticosteroids are decreased or discontinued. Because of the changes in corneal curvature and/or corneal thickness, Goldmann tonometry readings after PRK are artifactually reduced (see Chapter 11). Measurement of IOP from the temporal rather than the central cornea may be more accurate, and pneumotonometry and Tonopen readings are also more reliable. Other corticosteroid-associated complications that have been reported after PRK are corticosteroid-induced herpes simplex virus keratitis, corticosteroid-induced ptosis, and corticosteroid-induced cataracts.

Dry eye

Dry eye conditions after PRK occur as a result of denervation, as also happens after LASIK, although generally with less severity and duration. See the discussion under LASIK complications.

Endothelial effects

Unlike with radial keratotomy, no significant change occurred in central endothelial cell density after PRK in most studies. In fact, the polymegathism associated with contact lens use typically improves after PRK, as demonstrated by the significant decrease in the peripheral coefficient of variation of cell size 2 years postoperatively.

Carones F, Vigo L, Scandola E, et al. Evaluation of the prophylactic use of mitomycin-C to inhibit haze formation after photorefractive keratectomy. *J Cataract Refract Surg.* 2002;28:2088–2095.

Corbett MC, Prydall JI, Verma S, et al. An in vivo investigation of the structures responsible for corneal haze after photorefractive keratectomy and their effect on visual function. *Ophthalmology.* 1996;103:1366–1380.

Donnenfeld ED, O'Brien TP, Solomon R, et al. Infectious keratitis after photorefractive keratectomy. *Ophthalmology.* 2003;110:743–747.

Krueger RR, Saedy NF, McDonnell PJ. Clinical analysis of steep central islands after excimer laser photorefractive keratectomy. *Arch Ophthalmol.* 1996;114:377–381.

Matta CA, Piebenga LW, Deitz MR, et al. Excimer retreatment for myopic photorefractive keratectomy failures. Six- to 18-month follow-up. *Ophthalmology.* 1996;103:444–451.

Wilson SE. Analysis of the keratocyte apoptosis, keratocyte proliferation, and myofibroblast transformation responses after photorefractive keratectomy and laser in situ keratomileusis. *Trans Am Ophthalmol Soc.* 2002;100:411–433.

Conclusion

Photorefractive keratectomy and LASEK are reasonably safe, effective, and predictable techniques for correcting low to moderate myopia, astigmatism, and low hyperopia. The primary disadvantages of PRK and LASEK are the degree of postoperative discomfort, the length of time required for visual recovery, and the increase in corneal haze with treatment of higher refractive errors. Wound-modulating agents such as mitomycin are expanding the range of refractive errors that can be treated. Surface ablation may be preferable to LASIK in patients with epithelial basement membrane disease and in patients with thin corneas. PRK and LASEK avoid the increase of higher-order aberrations associated with creation of a LASIK flap. Consequently, with the advent of wavefront-guided laser ablation, surface ablation may return as the procedure of choice.

McColgin AZ, Steinert RF, Bafna S. Photorefractive keratectomy. In: Tasman W, Jaeger E, eds. *Duane's Clinical Ophthalmology.* Philadelphia: Lippincott; 2001.

Laser In Situ Keratomileusis (LASIK)

The term *keratomileusis* comes from the Greek words for "cornea" and "to carve." Laser in situ keratomileusis, which combines keratomileusis with excimer laser stromal ablation, has become the most popular refractive procedure performed today because of its safety, efficacy, quick visual recovery, and minimal patient discomfort.

Background

Barraquer first described corneal lamellar surgery for the correction of refractive error in 1949. The microkeratomes in use today employ many of the same general principles as Barraquer's original design of a manually advancing electric microkeratome for creating a corneal cap. Barraquer also invented a cryolathe that froze the corneal cap for precise lenticular reshaping of corneal tissue. This cryolathe did not gain popularity because it was technically difficult to use. In addition, the freezing process and subsequent suturing often resulted in irregular astigmatism and loss of BCVA.

Barraquer, Krumeich, and Swinger later developed a technique for removing corneal tissue without the complex cryolathe. After the corneal cap was cut by the microkeratome, it was stabilized with suction in the inverted position on a forming die. The refractive cut was made by a second pass of the microkeratome on the stromal side of the corneal cap, and then the reshaped free cap was turned back over and sutured back onto the patient's corneal stromal bed. This procedure avoided the technical difficulties encountered with the cryolathe, but unpredictability and irregular astigmatism remained as major obstacles.

In the late 1980s, Ruiz and Rowsey introduced the concept of tissue removal from the stromal bed rather than from the free corneal cap, referred to as in situ keratomileusis. In this technique, the microkeratome removed the corneal cap in a first pass and then the suction ring was changed in order to excise a free lenticule of tissue with a second pass of the microkeratome. The dimensions of the ring used in the second pass determined the thickness, and thus the dioptric power, of the lenticule removed. Although this technique involved less trauma to the corneal cap, the results remained suboptimal because of unpredictable refractive changes and irregular astigmatism. To improve the predictability of the microkeratome cut, Ruiz developed an automated microkeratome in the late 1980s. This procedure, automated lamellar keratoplasty, combined the advantages of an automated advancement of the microkeratome head with an adjustable suction ring for control of the second microkeratome cut. However, unacceptable optical aberrations often resulted because of the lack of predictable tissue removal in the second pass and the small optical zone of the excised refractive lenticule.

In 1990, Pallikaris performed the first LASIK procedure when he used the excimer laser instead of the second microkeratome pass for the removal of tissue to induce the refractive change. The excimer laser produced better optical results for three reasons: (1) the excimer laser ablates tissue with submicron accuracy; (2) the laser does not deform the tissue during the refractive reshaping; and (3) larger optical zones are achieved.

Modification in the microkeratome to stop the pass just short of creating a full free cap further improved results. By leaving a narrow hinge of tissue, the outer cornea becomes a flap which is reflected out of the way during the laser exposure. After it is returned to its original position, natural corneal dehydration causes the flap to adhere to the underlying stromal bed. Repositioning of the flap in its original position avoids the distortion induced by sutures and reduces irregular astigmatism.

Instrumentation

The microkeratome

The basic principles of the microkeratome and the role of the suction ring and cutting head are illustrated (Fig 6-9). The suction ring has two functions: (1) to adhere to the globe, providing a stable platform for the microkeratome cutting head; and (2) to raise the IOP to a high level, which stiffens the cornea so that it cannot move away from the cutting blade. The dimensions of the suction ring determine the diameter of the flap and the size of the stabilizing hinge. The suction ring is connected to a vacuum pump, which typically is controlled by an on-off foot pedal.

The cutting head has several key components. The highly sharpened disposable cutting blade is discarded after each patient, either after a single eye or after bilateral treatment. The applanation plate flattens the cornea in advance of the cutting blade; the length of the blade that extends beyond the applanation plate is a principal determinant of flap thickness. The motor, either electrical or gas-driven turbine, oscillates the blade rapidly, typically between 6,000 and 15,000 cycles per minute. The same motor or a second motor is often used to mechanically advance the cutting head, attached to the suction ring, across the cornea, although in several models, the surgeon manually controls the advance of the cutting head.

The Barraquer-designed sliding microkeratomes approached the cornea temporally for easy access, leaving a nasal hinge because this was the last area cut. Subsequently, several popular microkeratomes were introduced that allowed the microkeratome head to pivot on a post, resulting in an arcing path with a superior hinge because the superior zone was the last to be cut. A superior hinge has the potential advantage of the up-down wiping motion of the eyelid helping to avoid flap displacement. A nasal hinge does not have this advantage and also has the drawback that many pupils are located somewhat nasal of the corneal center. As a result, the nasal hinge, even if shifted maximally to the nasal limbus, might impinge on a large treatment zone. It is controversial which hinge

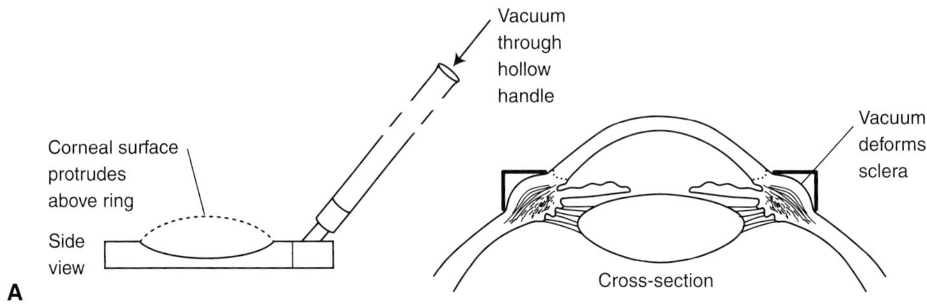

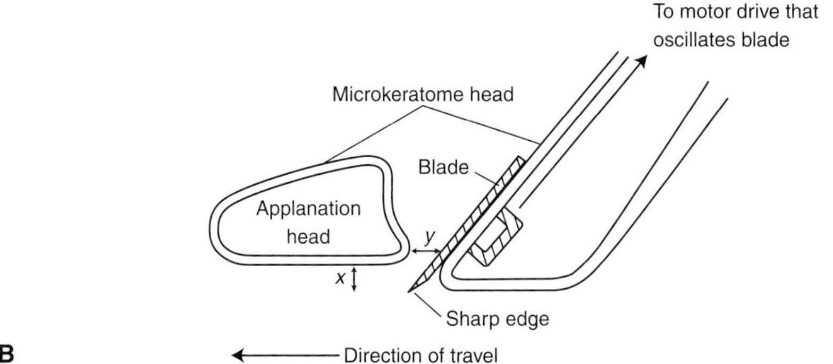

Figure 6-9 Schematic representation of the principles of a microkeratome. **A,** The suction ring serves as a platform for the microkeratome head, gripping the conjunctiva and sclera adjacent to the limbus. As the ring grips the globe, the vacuum deforms the scleral wall, increasing IOP by decreasing intraocular volume. By raising the IOP, the cornea is stiffened to prevent it from deforming away from the microkeratome blade when the flap is cut. The vertical dimension of the ring is a major factor in how much cornea protrudes to be exposed to the microkeratome blade, which determines the diameter of the flap. **B,** Simplified cross-section schematic of a typical microkeratome head. The protrusion of the cutting edge of the blade beyond the applanating head of the microkeratome is the major determinant of flap thickness. Specifically, the distance *x* between the applanation head that flattens the cornea and the cutting edge of the blade is the first-order determinant of the flap thickness. The dimension *y* is necessary to allow the flap to curl up as it is cut. When *y* is larger than *x,* the flap will tend to be thicker as corneal tissue bunches up into this space. When *y* is the same as *x,* it will tend to cause epithelial abrasions. **C,** Creation of the flap. When the microkeratome head passes across the cornea, the applanating surface of the head flattens the cornea in advance of the blade. The elevated IOP in the eye forces the cornea firmly against the cutting blade. **D,** Cross-section of the flap after the cut. The resultant flap has a beveled edge and then a relatively flat lamellar separation of the flap from the underlying stromal bed. The bevel occurs when the blade cuts the edge of the flattened corneal dome. The flap and bed should be of uniform thickness. The advancement of the blade is halted short of full transection, leaving a hinge of tissue connecting the flap to the peripheral cornea. *(Continues)*

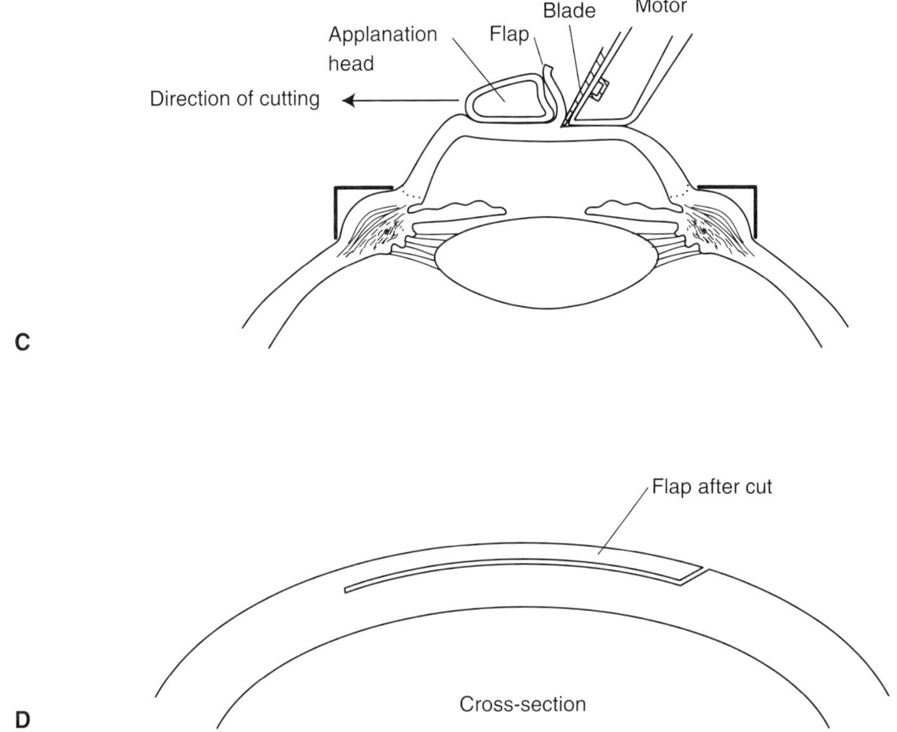

Figure 6-9 *(Continued) (Illustration by Jeanne Koelling.)*

position causes more prolonged corneal denervation and associated postoperative dry eye. While nasal hinge location spares some innervation of the flap because it does not transect the nasal long ciliary nerves as they enter the cornea, one study found more rapid recovery of corneal sensation in patients with superior hinges as compared with nasal hinges. Nevertheless, both patients with nasal or superior hinges recovered sensation to the preoperative levels within 6 to 12 months after surgery.

Prior to surgery, the microkeratome and vacuum unit are assembled, carefully inspected, and tested to ensure proper function. The importance of meticulous maintenance of the microkeratome and of carefully following the manufacturer's recommendations cannot be overemphasized. Corneal perforation can result when certain microkeratome models are incorrectly assembled, for example, when the depth plate is omitted in the Automatic Corneal Shaper (Chiron).

Regardless of the nominal flap thickness of a specific device, the surgeon should be aware that the actual flap thickness varies with the type of microkeratome, the patient age, the primary corneal thickness, the preoperative keratometry, the preoperative astigmatism, and the corneal diameter.

Creation of the flap by femtosecond laser

A femtosecond Nd:YAG laser (IntraLase) can create flaps by performing a lamellar dissection within the stroma. Each laser pulse creates a discrete area of photodisruption of the collagen. Thousands of adjacent pulses are scanned across the cornea in a controlled pattern that results in a flap, where the computer control is programmed for flap diameter, depth, and hinge location and size. It is unclear what, if any, effect the removal of tissue with photodisruption rather than the cutting of tissue with the traditional microkeratome will have on the seating of the corneal flap. Advocates cite the potential for better depth control, lessening or avoiding of such complications as buttonhole perforations, and precise control of flap dimension and location. The outcome of a randomized trial comparison with the metal blade microkeratome is pending. One study of 208 eyes that underwent femtosecond laser flap creation showed that 1.9% had a loss of suction during femtosecond laser flap creation but that all had successful flap performance 5 to 45 minutes after reapplanation of the eye.

Kumano Y, Matsui H, Zushi I, et al. Recovery of corneal sensation after myopic correction by laser in situ keratomileusis with a nasal or superior hinge. *J Cataract Refract Surg.* 2003;29:757–761.

Lee KW, Joo CK. Clinical results of laser in situ keratomileusis with superior and nasal hinges. *J Cataract Refract Surg.* 2003;29:457–461.

Nordan LT, Slade SG, Baker RN, et al. Femtosecond laser flap creation for laser in situ keratomileusis: 6-month follow-up of initial U.S. clinical series. *J Refract Surg.* 2003;19:8–14.

Pallikaris IG, Papatzanaki ME, Siganos DS, et al. A corneal flap technique for laser in situ keratomileusis: human study. *Arch Ophthalmol.* 1991;145:1699–1702.

Preoperative inspection of the excimer laser

Prior to the LASIK procedure, the excimer laser beam should be tested for proper homogeneity and fluence in an identical fashion to preparation for PRK.

Patient Selection

The preoperative evaluation of patients prior to LASIK is similar to the evaluation prior to PRK. This section will be limited to the differences in evaluating a patient for LASIK surgery. The full preoperative evaluation of refractive surgery patients is discussed in Chapter 3.

As with PRK, careful attention must be given to preexisting systemic or ocular conditions that may interfere with healing. However, because LASIK violates the corneal surface less than PRK and does not provoke a lengthy healing response of the epithelium and superficial keratocytes, a history of keloid formation is not necessarily a contraindication to LASIK. In addition, a history of quiescent herpes or controlled connective tissue disease may be less problematic in LASIK.

Many reports indicate that postoperative dry eye is more common with LASIK than with PRK. Preoperative evaluation for dry eyes is performed by assessment of history, the tear meniscus, rose bengal staining, and/or Schirmer testing. Dry eyes should be treated preoperatively with artificial tear supplementation, topical anti-inflammatory medications (corticosteroids or cyclosporine), and/or punctal occlusion, in order to limit keratopathy that can lead to postoperative flap irregularity.

When evaluating the cornea prior to LASIK, it is of particular importance to look for signs of a basement membrane dystrophy that could predispose the patient to epithelial defects with the microkeratome pass. These patients are usually best served by having PRK, if their refractive error permits.

Corneal topography must be performed to quantitate corneal cylinder and to rule out the presence of forme fruste keratoconus, pellucid marginal degeneration, or contact lens–induced corneal warpage. Corneas steeper than 48 D are more likely to have thin flaps or frank buttonholes (central perforation of the flap). Corneas flatter than 40 D are likely to have a smaller-diameter flap and are at increased risk for creation of a free cap due to transection of the hinge. These issues may be reduced or eliminated by the use of a smaller flap diameter, slower passage of the microkeratome, higher suction levels and higher IOP, use of a microkeratome head designed to create thicker flaps, or, in theory, the selection of an ultra-short-pulsed femtosecond laser to create the lamellar flap. The surgeon must be aware that use of the same blade for creation of the flap in the second eye of a patient will typically result in a flap that is 10 to 20 μm thinner than the flap in the first eye.

Preoperative pachymetric measurement of corneal thickness is mandatory because an adequate stromal bed must remain to decrease the possibility of postoperative corneal ectasia. The following formula is used to calculate the corneal thickness:

$$\text{Central corneal thickness} - \text{thickness of flap} - \text{depth of ablation} = \text{residual bed thickness}$$

In calculating the likely residual stromal thickness, the surgeon must use the ablation depth based on the intended total correction, not the value of the nomogram-adjusted refractive error that is programmed into the laser. The true tissue ablation depth will be closer to the value needed to achieve the refractive shift. A nomogram adjustment to a lower refractive error that is programmed into the laser does not mean that there is less tissue removed.

While most practitioners use as a guideline a minimum residual corneal bed thickness of 250 μm, this is a clinically derived figure and is not based on any definitive laboratory investigations. Even 250 μm remaining in the stromal bed after ablation does not guarantee that postoperative corneal ectasia will not develop. In a retrospective study of 10 eyes from 7 patients who developed corneal ectasia after LASIK, 30% had a residual stromal bed thickness ≥250 μm. In this series, 88% of patients had previously undiagnosed forme fruste keratoconus. It is possible that the actual LASIK flap may be thicker than the nominal expected thickness, making the stromal bed less than the calculated minimum of 250 μm. An increasing number of surgeons are using intraoperative pachymetry, especially for high myopic corrections, enhancements, or thin corneas, to determine the actual flap thickness.

Randleman JB, Russell B, Ward MA, et al. Risk factors and prognosis for corneal ectasia after LASIK. *Ophthalmology.* 2003;110:267–275.

The surgeon should preoperatively inform patients with thinner corneas or higher corrections that future enhancement may not be possible because of inadequate residual corneal bed thickness.

Excessive corneal flattening or steepening after LASIK may reduce the visual quality and increase the aberrations. Although no controlled studies have established specific limits, many surgeons avoid creating a postoperative corneal power below about 34 D or above about 50 D because of the high amount of spherical aberration that results from excessive corneal flattening or steepening. The surgeon should anticipate the postoperative keratometry by estimating a flattening of 0.8 D for every diopter of myopia treated and a steepening of 1.0 D for every diopter of hyperopia treated (see Chapter 3).

If wavefront-guided laser ablation is planned, wavefront error is measured preoperatively, as discussed in Chapter 1. Although the wavefront data are used to program the laser, the surgeon must still compare these data to the manifest refraction prior to surgery to prevent data input errors. One company specifies that the safety and effectiveness of the wavefront-guided laser (VISX Star4 Custom Vue) has not been established if the difference between the wavefront calculated power and the manifest power of sphere or cylinder is more minus than 0.50 D or more plus than 0.75 D or if the difference in manifest cylinder axis is greater than 15°. In such cases the wavefront data and manifest refraction must be rechecked to detect and correct potential errors prior to performing wavefront-guided ablation. In addition, a minimum scotopic pupil size (eg, 5.0 mm for the VISX Custom Vue) may be necessary to obtain adequate wavefront measurement data prior to the ablation.

Surgical Technique

Preoperative preparation of the patient

A mild sedative, such as oral diazepam 5 to 10 mg, may be administered to the patient approximately 30 minutes prior to the procedure. Topical anesthetic drops are instilled and the skin is usually prepped with povidone-iodine or another skin antiseptic. Preoperative topical antibiotic may be used.

Many surgeons drape the skin or eyelashes with a plastic drape or with Steri-Strips, while others consider this unnecessary and a potential source of material that might jam the microkeratome. An eyelid speculum is placed that has a configuration to accommodate the suction device and the path of the microkeratome. The cornea may be marked with an optical zone marker to assist in proper centration of the suction ring, and one or more pararadial lines are usually placed to ensure proper realignment of the flap.

Programming the laser

The actual treatment value programmed into the laser is typically an adjustment of the final refractive goal, derived from each surgeon's individual nomogram as developed by monitoring outcomes. Major variables that some but not all surgeons find to be important include: specific laser, individual surgeon, amount of correction, gender, and age. In addition, the size of the ablation zone and whether to include a blend will be determined by the patient's refractive error, the calculated residual stromal bed, and the pupillary diameter.

Creation of the flap by the microkeratome

The diameter of the flap is determined by the surgeon based on such variables as the type of refractive error to be treated (hyperopic corrections and wavefront-guided treatments require a larger flap because of the larger ablation diameter), the corneal curvature and microkeratome suction ring dimensions (flatter corneas result in a smaller flap for the same size ring), the patient's anatomy (peripheral corneal blood vessels and corneal diameter), and the surgeon's preference. Depending on the manufacturer, the suction ring is usually centered over the entrance pupil (Fig 6-10), but if a suction ring is being used that creates a flap less than 9.5 mm in diameter, some surgeons prefer to skew it toward the hinge to ensure that the hinge will not be located within the laser optical zone.

Thinner flaps leave more stromal bed thickness for the ablation and possible enhancements. However, thicker flaps have a lower risk of unexpected buttonholes and flap folds and may be more stable. Each type of microkeratome characteristically creates a flap with a range of thickness that the surgeon must know and include in the surgical plan to make sure there is an adequate residual stromal bed.

Once the ring is properly positioned, suction is activated. The IOP should be assessed at this point, because low IOP can result in a poor-quality, thin, or incomplete flap. It is essential to have both excellent exposure of the eye, allowing free movement of the microkeratome, and proper suction ring fixation. Inadequate suction may result from blockage of the suction ports from eyelashes under the suction ring or from redundant or scarred conjunctiva. To avoid the possibility of pseudosuction, the surgeon can confirm that true suction is present by observing that the eye moves when the suction ring is gently moved and that the patient can no longer see the fixation light. Methods employed to assess whether the IOP is adequately elevated include use of the Barraquer plastic applanator, use of a pneumotonometer, or palpation of the eye by the surgeon. Beginning surgeons are advised to use an objective rather than a subjective method.

Prior to making the lamellar cut, the surface of the cornea is moistened with proparacaine containing glycerin or with nonpreserved artificial tears. Balanced salt solution is avoided at this point due to the possibility of creating mineral deposits within the microkeratome that can interfere with its proper function. The microkeratome is placed on the suction ring and its path is checked to make sure it is free of obstacles such as the eyelid speculum, drape, or overhanging eyelid. The microkeratome is then activated, passed over the cornea (Fig 6-11) until halted by the hinge-creating stopper, and then

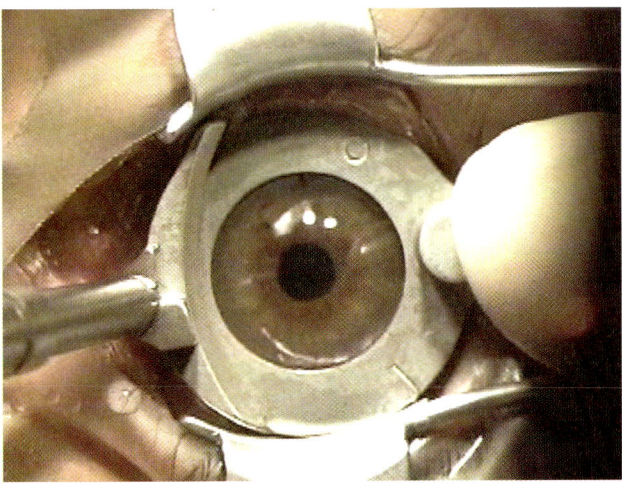

Figure 6-10 Placement of a suction ring. *(Photograph courtesy of Roger F. Steinert, MD.)*

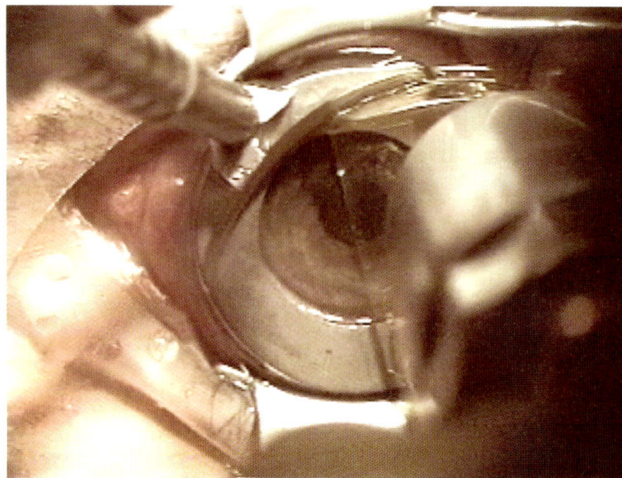

Figure 6-11 Movement of the microkeratome head across the cornea. *(Photograph courtesy of Roger F. Steinert, MD.)*

reversed off the cornea. With some models, some surgeons feel that epithelial defects may be reduced by lowering the vacuum or discontinuing the suction during the reversal; other models require the vacuum to remain at full pressure during reversal. Improvements in microkeratomes have decreased the incidence of epithelial defects. If a patient develops an epithelial defect in one eye during a microkeratome pass, an epithelial defect will usually develop when the second eye is treated regardless of alterations in the microkeratome vacuum level. This implies that there may be a subclinical epitheliopathy such as epithelial basement membrane disease that is made manifest by the microkeratome pass.

The ablation

The excimer laser system is then focused and centered over the pupil and the patient is asked to look at the fixation light. The flap is reflected (Fig 6-12) and the patient is asked to continue to fixate. The lights in the room and laser may need to be adjusted to allow the patient to be able to continue to visualize the fixation light through the irregular stromal surface after the flap has been lifted. If excess moisture is noted, the stromal bed is dried with a microsurgical debris-free sponge. The laser is refocused on the stromal bed and centered, most commonly on the pupil. A tracking system, if present, is activated. Once the patient confirms that the fixation light of the excimer laser is still visible and that the patient is looking directly at it, ablation is begun (see Figure 6-4). With or without a tracking device, the surgeon must monitor the patient to make sure that the patient's fixation is maintained throughout the laser exposure. It is important to initiate the stromal ablation promptly, before excessive stromal dehydration has taken place. If centration is lost, however, the ablation should be halted immediately, and fixation regained prior to finishing the treatment. During larger-diameter ablations, a flap protector may be needed to shield the underside of the flap near the hinge from the laser pulses.

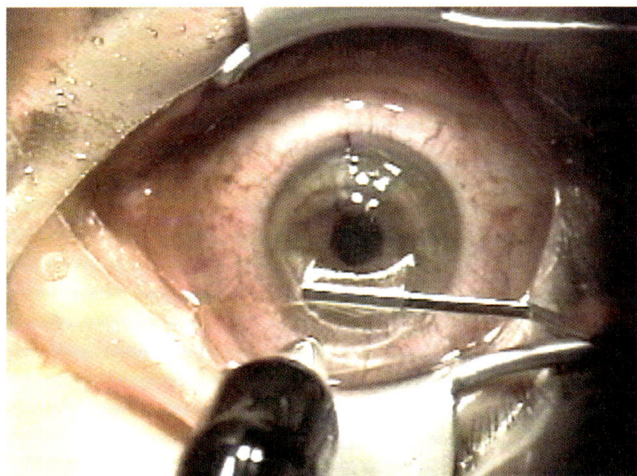

Figure 6-12 Reflecting the LASIK flap. *(Photograph courtesy of Roger F. Steinert, MD.)*

Replacing the flap

After the ablation is completed, the flap is replaced onto the stromal bed. The interface is irrigated until any interface debris is eliminated (which is better visualized with oblique rather than coaxial illumination). The surface of the flap is stroked with a smooth instrument, such as the irrigation cannula or a moistened microsurgical spear sponge, from the hinge to the periphery to ensure that wrinkles are eliminated and that the flap settles back into its original position, as indicated by the radial marks made earlier. The physiologic dehydration of the stroma by the endothelial pump will begin to secure the flap in position within several minutes. If a significant epithelial defect is present, a bandage contact lens should be placed. Once the flap is adherent, the eyelid speculum is carefully removed (taking care not to move the flap). Most surgeons place a drop of antibiotic and corticosteroid over the eye at the conclusion of the procedure. The flap is usually rechecked at the slit lamp before the patient leaves to make sure it has remained in proper alignment. A clear shield or protective goggles are often placed to guard against accidental trauma that could displace the flap.

Many surgeons instruct their patients to use topical antibiotics and corticosteroids postoperatively for 5 to 7 days. In addition, it is very important to keep the surface of the flap well lubricated in the early postoperative period. Patients may be told to use the protective shield when they shower or sleep for 1 day to 1 week and to avoid swimming or hot tubs for 2 weeks. The patient is examined 1 day after surgery to make sure that the flap has remained in proper alignment and that there is no evidence of infection or excessive inflammation. In the absence of complications, the next examinations are typically at approximately 1 week, 1 month, 3 months, 6 months, and 12 months postoperatively.

Lui MM, Silas MA, Fugishima J. Complications of photorefractive keratectomy and laser in situ keratomileusis. *J Refract Surg.* 2003;19:S247–S249.

Price FW. LASIK. In: *Focal Points: Clinical Modules for Ophthalmologists.* San Francisco: American Academy of Ophthalmology; 2000: vol 18, no 3.

Outcomes

LASIK studies vary considerably in the techniques employed, the degree of refractive error treated, the postoperative follow-up, and the variables analyzed. Consequently, it is often difficult to compare outcomes of different studies. While some trials separate results for low, moderate, and higher myopes, other studies merge the postoperative visual acuity results for all refractive error.

The improvement of visual results with the evolution of laser technology has been substantial. A 1999 clinical trial using a conventional laser for myopic astigmatic LASIK yielded postoperative UCVA of 20/20 in 47% of eyes. The more recent 2003 clinical trials of wavefront-guided ablation for myopic astigmatic LASIK achieved UCVA of 20/20 in 79% to 98% of eyes. The following section describes LASIK outcomes using results from FDA clinical trials and publications.

Boxer Wachler BS. Effect of pupil size on visual function under monocular and binocular conditions in LASIK and non-LASIK patients. *J Cataract Refract Surg.* 2003;29:275–278.

El-Maghraby A, Salah T, Waring III GO, et al. Randomized bilateral comparison of excimer laser in situ keratomileusis and photorefractive keratectomy for 2.50 to 8.00 diopters of myopia. *Ophthalmology.* 1999;106:447–457.

Mutyala S, McDonald MB, Scheinblum KA, et al. Contrast sensitivity evaluation after laser in situ keratomileusis. *Ophthalmology.* 2000;107:1864–1867.

Pop M, Payette Y. Photorefractive keratectomy versus laser in situ keratomileusis: a control-matched study. *Ophthalmology.* 2000;107:251–257.

Reviglio VE, Bossana EL, Luna JD, et al. Laser in situ keratomileusis for myopia and hyperopia using the Lasersight 200 laser in 300 consecutive cases. *J Refract Surg.* 2000;16:716–723.

Low myopia

Series of eyes treated with conventional (non–wavefront-guided) LASIK for low myopia (less than 6.0 D) in FDA clinical trials report that 67% to 86% of eyes achieved UCVA of 20/20 or better, 93% to 100% achieved 20/40 or better, and 94% to 100% obtained a postoperative refraction within 1.0 D of the intended refraction. Up to 2.1% of eyes lost 2 or more lines of BCVA.

El Danasoury MA, El-Maghraby A, Klyce SD, et al. Comparison of photorefractive keratectomy with excimer laser in situ keratomileusis in correcting low myopia (from −2.00 to −5.50 diopters): a randomized study. *Ophthalmology.* 1999;106:411–420.

Fernandez AP, Jaramillo J, Jaramillo M. Comparison of photorefractive keratectomy and laser in situ keratomileusis for myopia of −6 D or less using the Nidek EC-5000 laser. *J Refract Surg.* 2000;16:711–715.

Tole DM, McCarty DJ, Couper T, et al. Comparison of laser in situ keratomileusis and photorefractive keratectomy for the correction of myopia of −6 diopters or less. Melbourne Excimer Laser Group. *J Refract Surg.* 2001;17:46–54.

Moderate myopia

In patients with moderate myopia (approximately −6.0 to −12.0 D), results from large published series and FDA clinical trials report that 26% to 71% of eyes achieved an UCVA of 20/20 or better, 55% to 100% reached at least 20/40, and 41% to 96% were within 1.0 D of intended correction. The percentage of eyes losing 2 or more lines of BCVA ranged from 0% to 4.5%. The poorer outcomes usually reflect earlier studies using older laser technology.

High myopia

High myopia is most often defined as myopia greater than −12.0 D, with several studies reporting treatment results in patients with up to −29.0 D. In this range, the predictability of the procedure is markedly reduced, with 26% to 65% of eyes achieving at least 20/40 UCVA and 32% to 65% attaining a postoperative refraction within 1.0 D of the intended correction. In addition, when treating such high amounts of myopia, there was a higher incidence of loss of BCVA than in the correction of lower levels of myopia. However, patients with high myopia often gain BCVA after LASIK, probably due to decreased image minification compared with preoperative spectacles.

As experience with LASIK has accumulated, an increasing number of surgeons choose to rarely, if ever, perform LASIK or PRK for corrections above −12.0 D. The required ablation depths for high corrections may leave an inadequate stromal bed (less than 250 μm at a minimum) for long-term structural stability of the cornea. While some studies have reported no eyes with loss of 2 or more lines of BCVA, other series have reported up to 27% loss of 2 or more lines of BCVA for this range of myopic LASIK. High corrections have poor predictability for achieving good high-contrast UCVA. In addition, high corrections have an unacceptably high level of side effects, including glare, haloes, and loss of contrast sensitivity. These difficulties are attributable to the induction of high-order aberrations, particularly spherical aberration, because of the marked flattening of the central cornea compared with the midperipheral cornea.

Hersh PS, Brint SF, Maloney RK, et al. Photorefractive keratectomy versus laser in situ keratomileusis for moderate to high myopia: a randomized prospective study. *Ophthalmology.* 1998;105:1512–1522.

Kawesh GM, Kezerian GM. Laser in situ keratomileusis for high myopia with the VISX Star laser. *Ophthalmology.* 2000;107:653–661.

Pallikaris IG, Siganos DS. Excimer laser in situ keratomileusis and photorefractive keratectomy for correction of high myopia. *J Refract Surg.* 1994;10:498–510.

Myopia with astigmatism

Overall, the results for toric LASIK ablations are not as predictable as for spherical LASIK ablations. Most often, the procedure undercorrects the cylinder, which may simply indicate the need for improved nomograms or may indicate an inaccuracy of the axis ablated. Often it is difficult to determine the outcome of treatment for myopic astigmatism when reviewing large series of patients. Some clinical trials summarize the final outcome for all patients and do not distinguish between results for myopia and for myopic astigmatism.

In FDA clinical trials, including patients undergoing LASIK for myopic astigmatism, 43% to 87% of eyes achieved UCVA of 20/20 or better and 84% to 99% achieved UCVA of 20/40 or better, with 82% to 92% within ±1.0 D of the intended refraction. Up to 1.8% lost 2 or more lines of BCVA.

Casebeer JC, Kezerian GM. Outcomes of spherocylinder treatments in the comprehensive refractive surgery LASIK study. *Sem Ophthalmol.* 1998;13:71–78.

McDonald MB, Carr JD, Frantz JM, et al. Laser in situ keratomileusis for myopia up to −11 diopters with up to −5 diopters of astigmatism with the Summit Autonomous LADAR-Vision excimer laser system. *Ophthalmology.* 2001;108:309–316.

Hyperopia

In contrast to a myopic ablation, where the central cornea is ablated and flattened, a hyperopic ablation steepens the central cornea by ablating a doughnut-shaped area in the midperiphery. Initial problems with hyperopic treatment included decreased predictability and stability in comparison with myopic treatment as well as loss of BCVA (partially secondary to decentrations with small ablation zones). With enlargement of both the optical zone and the peripheral blend zone, as well as improved centration with the assistance of tracking devices, studies of hyperopic LASIK with longer follow-up periods have shown improved outcomes.

In FDA clinical trials of LASIK for hyperopia up to 6.0 D, 49% to 59% of eyes achieved postoperative UCVA of 20/20 or better, 93% to 96% achieved postoperative UCVA of 20/40 or better, 86% to 87% were within 1.0 D of emmetropia postoperatively, and up to 3.5% of eyes lost 2 or more lines of BCVA. Overall, studies with larger ablation zones have demonstrated good results for refractive errors up to +4.0 to +5.0 D, but predictability and stability are markedly reduced with hyperopic treatments above this level. Consequently, most refractive surgeons do not treat up to the highest levels of hyperopia that have been approved by the FDA.

Davidorf JM, Eghbali F, Onclinx T, et al. Effect of varying the optical zone diameter on the results of hyperopic laser in situ keratomileusis. *Ophthalmology.* 2001;108:1261–1265.

Tabbara KF, El-Sheikh HF, Islam SM. Laser in situ keratomileusis for the correction of hyperopia from +0.50 to +11.50 diopters with the Keracor 117C laser. *J Refract Surg.* 2001;17:123–128.

Hyperopic astigmatism

In several FDA clinical trials of hyperopic astigmatic correction, 37% to 65% of eyes achieved postoperative UCVA of 20/20 or better, 91% to 99% had UCVA of 20/40, 87% to 91% were within 1.0 D of emmetropia, and 3.8% to 5.8% lost 2 or more lines of BCVA. Efficacy was decreased with higher refractive errors.

Salz JJ, Stevens CA, and the LADARVision LASIK Hyperopia Study Group. LASIK correction of spherical hyperopia, hyperopic astigmatism, and mixed astigmatism with the LADAR-Vision excimer laser system. *Ophthalmology.* 2002;109:1647–1656.

Mixed astigmatism

Mixed astigmatism is defined as refractive error with cylinder greater than sphere and of opposite sign. LASIK has been approved by the FDA for mixed astigmatism of up to 6.0 D of sphere and cylinder. The outcomes of LASIK for mixed astigmatism are similar to the results for hyperopia and hyperopic astigmatism. From 46% to 62% of eyes had UCVA of 20/20 or better, 93% to 99% had postoperative UCVA of 20/40 or better, 88% to 96% were within 1.0 D of emmetropia, and up to 2% lost 2 or more lines of BCVA.

Retreatment

Although LASIK reduces refractive error and improves UCVA in almost all cases, some patients have residual refractive error that requires retreatment. The degree of refractive error that warrants retreatment varies, depending on the patient's lifestyle and expectations. Retreatment rates vary, depending partially on the degree of refractive error being treated, the laser and nomograms used, and the expectations of the patient population. One study showed that rates of retreatment are higher with higher initial correction, with residual astigmatism, and for patients older than 40 years. One advantage of LASIK compared with PRK is that refractive stability generally occurs earlier, allowing earlier enhancements, typically within the first half year after LASIK, whereas in PRK the ongoing activation of keratocytes and the risk of haze after enhancement usually requires a wait of at least 3 to 6 months before an enhancement PRK can be safely performed. Typically, retreatment rates are higher in hyperopia and higher myopia than in other indications.

One study reported the overall retreatment rate as 10.5% after LASIK for myopia, hyperopia, or astigmatism. Risk factors for LASIK retreatment include higher initial correction, astigmatism, and older age. Retreatment is usually performed by lifting the preexisting lamellar flap and applying additional ablation to the stromal bed. In many cases the flap can be lifted even several years after the original procedure. Alternatively, if a strong Bowman's layer scar has formed, a new flap can be created with the microkeratome. When lifting a preexisting flap, it is important to minimize epithelial disruption. A jeweler's forceps or 27-gauge needle can be used to localize the edge of the previous flap. Because the edge of the flap can be seen more easily at the slit lamp than with the diffuse illumination of the operating microscope of the laser, it may be easier to begin a flap lift at the slit lamp and then to complete it at the excimer laser. A careful circumferential epithelial dissection is performed so that the flap can then be lifted without tearing the epithelial edges. Alternatively, the surgeon can often visualize the edge of the flap under the diffuse illumination of the operating microscope by applying pressure with a small Sinskey hook or a similar device; the edge of the flap will dimple and disrupt the light reflex (Fig 6-13).

Once the ablation has been performed, the flap is repositioned and the interface is irrigated as in the initial LASIK procedure. Special care must be taken to make sure that no loose epithelium is trapped beneath the edge of the flap that could lead to epithelial ingrowth.

Occasionally PRK is considered to enhance a previous primary LASIK treatment. PRK performed on a LASIK flap carries an increased risk of haze formation and irregular astigmatism. On the other hand, PRK is an appealing alternative when the residual stromal bed is insufficient for further ablation, or in other situations such as a buttonhole flap. Recently, some surgeons have investigated the concomitant use of antiscarring agents such as mitomycin to improve the results of PRK performed on LASIK flaps.

Carones F, Vigo L, Carones A, et al. Evaluation of photorefractive keratectomy retreatments after regressed myopic laser in situ keratomileusis. *Ophthalmology.* 2001;108:1732–1737.

Davis EA, Hardten DR, Lindstrom M, et al. LASIK enhancements: a comparison of lifting to recutting the flap. *Ophthalmology.* 2002;109:2308–2313.

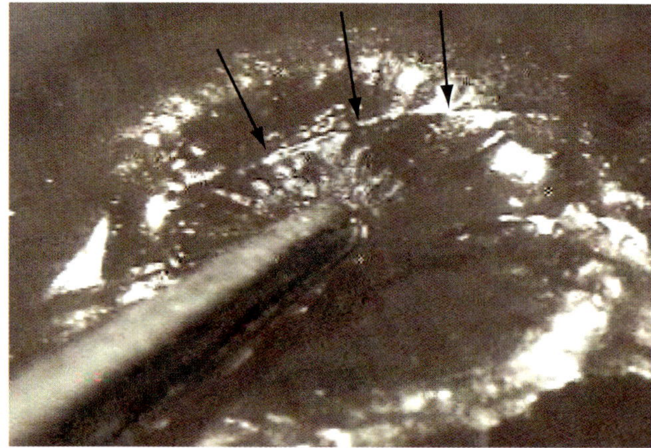

Figure 6-13 Indenting the cornea with forceps to visualize the edge of the flap *(arrows)* through an operating microscope prior to an enhancement procedure. *(Photograph courtesy of Roger F. Steinert, MD.)*

Hersh PS, Fry KL, Bishop DS. Incidence and associations of retreatment after LASIK. *Ophthalmology.* 2003;110:748–754.

Complications

Microkeratome complications

In the past, the more severe complications associated with LASIK have been related to problems with the microkeratome. Previously, abandonment of the planned LASIK procedure was reported to occur in 0.6% to 1.6% of cases. Advances in microkeratome technology have significantly reduced the incidence of severe, sight-threatening complications. However, it is still imperative that meticulous care be taken in the cleaning and assembly of the microkeratome to ensure that a smooth, uninterrupted keratectomy is performed.

Defects within the blade, poor suction, or uneven progression of the microkeratome across the cornea can produce an irregular, thin, or buttonholed flap, which can result in irregular astigmatism with loss of best-corrected vision. A steep corneal curvature is a risk factor for the development of these intraoperative flap complications. If a thin or buttonholed flap is created, it should be replaced without performing the ablation. Similarly, if an incomplete flap does not provide a sufficient- size corneal stromal surface to perform the laser ablation, it should be replaced without performing the ablation. Significant visual loss can be prevented if the ablation is not performed at the time and the flap is allowed to heal down before another LASIK procedure is attempted months later. In such a case, a bandage soft contact lens is applied to stabilize the flap, typically for several days to 1 week. A new flap can be cut after at least 3 months of healing, preferably with a different microkeratome head designed to produce a deeper cut, and the ablation can be applied at that time. Alternatively, some surgeons prefer surface PRK once the defective flap is judged to be healed.

Occasionally a free cap is created instead of the hinged flap (Fig 6-14). In these cases, the laser treatment to the corneal stroma can still be applied after placing the corneal cap in a moist chamber. It is important to replace the cap epithelial side up and to properly position it using the previously placed radial marks. A temporary 10–0 nylon suture can be placed to create an artificial "hinge," but the physiologic dehydration of the stroma by the endothelial pump generally will keep the cap secured in proper position. A bandage soft contact lens can help to protect the cap. A flat corneal curvature (less than 40 D) is a risk factor for cutting of a free cap because the flap diameter is often smaller than average in flat corneas.

Corneal perforation is a rare but devastating intraoperative complication that can occur if the microkeratome is not properly assembled, or if the depth plate of the microkeratome is not properly placed in an older-model microkeratome. Therefore, it is imperative that the surgeon doublecheck that the microkeratome has been properly assembled prior to proceeding. Most newer microkeratomes are made with a prefixed depth plate so that this source of error is eliminated. Corneal perforation can also occur when LASIK is performed on an excessively thin cornea. Therefore, corneal thickness must be measured with pachymetry prior to the LASIK procedure, especially in patients who are undergoing retreatment. Intraoperative pachymetry should especially be considered during a retreatment of a patient who had LASIK by another surgeon. In such a case, the surgeon does not know the thickness of the stromal bed after the flap is lifted because he or she may not have access to information about the prior flap thickness.

Jacobs JM, Taravella MJ. Incidence of intraoperative flap complications in laser in situ keratomileusis. *J Cataract Refract Surg.* 2002;8:23–28.

Lin RT, Maloney RK. Flap complications associated with lamellar refractive surgery. *Am J Ophthalmol.* 1999;127:129–136.

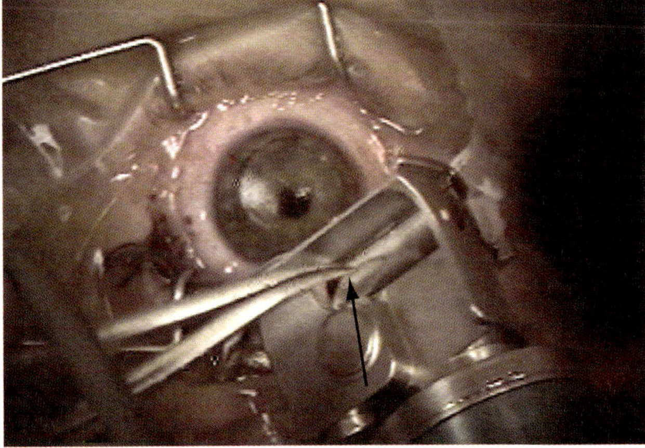

Figure 6-14 A free cap due to transection of the hinge. The cap is being lifted with forceps from the microkeratome *(arrow)*, taking care to maintain the orientation of the epithelial external layer, to prevent accidental inversion of the cap when it is replaced. *(Photograph courtesy of Roger F. Steinert, MD.)*

Epithelial erosions

The friction of microkeratome passage across the pressurized cornea may loosen the epithelium ("epithelial slider") or cause a frank epithelial defect. While patients with anterior basement dystrophy are at particular risk, in which case PRK rather than LASIK is advisable, other patients show no preoperative abnormality. Risk of epithelial erosion during LASIK correlates with older age. In bilateral LASIK procedures, the second eye has a greater likelihood of sustaining an epithelial defect (57%) if the first eye developed an intraoperative epithelial defect. Techniques suggested to decrease the erosion rate include limitation of toxic topical medication, having the patient keep the eyes closed after administration of topical anesthetic, frequent use of corneal lubricating drops, meticulous microkeratome maintenance, and shutting off of suction on the microkeratome reverse pass. A bandage soft contact lens is often applied immediately postoperatively and retained until stable re-epithelialization occurs, with subsequent use of intensive lubricants and occasionally punctal occlusion. In recalcitrant cases, persistent abnormal epithelium with recurrent erosions or loss of BCVA may require debridement and even superficial phototherapeutic keratectomy using the technique employed for treatment of recurrent erosions (see BCSC Section 8, *External Disease and Cornea*).

Tekwani NH, Huang D. Risk factors for intraoperative epithelial defect in laser in-situ keratomileusis. *Am J Ophthalmol.* 2002;134:311–316.

Striae

Flap folds are a major cause of decreased visual acuity after LASIK. Some 56% of flap folds occur on the first postoperative day, and 95% occur within the first week. Risk factors for development of folds include excessive irrigation under the flap during LASIK, thin flaps, and deep ablations with flap–bed mismatch.

While there is no consensus on definitions and treatments for flap folds, there are certain facts on which there is agreement. Flap folds are painless and may be asymptomatic. Recognition of visually significant folds is important because the success rate of treating folds falls dramatically with time. Early intervention is often critical in treating folds that cause loss of BCVA and/or visual distortion.

The first part of the evaluation of the patient with corneal folds is determination of the BCVA. Even if folds are noted on the slit-lamp exam, these are not treated if the BCVA and the subjective visual acuity are excellent. In fact, frequently the subjective vision does not correlate with the number and severity of folds. However, visually significant folds often induce irregular astigmatism and may be associated with hyperopic astigmatic refractive errors.

Slit-lamp examination should be performed using direct illumination, retroillumination, and fluorescein staining. Circumferential folds may be associated with high myopia and typically resolve with time. Folds that are parallel and grouped in the same direction may indicate a flap slippage, which requires prompt intervention. Corneal topography is typically not helpful in diagnosis of folds.

The challenge for the ophthalmologist is to determine which folds are visually significant and will not resolve with time. These folds should be promptly treated with flap massage at the slit lamp or by stretching the flap with sponges and forceps with or without lifting. Folds that are visually insignificant or those that cause minimal symptoms and resolve with time (eg, circumferential folds after a large myopic ablation) do not need intervention.

Some ophthalmologists have attempted to use specific clinical characteristics to classify the folds into folds that involve the entire thickness of the flap, called macrostriae or macrofolds, and superficial folds that are mostly in Bowman's layer, called microstriae or microfolds (Table 6-1). This classification system can be helpful in guiding treatment. Macrostriae typically require prompt flap repositioning to prevent permanent visual distortion or loss of BCVA. Microstriae frequently resolve with time and do not require intervention.

Despite this logical classification system, at times it may be difficult to determine if the folds present are macrostriae or microstriae. The surgeon may observe a few folds in the visual axis and may not be certain whether these are superficial or deep. While the classification system should be used when it is a helpful guide, it should not be used to arbitrarily dictate treatment. Some ophthalmologists have abandoned the use of the terms macrostriae and microstriae.

For example, prompt intervention can be considered for a patient who complains of decreased vision in one eye on the first postoperative day after bilateral LASIK and who has an asymmetric decrease in BCVA, hyperopic astigmatic refraction, and a few folds in the visual axis. Even if the surgeon believes the folds are microstriae, a flap smoothing has the potential of providing quick resolution of this problem in this unhappy patient. Ultimately, the patient's clinical situation must always be the most important factor in guiding treatment.

The following discussion uses the classic description of macrostriae and microstriae. When deciding whether or not to intervene, the ophthalmologist should always be guided by the individual clinical situation rather than just a rigid template.

Macrostriae represent full-thickness, undulating stromal folds. These folds invariably occur because of initial flap malposition or postoperative flap slippage (Fig 6-15A). Current approaches to smoothing the flap and avoiding striae at the end of the LASIK procedure vary widely. No matter which technique is employed, however, the surgeon must carefully examine for the presence of striae once the flap is repositioned. Coaxial and oblique illumination should be used at the operating microscope. Checking the patient in the early postoperative period is important to detect flap slippage. A protective plastic shield for the first 24 hours is often used to discourage touching of the eyelids and inadvertent disruption of the flap.

Flap subluxation has been reported to occur in up to 1.4% of eyes. Careful examination should disclose a wider gutter on the side where the folds are most prominent. Flap slippage should be rectified as soon as it is recognized, because the folds rapidly become fixed. Under the operating microscope or at the slit lamp, an eyelid speculum is placed, the flap is lifted, copious irrigation is used in the interface, and the flap is stroked repeatedly until the striae resolve. Hypotonic saline or sterile distilled water as the interface irrigating solution will swell the flap and may initially reduce the striae, but swelling reduces the flap diameter, which widens the gutter, delays flap adhesion due to prolonged endothelial dehydration time, and may leave worse striae after the flap dehydrates. If the macrostriae have been present for more than 24 hours, reactive epithelial hyperplasia in the valleys and hypoplasia over the elevations of the macrostriae will tend to fix the folds

Table 6-1 Differentiation of Macrostriae and Microstriae in LASIK Flaps

Characteristic		Macrostriae	Microstriae
Pathology		Large folds involving entire flap thickness	Fine folds, principally in Bowman's layer
Cause		Flap slippage	Mismatch of flap to new bed; contracture of flap
Slit-lamp appearance	Direct illumination	Broad undulations as parallel or radial converging lines; widened flap gutter may be seen	Fine folds, principally in Bowman's layer; gutter usually symmetric
	Retroillumination	Same as above	Folds more obvious on retroillumination
	Fluorescein	Same as above	Folds more obvious on fluorescein staining
Analogy		Wrinkles in skewed carpet	Dried cracked mud
Topography		Marked disruption over striae	Color map may be normal or slightly disrupted; Placido disc mires show fine irregularity
Vision		Markedly decreased BCVA and/or multiplopia if central	Subtle decreased BCVA or multiplopia if clinically significant; microstriae masked by epithelium are universal and asymptomatic
Treatment options	Acute	Refloat/reposition flap immediately	Observe; support surface with aggressive lubrication
	Established	Refloat, de-epithelialize over striae, hydrate and stroke, apply traction, or suture Phototherapeutic keratectomy	If visually significant, refloat; try hydration, stroking, tight suture Phototherapeutic keratectomy

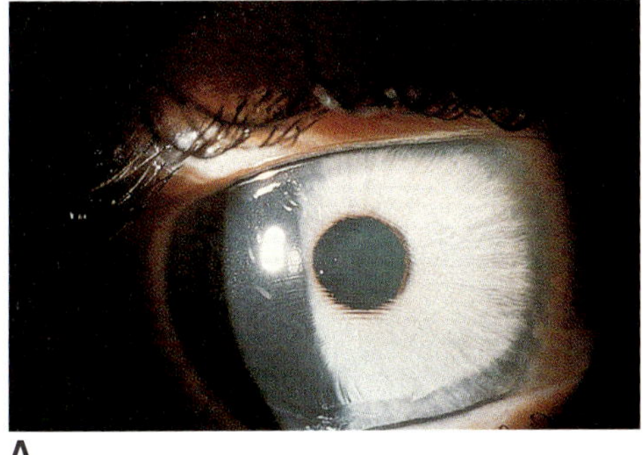

A

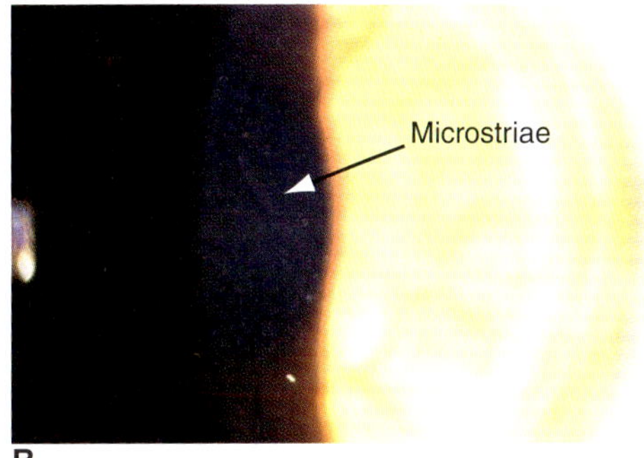

B

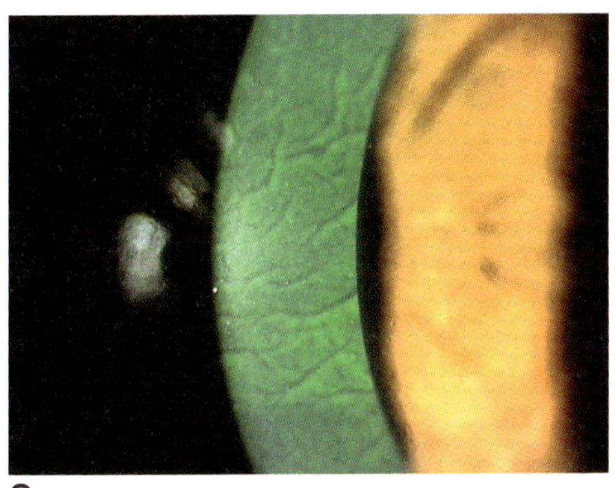

C

Figure 6-15 **A,** Retroillumination of multiple horizontal parallel macrostriae in the visual axis from mild flap dislocation. **B,** Diffuse illumination of visually insignificant microstriae in the visual axis after LASIK. **C,** Numerous randomly directed microstriae on fluorescein staining. These resemble multiple cracks in a piece of ice, are seen on the first postoperative day after LASIK, and usually resolve without intervention. *(A reprinted with permission from* External Disease and Cornea: A Multimedia Collection. *San Francisco: American Academy of Ophthalmology; 2000. B courtesy of Jayne S. Weiss, MD. C courtesy of Steven C. Schallhorn, MD.)*

into position. In such a case, in addition to refloating the flap, the central 6 mm of the flap over the macrostriae may be de-epithelialized to remove this impediment to smoothing the wrinkles. A bandage soft contact lens should always be employed to stabilize the flap and to protect the surface until full re-epithelialization occurs. In severe cases of intractable macrostriae, a tight 360° antitorque running 10-0 nylon suture or multiple interrupted sutures may be placed for several days, but irregular astigmatism may be present after suture removal.

Microstriae are fine, hairlike optical irregularities that are best seen on red reflex illumination or light reflected off the iris (Fig 6-15B and C). Microstriae are fine folds in Bowman's layer; this anterior location of the microstriae accounts for the disruption of best-corrected visual acuity. Computer topographic color maps do not usually show these fine irregularities. Disruption of the surface contour usually results in irregularity of the topographer's Placido disk image. In addition, application of dilute fluorescein will reveal so-called negative striae, where the elevated striae disrupt the tear film with loss of fluorescence over the elevated striae.

A few striae may not be visually significant. In addition, mild loss of visual acuity and other optical symptoms such as ghost images usually improve over time as the epithelial thickness adjusts to the folds and restores a more regular anterior tear film. The ocular surface should be supported with frequent administration of nonpreserved artificial tears and/or a bandage soft contact lens to encourage remodeling of a smooth corneal surface.

Persistent, optically significant striae must be addressed, however, if they cause loss of BCVA or unacceptable symptoms such as multiplopia. In many cases the surgeon can counsel a patient to wait several months, if possible, before intervention for microstriae, because epithelial remodeling may reduce or eliminate the optical effects of the microstriae. During this period, the epithelium should be supported with frequent artificial tear substitutes. However, as always the surgeon must be guided by the individual clinical findings to determine if prompter intervention is indicated.

Many interventions for microstriae have been recommended, with variable results. Some surgeons advocate hydration of Bowman's layer. While hydration will eventually occur with prolonged stroking of the epithelial surface with a moistened surgical spear sponge or irrigating cannula, microstriae also usually disappear within minutes of deliberate de-epithelialization of the area over the microstriae, followed by application of several drops of sterile distilled water. A hypotonic solution applied directly to Bowman's layer speeds the disappearance of the microstriae. If the striae persist, then the flap should be lifted and the interface irrigated with balanced salt solution to allow the flap to reposition. In severe cases, traction with fine-tooth forceps may also be helpful. Care must be taken not to tear the fragile flap. A bandage soft contact lens is then applied and topical antibiotic and corticosteroid drops are prescribed until re-epithelialization is established.

If optically significant microstriae persist, the flap may be sutured to attempt to reduce the striae through tension. As with macrostriae discussed above, suturing has the potential of inducing new irregular astigmatism. An alternative procedure is phototherapeutic keratectomy. Pulses from a broad-beam laser, set to a maximal diameter of 6.5 mm, are applied initially to penetrate the epithelium in about 200 pulses. The epithelium will act as a masking agent, exposing the elevated striae before the valleys between the striae. After the transepithelial ablation, additional pulses are applied, with the administration of a thin film of medium-viscosity artificial tears every 5 to 10 pulses, up to a maximum of 100 additional pulses. If these guidelines are followed, little to no haze results and an average hyperopic shift of less than +1 D occurs, due to the minimal tissue removal.

Jackson DW, Hamill MB, Koch DD. Laser in situ keratomileusis flap suturing to treat recalcitrant flap striae. *J Cataract Refract Surg.* 2003;29:264–269.

Steinert RF, Ashrafzadeh A, Hersh P. Phototherapeutic keratectomy for the treatment of flap striae after laser in-situ keratomileusis. *Ophthalmology* (in press).

Traumatic flap dislocation

Flap subluxation has been reported to occur in up to 1.4% of eyes. Dislocation of the LASIK flap is not uncommon on the first postoperative day, when dryness and adhesion of the flap to the upper tarsal conjunctiva is sufficient to cause slippage of the flap, which is stabilized only by the negative (suction) pressure of the corneal endothelial pump. After the first day, however, the re-epithelialization of the gutter begins the process of increasing flap stability. Within several weeks, keratocytes begin to lay down new collagen at the cut edge of Bowman's layer and eventually establish a fine scar at the edge of the flap. Minimal healing occurs across the stromal interface for several years, however, allowing flap lifting for enhancement procedures. Late traumatic dislocation from blunt trauma has been reported more than 1 year after LASIK and can also occur if the shearing force exceeds the strength of the peripheral Bowman's layer–level healing.

Dry eye and corneal sensation

Dry eye is one of the most frequent side effects of LASIK and has been reported in up to 33% of patients in some studies. The surgeon must carefully monitor the patient postoperatively for signs of punctate keratitis or more severe manifestations of neurotrophic epitheliopathy. While awaiting the return of innervation, treatment includes nonpreserved artificial tears, gels, and ointments, and when necessary, punctal occlusive plugs. Ointments should not be used in the early postoperative period, to avoid the potential of migration under the flap. (See also Chapter 10.)

Both the surgeon and the patient must remain aware that many patients seeking laser vision correction do so because of contact lens intolerance, and dry eyes are one of the most common reasons for that intolerance. Such dryness will persist, of course, and will be transiently worsened during the recovery by the denervation of the flap. The patient may feel that long-term, persistent dryness has worsened and may blame the LASIK procedure.

Central islands and decentration

See the discussion in the PRK section of this chapter.

Interface inflammation

Sterile interface inflammation has been referred to as diffuse lamellar keratitis (DLK), "sands of the Sahara" (SOS), or, perhaps most accurately, diffuse interface keratitis (Fig 6-16). This syndrome can range from asymptomatic interface haze near the edge of the flap to marked diffuse haze with diminished BCVA. The condition appears to be a nonspecific inflammatory response to a variety of toxic insults. The interface is a potential space; any cause of anterior stromal inflammation may cause white blood cells to accumulate in that space. DLK has been reported in association with epithelial defects that occur during primary LASIK or during enhancement or even months after the LASIK procedure. Other reported inciting factors include foreign material on the surface of the microkeratome blade or motor, meibomian gland secretions, povidone-iodine solution, substances produced by laser ablation, contamination of the sterilizer with gram-negative endotoxin, and red blood cells in the interface. The inflammation generally resolves on its own without sequelae, but severe cases can lead to scarring or flap melting.

DLK is usually classified by the stages described (Table 6-2). Although stages 1 and 2 usually respond to frequent topical corticosteroids, stages 3 and 4 usually require lifting the flap and irrigating, followed by intensive topical corticosteroid treatment. Systemic corticosteroids may be used adjunctively in severe cases. Some surgeons use topical and systemic corticosteroids in stage 3 DLK instead of lifting the flap. Recovery of vision in DLK is usually excellent if the condition is detected and treated promptly.

Late-onset interface opacity similar to DLK and water cleft accumulation have been reported as a result of elevated IOP; the surgeon must be aware of this unusual manifestation in order to properly diagnose and treat it.

Belin MW, Hannush SB, Yau CW, et al. Elevated intraocular pressure–induced interlamellar stromal keratitis. *Ophthalmology.* 2002;109:1929–1933.

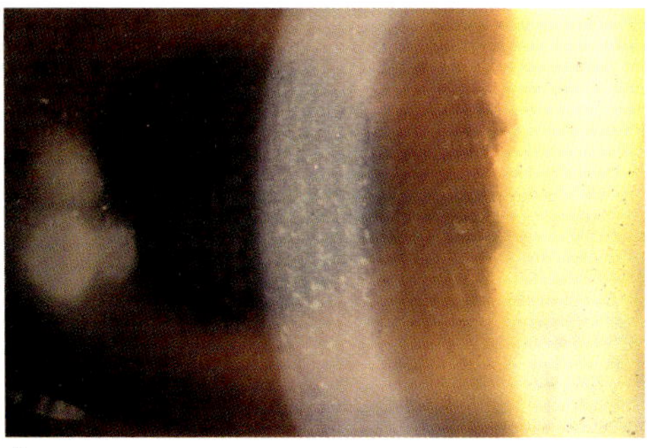
A

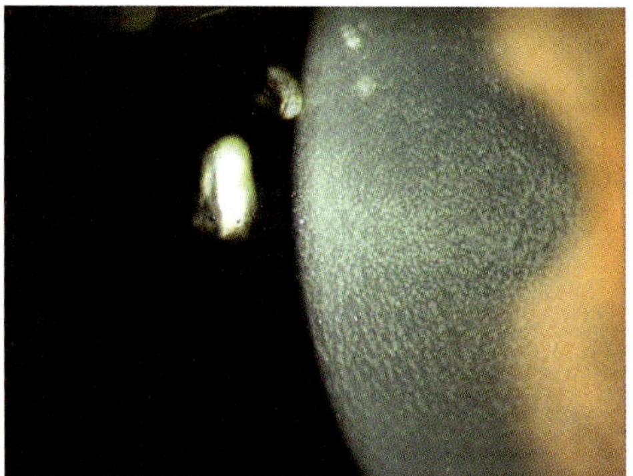
B

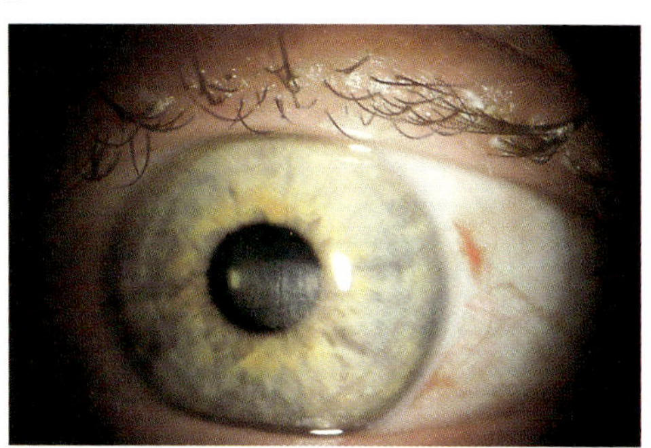
C

Figure 6-16 Diffuse lamellar keratitis. **A,** High magnification of stage 2 DLK (note accumulation of inflammatory cells in the fine ridges created by the oscillating microkeratome blade). **B,** Stage 3 DLK (dense accumulation of inflammatory cells centrally). **C,** Stage 4 DLK with central scar and folds. *(A and B courtesy of Roger F. Steinert, MD; C courtesy of Jayne S. Weiss, MD.)*

Table 6-2 Staging of Diffuse Lamellar Keratitis

Stage	Findings
1	Peripheral faint white blood cells; granular appearance
2	Central scattered white blood cells; granular appearance
3	Central dense white blood cells in visual axis
4	Permanent scarring or stromal melting

Hoffman RS, Fine IH, Packer M. Incidence and outcomes of LASIK with diffuse lamellar keratitis treated with topical and oral corticosteroids. *J Cataract Refract Surg.* 2003;29: 451–456.

Holland SP, Mathias RG, Morck DW, et al. Diffuse lamellar keratitis related to endotoxins released from sterilizer reservoir biofilms. *Ophthalmology.* 2000;107:1227–1233.

Smith RJ, Maloney RK. Diffuse lamellar keratitis: a new syndrome in lamellar refractive surgery. *Ophthalmology.* 1998:105:1721– 1726.

Steinert RF, McColgin AZ, White A, et al. Diffuse interface keratitis after laser in situ keratomileusis (LASIK): a nonspecific syndrome. *Am J Ophthalmol.* 2000;129:380–381.

Infectious keratitis

It is important to differentiate sterile interface inflammation from potentially devastating infectious inflammation. Infection within the interface can lead to flap melting, severe irregular astigmatism, and corneal scarring that requires penetrating keratoplasty. If infection is suspected, the flap should be lifted and the interface cultured and irrigated with antibiotics. The most common infections are from gram-positive organisms, followed closely in frequency by atypical mycobacteria. A more rapid diagnosis for mycobacteria may be made by acid-fast and fluorochrome stains while waiting for cultures. Onset of symptoms occurs earlier with bacteria and is more delayed with mycobacteria, fungi, and *Acanthamoeba*. Infection from virtually all organisms has been reported; fungal infection is particularly difficult to treat. If the infection does not respond to treatment, amputation of the flap may be necessary to improve antibiotic or antifungal penetration. The fourth-generation fluoroquinolones gatifloxacin and moxifloxacin have excellent efficacy against the more common bacteria that cause post-LASIK infections, including some atypical mycobacteria. Topical and oral clarithromycin (500 mg BID) have also been used for the treatment of mycobacterial infections. An infected LASIK flap may occur after a recurrent abrasion (Fig 6-17).

Freitas D, Alvarenga L, Sampaio J, et al. An outbreak of *Mycobacterium chelonei* infection after LASIK. *Ophthalmology*. 2003;110:276–285.

Karp CL, Tuli SS, Yoo SH, et al. Infectious keratitis after LASIK. *Ophthalmology*. 2003;110:503–510.

Epithelial ingrowth

Epithelial ingrowth occurs in less than 3% of eyes (Fig 6-18). Isolated nests of epithelial cells in the lamellar interface that are not advancing do not need to be treated. However, if the epithelium is advancing toward the visual axis, is associated with irregular astigmatism (Fig 6-19), or triggers overlying flap melting, it should be removed by lifting the flap and scraping the epithelium from the underside of the flap as well as from the stromal bed prior to repositioning the flap. The incidence of epithelial ingrowth is greater in patients who develop an epithelial defect at the time of the procedure and in those undergoing a retreatment with lifting of a preexisting flap. Therefore, in these instances special care should be taken to make sure that no epithelium becomes caught under the

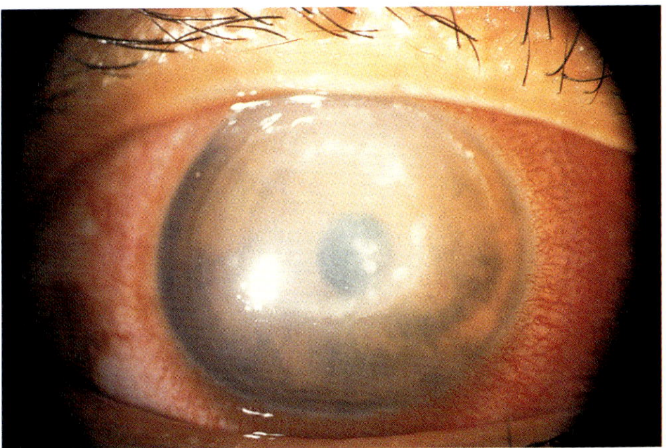

Figure 6-17 Infectious keratitis in a LASIK flap after recurrent epithelial abrasion. *(Photograph courtesy of Jayne S. Weiss, MD.)*

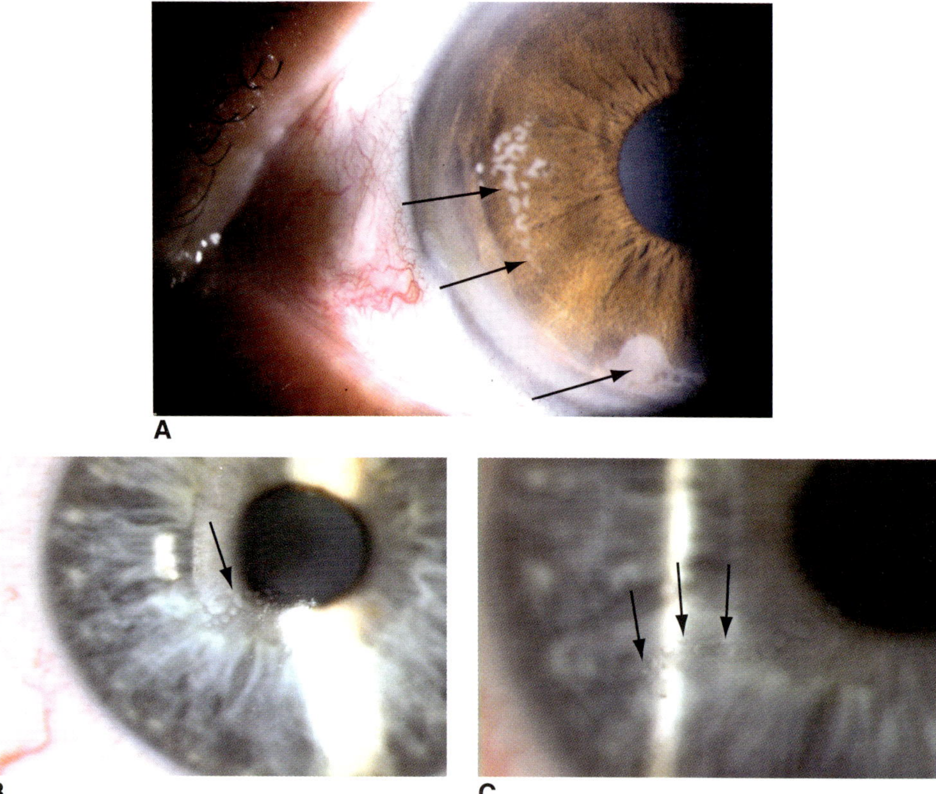

Figure 6-18 Epithelial ingrowth in the interface under a LASIK flap. **A,** Peripheral ingrowth of 1 to 2 mm *(arrows)* is common and inconsequential and does not require intervention unless it induces melting of the overlying flap. **B,** Central nests of epithelial cells *(arrow)* disrupt the patient's vision by elevating and distorting the flap. The flap must be lifted and the epithelium debrided. **C,** Inspection of the midperiphery shows the track followed by the invading epithelium from the periphery toward the center *(arrows)*. *(Photographs courtesy of Roger F. Steinert, MD.)*

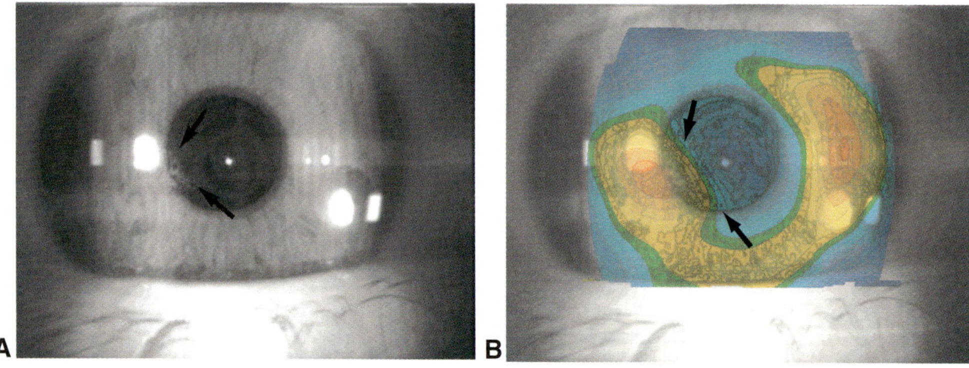

Figure 6-19 **A,** Epithelial ingrowth in visual axis *(arrows)*. **B,** Corresponding topographic steepening and irregularity on Orbscan topography. *(Topography scans courtesy of Jayne S. Weiss, MD.)*

edge of the flap when it is repositioned. Placement of a bandage contact lens at the conclusion of the procedure may also decrease the incidence of epithelial ingrowth for patients at higher risk of developing this complication.

Asano-Kato N, Toda I, Hori-Komai Y, et al. Epithelial ingrowth after laser in situ keratomileusis: clinical features and possible mechanisms. *Am J Ophthalmol.* 2002;134:801–807.

Interface debris

Debris in the interface is occasionally seen postoperatively. The principal indication for intervention, with flap lifting, irrigation, or manual removal of debris, is an inflammatory reaction elicited by the foreign material. Small amounts of lint, nondescript particles, or tiny metal particles from stainless steel surgical instruments are usually well tolerated. On the other hand, while a small amount of blood that has oozed into the interface from transected peripheral vessels may be tolerated, any significant amount of blood will usually elicit an inflammatory cell response and should be irrigated from the interface at the time of the LASIK procedure (Fig 6-20). Use of a topical vasoconstrictor such as epinephrine to facilitate coagulation at the time of replacing the flap will help minimize this problem. The surgeon should be aware, however, that application of epinephrine prior to laser ablation can result in pupillary dilation and decentration. Blood remaining in the interface will typically resolve spontaneously with time.

Ectasia

The importance of an adequate residual stromal bed to prevent structural instability and postoperative corneal ectasia is discussed in the section on preoperative evaluation. Current standards recommend a minimum residual stromal bed of at least 250 µm after completion of the ablation (see Chapter 3). Although keratectasia is usually associated with LASIK performed for higher myopic corrections, in thin corneas or in patients who have had multiple laser ablations, cases of ectasia have been reported in corrections as low as −4 D where the residual stroma was believed to be thicker than 250 µm. In many of these cases, later examinations have shown that the microkeratome created a flap thicker than expected, resulting in a thinner residual stromal bed. In other cases,

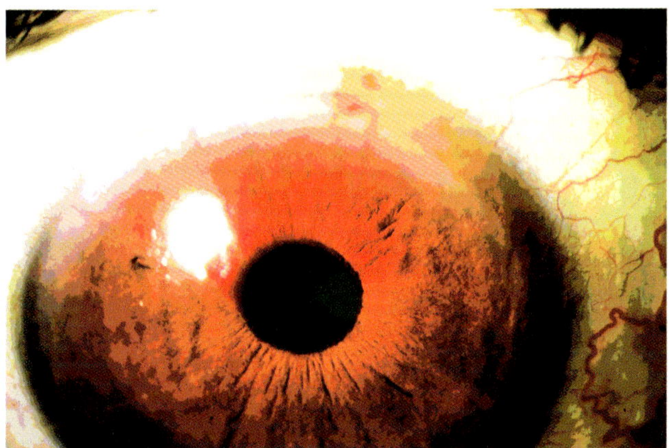

Figure 6-20 Blood in the LASIK interface. *(Photograph courtesy of Jayne S. Weiss, MD.)*

preoperative subtle keratoconus or other ectasias may have been present. In a retrospective study of 10 eyes from 7 patients who developed corneal ectasia after LASIK, all patients had either preoperative undiagnosed forme fruste keratoconus (88%) or a residual stromal bed of less than 250 μm (70%). Often, good vision can be restored with a rigid gas-permeable contact lens. The implantation of symmetrical or asymmetrical intrastromal polymethylmethacrylate ring segments (Intacs) to reduce the irregular astigmatism is being studied. In extreme cases, penetrating keratoplasty may be required.

Fogla R, Rao SK, Padmanabhan P. Keratoectasia in 2 cases with pellucid marginal corneal degeneration after laser in situ keratomileusis. *J Cataract Refract Surg.* 2003;29:788–791.

Ou RJ, Shaw EL, Glasgow BJ. Keratectasia after laser in situ keratomileusis (LASIK): evaluation of the calculated residual stromal bed thickness. *Am J Ophthalmol.* 2002;134:771–773.

Randleman JB, Russell B, Ward MA, et al. Risk factors and prognosis for corneal ectasia after LASIK. *Ophthalmology.* 2003;110:267–275.

Rare complications

Rare complications include optic nerve ischemia, premacular subhyaloid hemorrhage, macular hemorrhage associated with preexisting lacquer cracks or choroidal neovascularization, choroidal infarcts, postoperative corneal edema associated with preoperative corneal guttata, and ring scotoma. Diplopia is a rare complication and is related to technical problems, prior need for prisms, aniseikonia, iatrogenic monovision, and improper control of accommodation in patients with strabismus.

Gimbel HV, Anderson Penno EE, van Westenbrugge JA, et al. Incidence and management of intraoperative and early postoperative complications in 1000 consecutive laser in situ keratomileusis cases. *Ophthalmology.* 1998;105:1839–1848.

Kushner BJ, Kowal L. Diplopia after refractive surgery: occurrence and prevention. *Arch Ophthalmol.* 2003;121:315–321.

Stulting RD, Carr JD, Thompson KP, et al. Complications of laser in situ keratomileusis for the correction of myopia. *Ophthalmology.* 1999;106:13–20.

Sugar A, Rapuano CJ, Culbertson WW, et al. Laser in situ keratomileusis for myopia and astigmatism. *Ophthalmology.* 2002;109:175–187.

Tabbara KF, El-Sheikh HF, Vera-Cristo CL. Complications of laser in situ keratomileusis (LASIK). *Eur J Ophthalmol.* 2003;13:139–146.

Conclusion

Although LASIK is the most popular refractive surgery procedure performed today, it does have limitations. Many surgeons will not use LASIK to treat higher levels of myopia (>−12.0 D) and hyperopia (>+4.0 D) because of poorer predictability and an increased possibility of complications.

Although LASIK has rapidly surpassed PRK in popularity for the treatment of many refractive errors, visual results are actually very similar between the procedures. A study of patients treated for myopia of −1.0 to −9.5 D showed equal refractive outcomes. Another study of treatment of myopia between −6.0 and −15.0 D showed a slightly decreased incidence of postoperative optical symptoms in LASIK compared with PRK. However, in a randomized bilateral comparison of LASIK and PRK in patients with −2.5 to −8.0 D, almost twice as many were highly satisfied with their LASIK eye as compared with their PRK eye 1 year after treatment. In addition to having less postoperative pain and more rapid visual recovery, the LASIK eyes were more likely to achieve UCVA of 20/20 or better and less likely to have postoperative topographic irregularities.

The incidence of complications in LASIK decreases with surgeon experience and, as with any surgical procedure, it is preferable to optimize surgical technique in order to attempt to avoid complications. When recognized and properly treated, however, the majority of complications will not result in loss of BCVA. Irregular astigmatism is a common cause of decreased BCVA. Often epithelial hyperplasia and hypoplasia occur, which smooths the corneal surface over time, reducing the irregular astigmatism and improving the visual acuity. If significant symptoms persist, however, the patient may benefit from selective surface treatments.

Technological advances will continue to improve visual outcomes. Wavefront-guided laser ablation, discussed following and in Chapter 1, offers the potential for improvement in visual quality. PRK may again become more popular in conjunction with the wavefront-guided lasers because surface ablation avoids the higher-order aberrations induced by the corneal flap in LASIK. Future advances in laser technology may eventually afford true custom ablation, including treatment of such entities as irregular astigmatism for which there is currently no effective refractive surgical procedure.

McColgin AZ, Steinert RF. *LASIK.* In: Tasman W, Jaeger E, eds. *Duane's Clinical Ophthalmology.* Philadelphia: Lippincott; 2001.

Wavefront-Guided PRK and LASIK

Background

Conventional excimer laser ablation treats lower-order or spherocylindrical aberrations such as myopia, hyperopia, and astigmatism. These lower-order aberrations comprise approximately 90% of all aberrations, with higher-order aberrations making up the remainder. We are still learning about the visual impact of higher-order aberrations in the normal population. It is possible that the small amounts of higher-order aberration found in the normal population do not adversely affect vision. Higher-order aberrations are also a by-product of excimer laser ablation. Some higher-order aberrations can cause symptoms such as loss of contrast sensitivity and nighttime haloes and glare, decreasing the quality of vision.

Wavefront-guided ablation creates ablation profiles that are customized for an individual patient, in an effort to reduce preexisting aberrations and to reduce the induction of new aberrations. In addition to addressing higher-order aberrations, wavefront-guided treatments can correct the lower-order aberrations of spherical error and astigmatism.

Wavefront-guided ablation offers the potential advantage of better visual quality because of treatment of higher-order aberrations. When compared with conventional excimer laser ablation, wavefront-guided ablation appears to offer better contrast acuity and less induction of postoperative higher-order aberrations. However, patients undergoing wavefront-guided ablation may still have more higher-order aberrations postoperatively than they did preoperatively. Although there is the possibility that wavefront-guided ablation may offer better visual acuity results than conventional excimer laser ablation, the promise of "supernormal visual acuity" has yet to be realized.

Wavefront-guided ablation is not suitable for all patients. It is currently approved by the FDA for manufacturer-specific ranges of myopia and myopic astigmatism. Wavefront data may be impossible to obtain in very irregular corneas or with smaller pupillary diameters. The treatment is more costly than conventional excimer laser ablation because of the time required to collect the wavefront data that are needed to program the excimer laser. Wavefront technology is still in evolution and may lead to further expansion of refractive surgical indications and additional improvements in postoperative results. (See also the discussion in Chapter 1.)

Nuijts RM, Nabar VA, Hament WJ, et al. Wavefront-guided versus standard laser in situ keratomileusis to correct low to moderate myopia. *J Cataract Refract Surg.* 2002;28: 1907–1913.

Instrumentation

The wavefront mapping systems are unique to the specific wavefront-guided laser used. FDA-approved wavefront-guided excimer lasers include the Alcon CustomCornea, the VISX WaveScan, and the Bausch & Lomb Zyoptix systems. Calibration should be performed according to the manufacturer's specifications.

Preoperative Preparation

Preoperative wavefront analysis is first performed. Some systems require pupillary dilation to capture wavefront data, while others do not. The wavefront refraction indicated on wavefront analysis is compared with the manifest refraction and should be no greater than 0.75 D difference; otherwise the manifest refraction and the wavefront analysis should be repeated. The data are either electronically transferred to the laser or downloaded to a floppy disk and then transferred to the laser. Unlike a conventional excimer laser, where the refraction is used to program the laser, the wavefront-guided laser uses programmed wavefront data to create a custom ablation pattern.

The accuracy of the wavefront analysis may be somewhat dependent on the experience of the examiner obtaining the data. Wavefront analysis may not be possible in patients with extremely irregular corneas, for example, corneas with prior penetrating keratoplasty or corneal scars; such patients will not be candidates for wavefront-guided ablation.

Surgical Technique

The surgical technique is similar to conventional excimer laser treatment.

Outcomes

In its premarket approval application to the FDA, Alcon compared 139 eyes that had wavefront-guided custom ablation with 47 conventionally treated eyes at 6 months after surgery. All eyes had a preoperative myopic manifest refractive error under −7.0 D sphere and under 0.5 D cylinder. Of these, 79.9% of wavefront-treated eyes achieved UCVA of

20/20 or better, 91.5% achieved 20/25 or better, and 98.6% achieved 20/40 or better. Mean postoperative refractive spherical equivalent was ±0.5 D in 74.8% and ±1.0 D in 95.7%.

Higher-order aberrations increased by 20% in the wavefront-treated group vs 77% in the conventional group. Spherical aberrations increased by 22% for wavefront-treated eyes and 108% for conventionally treated eyes. Mean contrast sensitivity for wavefront-treated eyes improved by 0.1 to 0.2 log units relative to conventionally treated eyes. There was a statistically significant decrease in loss of low-contrast BCVA in the wavefront-treated group compared with those in the conventional treatment group.

Although there were no data supporting a statistically significant difference in UCVA between the two groups, BCVA and low-contrast visual acuity were both slightly better for wavefront-treated eyes than for conventionally treated eyes. Postoperative UCVA was as good or better than preoperative BCVA in 52% of the wavefront-guided ablation group, and 37% gained 1 or more lines of BCVA.

Both VISX and Bausch & Lomb have FDA approval for wavefront-guided laser ablation of up to −7.0 D sphere and 3.0 D cylinder. In the VISX clinical trials, after excluding eyes that required enhancement retreatment, 98% of the remaining eyes had UCVA of 20/20 or better at 12 months. Postoperative UCVA was equal to or better than preoperative BCVA in 80% of eyes; 10% of patients gained more than 1 line of BCVA, and 93% of eyes were within 0.5 D of intended correction. In the Bausch & Lomb clinical trials, 91.5% of eyes had UCVA of 20/20 at 6 months. Postoperative UCVA was equal to or better than preoperative BCVA in 78% of eyes; 75.9% of eyes were within 0.5 D of intended correction.

CHAPTER 7

Thermokeratoplasty

History

Using heat to alter the shape of the cornea was first proposed by Lans, a Dutch medical student, in 1898. Utilizing electrocautery to heat the corneal stroma, he noticed astigmatic changes in the cornea. Two years later, in 1900, Terrien reported the use of cautery to correct the severe astigmatism associated with Terrien marginal degeneration, and in 1928, Knapp used cautery to improve the visual acuity of patients with keratoconus.

In 1975, Gasset and Kaufman proposed a modified technique of thermokeratoplasty to treat keratoconus. They theorized that the hot cautery used in prior reports caused collagen necrosis, leading to tissue destruction and corneal melting. Their goal was to measure the heat applied to the cornea to control its application, in order to shrink collagen fibers without causing necrosis. The cornea was reportedly heated to 115°C in the region of the cone, resulting in an overall flattening of the cornea. They performed the procedure on eyes requiring penetrating keratoplasty in which the vision was not correctable with spectacles or contact lenses. Vision improved to 20/30 or better in most eyes, and penetrating keratoplasty was avoided in 95% of their 59 patients. Similar attempts by others during the 1970s proved less successful, and complications were encountered such as delayed epithelial healing, recurrent epithelial erosions, corneal neovascularization, aseptic stromal necrosis and melting, stromal scarring, iritis, and hypopyon.

The optimal temperature to avoid stromal necrosis while still obtaining collagen shrinkage is approximately 60 to 65°C, much lower than that used by Gasset and Kaufman. Human collagen fibrils can shrink by almost two thirds when exposed to temperatures in this range. The heat disrupts the hydrogen bonds in the supercoiled structure of collagen. In the cornea, the maximal shrinkage is approximately 7%. When higher temperatures are reached (>78°C), tissue necrosis occurs.

Various other approaches to heating the cornea have been proposed, none of which has met with long-term acceptance. In an attempt to reduce possible complications, Rowsey and co-workers in 1981 introduced an alternative method to heat the cornea using diathermy (radiofrequency current). This was thought to be more predictable and delivered less total energy. They used the Los Alamos keratoplasty unit in which the probe treated an area between 200 and 400 μm below the corneal epithelium. Although corneal changes were noted, marked regression occurred with this technique.

In 1984, Fyodorov introduced a technique of radial thermal keratoplasty using a handheld heated nichrome needle designed for deeper thermal keratoplasty. The handheld probe contained a retractable 34-gauge wire heated to 600°C. A motor advanced the wire to a preset depth of 95% of the corneal pachymetry for a duration of 0.3 second. He used different patterns to treat hyperopia and astigmatism. Excessive heating of the cornea resulted in necrosis and corneal remodeling. Regression of treatment and unpredictability limited its success.

Neumann A, Fyodorov S, Sanders D. Radial thermokeratoplasty for the correction of hyperopia. *J Refract Surg.* 1990;6:404–412.

Laser Thermokeratoplasty

In the 1990s, multiple lasers were tested for use in laser thermokeratoplasty (LTK), including CO_2, cobalt-magnesium-fluoride, erbium:glass, and holmium:yttrium-aluminum-garnet (Ho:YAG). Only the Ho:YAG laser reached commercial production and FDA approval. The Ho:YAG laser produces light in the infrared region at a wavelength of 2100 nm and has corneal tissue penetration to approximately 480 to 530 μm. Two different delivery systems were investigated, a contact system (Summit) and a noncontact laser, the Sunrise Hyperion (Sunrise Technologies).

The contact laser was originally developed as part of the integrated Summit workstation. The contact Ho:YAG handheld probe emitted a 300 μsec pulse at a repetition rate of 15 Hz and a pulse power of approximately 19 mJ. Laser applications were placed in a set pattern around the corneal periphery. High degrees of regression and induced astigmatism were noted. The system never received FDA approval for the correction of hyperopia and is no longer commercially available.

The noncontact Sunrise Hyperion system was approved by the FDA in 2000. This laser uses a slit-lamp delivery system and delivers 8 simultaneous spots at a wavelength of 2.1 μm at a frequency of 5 Hz and a pulse duration of 250 μsec. The laser places 8 circumferential applications in the corneal periphery at a set optical zone of 6.0 and/or 7.0 mm. The treatment consists of either one or two rings of spots. The system is approved for the temporary correction of 0.75 to 2.5 D of hyperopia with less than 1.0 D of astigmatism. One-year results indicated that 37.4% of study patients obtained an uncorrected visual acuity of 20/20 or better and 85.0% achieved 20/40 or better. A total of 16.4% were undercorrected by over 1.0 D. Patient satisfaction varied, with 8.0% of patients reporting being "very disappointed," and 35.7% reporting being "most satisfied." No patients had a best-corrected visual acuity below 20/40, and 2.3% had lost 2 lines or more of best-corrected visual acuity at the 12-month visit. While only low amounts of hyperopia are correctable, the procedure is quick and simple, each treatment ring taking just a few seconds.

Because the Ho:YAG lasers heat the surface of the cornea and rely on passive conduction of heat, even heating of the cornea is not possible. The surface of the cornea has to be heated above 65° C to obtain an adequate temperature rise in the midstroma. This leads to epithelial necrosis, initial patient discomfort, and inadequate heating of the deeper layers of the cornea. Strong initial interest in LTK has waned, partly because of the visual fluctuations and refractive regression and partly because of the high purchase price of the equipment. LTK has largely been superseded by conductive keratoplasty.

Aker AB, Brown DC. Hyperion laser thermokeratoplasty for hyperopia. *Int Ophthalmol Clin.* 2000;40:165–181.

Ogawa GSH, Azar DT, Koch DD. Laser thermokeratoplasty for hyperopia, astigmatism, and myopia. In: Azar DR, ed. *Refractive Surgery.* Stamford, Conn: Appleton & Lange; 1997: 491–499.

Thompson VM, McDonnell PJ. The holmium laser: thermokeratoplasty. In: Wu HK, Thompson VM, Steinert RF, et al, eds. *Refractive Surgery.* New York: Thieme; 1999.

Conductive Keratoplasty

In recent years, radiofrequency has again emerged as a method of heating the cornea. In 2002, the FDA approved the ViewPoint CK system (Refractec) for the temporary treatment of mild to moderate hyperopia (+0.75 to +3.00 D) with astigmatism of 0.75 D or less. In 2004, conductive keratoplasty received FDA approval for treatment of presbyopia in the nondominant eye of a presbyopic patient with an endpoint of −1.00 to −2.00 D.

Conductive keratoplasty (CK) is a nonablative, collagen-shrinking procedure. CK is based on the delivery of radiofrequency energy through a fine conducting tip that is inserted into the peripheral corneal stroma (Fig 7-1). Because of its electrolytic properties, the cornea conducts radiofrequency energy. As the current flows through the tissue surrounding the tip, resistance to the current creates localized heat. Collagen lamellae in the area surrounding the tip shrink in a controlled fashion and form a column of denatured collagen. The ViewPoint CK system consists of a portable console, an eyelid speculum that acts as the electrical return path, and a handpiece that holds the 450 μm long and 90 μm wide metal Keratoplast tip (Fig 7-2).

For hyperopia treatment, the surgeon first marks the cornea in a set pattern and then inserts the tip into the stroma in a ring pattern around the peripheral cornea (Fig 7-3) according to the supplied nomogram (Table 7-1). The CK unit delivers a set power and duration (0.6 seconds) when the foot pedal is depressed (for equipment sold internationally, both power and duration can be adjusted by the surgeon). The number and location of spots determines the amount of refractive change, with an increasing number of spots and rings used for higher amounts of hyperopia. The CK procedure is performed under topical anesthesia and typically takes less than 5 minutes. The collagen shrinkage leads to visible striae between the treated spots, which fade with time (Fig 7-4). The shortening of the collagen fibrils creates a band of tightening that increases the curvature of the central cornea.

CK and LTK differ in several respects. In LTK, heat is applied directly to the corneal surface, resulting in a thermal gradient in which treatment is hotter at the surface and cooler in the deeper stroma. CK-treated tissue is exposed to the same temperature at the tip of the probe (deep in the stroma) as at the back of the probe (corneal surface).

CK appears to have advantages both in cost and in allowing flexible (off-label) treatment patterns, since the tip can be placed anywhere on the cornea. CK is being evaluated for the treatment of astigmatism after LASIK or cataract surgery. When used to correct astigmatism, the spots are applied to the flatter meridian to induce steepening. More experience and long-term data will be required to determine how important CK will be in the refractive surgeon's armamentarium.

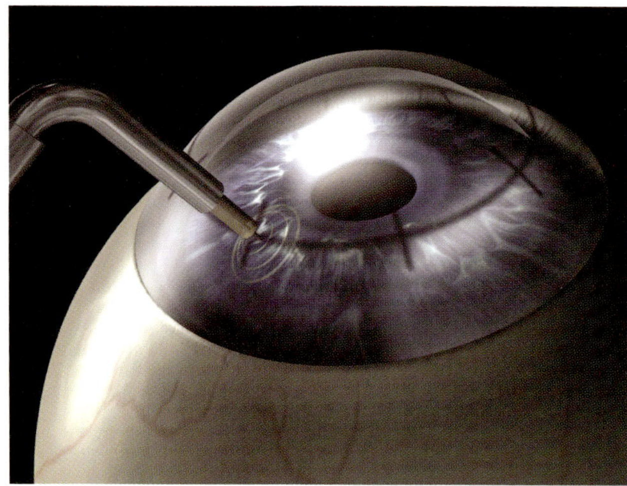

Figure 7-1 Conductive keratoplasty delivers radiofrequency energy to the cornea through a handheld probe that is inserted into the peripheral cornea. *(Courtesy of Refractec, Inc.)*

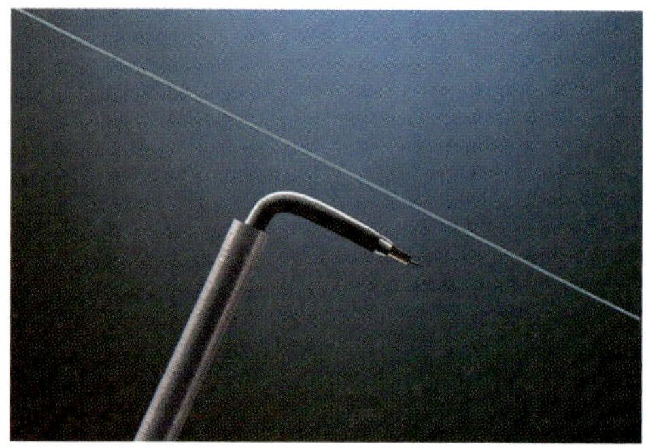

Figure 7-2 The CK probe (displayed next to a 10-0 nylon suture for comparison) consists of a thin conductive wire, 450 μm long and 90 μm wide. *(Courtesy of Refractec, Inc.)*

Patient Selection and Results

The Refractec system is approved for the temporary reduction of spherical hyperopia in patients 40 years or older with a spherical equivalent of +0.75 to +3.0 D and ≤0.75 D of astigmatism. The clinical trial consisted of 12-month data in 401 eyes with a mean cohort age of 55.3 years (range, 40.2 to 73.9 years). The mean cycloplegic spherical equivalent was +1.86 ± 0.63 D. By 12 months postoperatively, 92% of study patients had achieved uncorrected visual acuity of 20/40 or better, 57% were 20/25 or better, and 56% were 20/20 or better. There was a slow continued drift toward increasing hyperopia (0.02 D/month). This "loss of effect" is probably a combination of true regression and the normal hyperopic drift that is seen as patients age. Early reports of the ≥24-month data suggest that long-term stability is better than LTK and comparable to hyperopic LASIK.

McDonald MB, Hersh PS, Manche EE, et al. Conductive keratoplasty for the correction of low to moderate hyperopia: U.S. clinical trial 1-year results on 355 eyes. *Ophthalmology.* 2002;109:1978–1989.

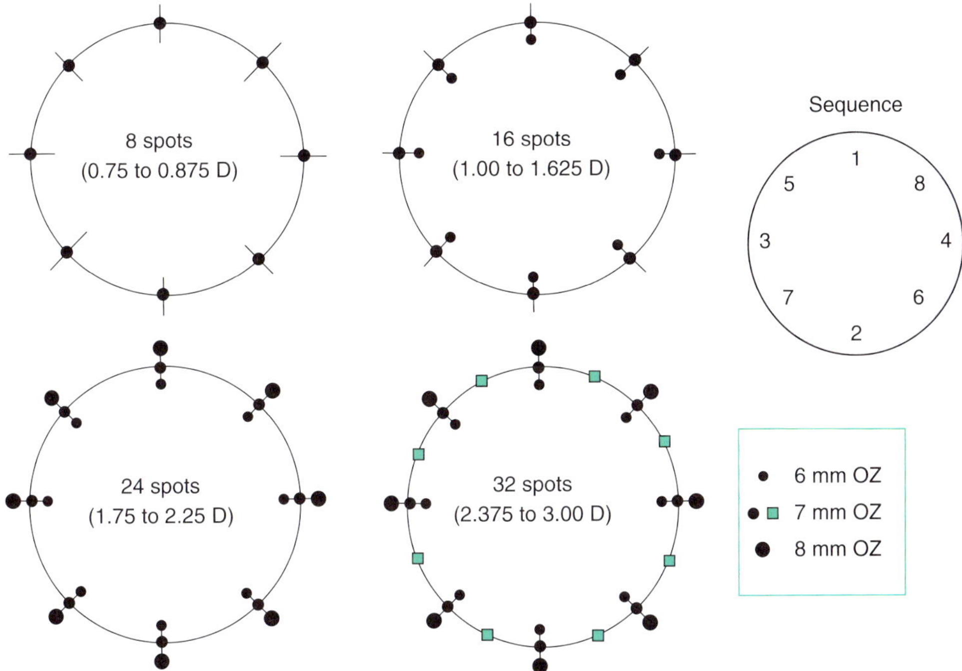

Figure 7-3 In CK, radiofrequency energy is delivered in a series of spots to the corneal periphery. More circles of spots are used for higher hyperopic corrections. When 32 spots are applied, the last 8 spots are placed in the intermediate areas (between existing spots) of the 7.0 mm ring. *(Courtesy of Refractec, Inc.)*

Table 7-1 Application Nomogram for Conductive Keratoplasty

Spherical Equivalent	Number of Spots	Treatment Diameter
0.75 to 0.875 D	8	7.0 mm
1.00 to 1.625 D	16	6.0 mm; 7.0 mm
1.75 to 2.25 D	24	6.0 mm; 7.0 mm; 8.0 mm
2.375 to 3.00 D	32	6.0 mm; 7.0 mm; 8.0 mm; intermediate 7.0 mm

CK is contraindicated in patients with RK, keratoconus, or ectatic disorders and with significant irregular astigmatism. The upper limit of +3.0 D appears to be the current treatment ceiling for this technology and multiple applications over time or more spots do not seem to enhance or increase that limit. Patients with a decentered apex (a significant difference between the corneal geometric apex and the corneal sighting point) may have less-optimal results with all hyperopic procedures.

Safety

While the efficacy results for CK appear to be similar to LASIK and LTK, the safety variables were superior. In the principal FDA clinical trial, no patient was worse than 20/40 and no patient lost more than 2 lines of vision. One patient out of 391 had >2.0 D

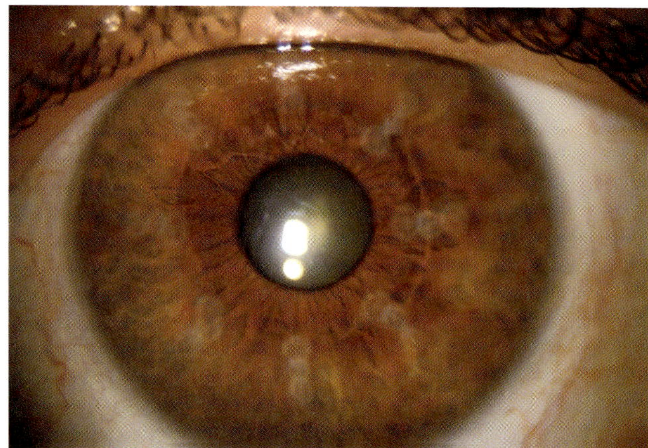

Figure 7-4 A month after a 24-spot CK treatment in a +2.0 D hyperope, the spots are beginning to fade. Three sets of 8 spots were applied at a 6.0 mm, 7.0 mm, and 8.0 mm optical zone. *(Courtesy of Refractec, Inc.)*

of induced cylinder, and no patient with a preoperative best-corrected visual acuity of ≥20/20 had <20/25 at 1 year. While induced cylinder of >2.0 D is an FDA safety variable, smaller amounts of induced cylinder were apparent. At 1 year, 6% of patients had >1.0 D of induced cylinder. The magnitude of the induced cylinder appears to diminish with time.

The advantage of CK over LASIK and PRK is that CK does not require making a flap, removing corneal tissue, or treating the central visual axis. CK may be advantageous in very flat corneas, since large flap creation can be problematic, and in patients with dry eyes, because CK does not cause any significant corneal denervation. The greatest drawback of this surgery is its narrow treatment range.

Other Applications

Conductive keratoplasty can be used to induce mild myopia of −1.00 to −2.00 D in emmetropic patients to relieve presbyopic symptoms. A number of potential off-label uses also exist for CK, but the nomograms are in evolution. CK is being investigated for the following purposes:

- Overcorrected myopic LASIK and myopic PRK, especially when the original flap is inadequate for a hyperopic correction. CK obviates the need to cut another flap.
- Postcataract or postkeratoplasty astigmatism. Because each spot is individually placed, CK can be used to steepen the flat axis. The overall effect is still a myopic shift, so CK is particularly useful when the spherical equivalent is hyperopic.

Additional time, data, and further studies will be required to determine the ultimate place of CK in the refractive practice.

Kolahdouz-Isfahani AH, McDonnell PJ. Thermal keratoplasty. In: Brightbill FS, ed. *Corneal Surgery: Theory, Technique, and Tissue.* St. Louis: CV Mosby; 1999.

CHAPTER 8

Intraocular Surgery

In its first two decades, refractive surgery was synonymous with corneal surgery, which compensates for refractive error by altering the contour of the anterior surface of the eye. Several factors expanded the range of refractive surgery to include intraocular surgery. Ophthalmologists became accustomed to cataract patients not only expecting to see clearly after their operation, but also becoming less dependent on glasses as a consequence of IOL surgery. Technology has helped to achieve this goal. Small-incision cataract surgery with self-sealing, astigmatism-neutral wounds has all but eliminated the high postoperative astigmatism that was previously common. New formulas and software have made IOL power selection more accurate. Foldable IOLs, multifocal IOLs, toric IOLs, and accommodating IOLs are now a reality. These technological advances have led to a renewed interest in clear lens surgery, particularly for correction of hyperopia in the presbyopic patient.

Phakic IOLs (PIOLs) represent a new category of IOL that expands the range of keratorefractive surgery, offering surgeons and their patients new options for vision correction. The combination of corneal and intraocular refractive surgery, so-called *bioptics*, may ultimately allow patients at the extremes of refractive error to achieve predictable outcomes by combining the advantages of the PIOL in treating large corrections with the adjustability of a keratorefractive technique. In addition, the optical quality may be improved by dividing the refractive correction between two different locations.

This chapter discusses the intraocular surgical techniques that are now or expected to be soon within the armamentarium of the refractive surgeon.

Phakic IOL (PIOL)

Background

The history of the PIOL to correct refractive error began in Europe in the 1950s with Strampelli, Dannheim, and Barraquer each separately attempting to design a PIOL that would be well tolerated in the eye. The lack of modern IOL-manufacturing capability, microsurgical techniques, and knowledge about the fragility of anterior segment structures resulted in a high incidence of corneal edema, iritis, cataract, and glaucoma. Ultimately, many of these IOLs were removed and, by the late 1960s, interest in PIOL implantation had waned.

In the middle 1980s there was renewed interest in PIOLs. Improvements in IOL manufacture, development of modern microsurgical technique, viscoelastic and topical corticosteroid availability, and improved knowledge of the corneal endothelium and anterior segment structures led to greater success. Worst modified his aphakic, iris-fixated "claw" IOL to correct both myopia and hyperopia. Baikoff worked on variations of the open-loop, flexible anterior chamber IOL to correct myopia, while Fyodorov experimented with a plate-haptic IOL for use in the posterior chamber.

Different PIOL designs were associated with different types of complications. Early versions of the Baikoff anterior chamber PIOLs were associated with significant endothelial cell loss. The PIOL placed in the ciliary sulcus over a clear lens was associated with pupillary block and cataract. Refinements in IOL design have reduced the incidence of complications, which has resulted in increasing the popularity of these PIOLs outside the United States. Within the United States, only 1 PIOL is currently FDA approved for myopia. Representative lenses in each category (Table 8-1) will be discussed.

Advantages

PIOLs have the advantage of treating a much larger range of myopic and hyperopic refractive errors than can be achieved with keratorefractive surgery. The skills required for insertion are, with a few exceptions, similar to those used in cataract surgery. The equipment is significantly less expensive than an excimer laser, and most or all of it is already used for cataract surgery.

The PIOL is removable; therefore the refractive effect should theoretically be reversible. However, any intervening pathology caused by the PIOL would most likely be irreversible.

Disadvantages

PIOL insertion is an intraocular procedure with all the potential risks associated with intraocular surgery. Each PIOL style has its own set of associated risks. In the case of PIOLs with polymethylmethacrylate (PMMA) optics, insertion requires a larger wound that may result in unintended postoperative astigmatism. There is less flexibility than with LASIK for fine-tuning the refractive outcome. If a patient eventually develops a visually significant cataract, the PIOL will have to be explanted at the time of cataract surgery, possibly through a larger-than-usual wound.

Patient Selection

Indications

Patients who are near or beyond the FDA-approved limits for laser correction may be candidates for a PIOL. Although the programmable upper limit of myopic excimer laser treatment is as high as −14.0 D, some surgeons have further reduced the upper limit of LASIK and PRK in their refractive practice because of reduced predictability, high rate of regression, increased incidence of microstriae, and night-vision problems that can occur with treatment of the high myope. Similarly, LASIK and PRK for hyperopia above +4.0 D and astigmatism correction above 4.0 D of cylinder are less accurate than at lower corrections. If PIOLs are approved by the FDA and surgeons become familiar with their

Table 8-1 Phakic IOLs

Position	Model	Available Power	Optic Size	Length	Material	Manufacturer
Angle-supported	NuVita MA20	7–20 D myopia	5.0 mm (4.5 mm effective diameter)	12.0, 12.5, 13.0, 13.5 mm	PMMA	Bausch & Lomb
	Vivarte	7–20 D myopia	5.5 mm	12.0, 12.5, 13.0 mm	Acrylic	CIBA Vision
	93A or ZSAL-4	6–22 D myopia	5.5 mm (5.0 mm effective diameter)	13.0 mm	PMMA	Morcher
	MCR 200 "phakic 6"	2–25 D myopia	6.0 mm	12.0, 12.5, 13.0, 13.5, 14.0 mm	PMMA	M&C
	MCR 200 "phakic 6"	2–10 D hyperopia	6.0 mm	12.0, 12.5, 13.0, 13.5, 14.0 mm	PMMA	M&C
Iris-supported*	Artisan model 204	3–15.5 D myopia	5.0 or 6.0 mm	8.5 mm	PMMA	Ophtec
	Artisan model 206	3–23.5 D myopia	5.0 or 6.0 mm	8.5 mm	PMMA	Ophtec
	Artisan model 203	3–12 D hyperopia	5.0 or 6.0 mm	8.5 mm	PMMA	Ophtec
	Artisan toric IOL	Custom combinations up to +7.0 D	5.0 or 6.0 mm	8.5 mm	PMMA	Ophtec
Sulcus-supported	ICL (for myopia)	3–23 D myopia	4.65–5.5 mm	11.0, 11.5, 12.0, 12.5, 13.0, 13.5 mm	Collamer	STAAR
	ICL (for hyperopia)	3–20 D hyperopia	5.5 mm	11.0, 11.5, 12.0, 12.5, 13.0 mm	Collamer	STAAR
	ICL (toric for myopia)		4.65–5.5 mm	11.0, 11.5, 12.0, 12.5, 13.0, 13.5 mm	Collamer	STAAR
	PRL	3–20 D myopia	4.75–5.5 mm	10.8 and 11.3 mm	Silicone	CIBA Vision
	PRL	4–15 D hyperopia	4.5 mm	10.6 mm	Silicone	CIBA Vision

* The Artisan lens (Ophtec), marketed as the Verisyse lens (AMO), has been FDA approved for use in the lens power range of −5.0 to −20.0 D.

use, it is possible that surgeons may choose to implant the PIOLs for refractive powers significantly lower than the programmable excimer laser limits.

Most myopic PIOLs can correct up to −20.0 D (see Table 8-1). The 6 mm optic Artisan iris-fixation PIOL (manufactured by Ophtec; to be distributed as the Verisyse PIOL by AMD) can correct up to −23.5 D. All three categories of PIOL are available for correction of hyperopia of at least +10.0 D. Ophtec and CIBA Vision are conducting clinical trials of toric PIOLs.

PIOLs can be an attractive alternative if PRK or LASIK is contraindicated. LASIK surgery is contraindicated if the resultant residual corneal stromal bed thickness would be <250 μm, because this could increase the risk of developing corneal ectasia. Because extremes of corneal curvature lead to induced aberrations and degradation of optical quality, a final corneal curvature flatter than 34.0 D in myopic corrections or steeper than 50.0 D in hyperopic corrections is also undesirable. More sophisticated measurement and treatment planning based on wavefront analysis may refine these limits.

Contraindications

PIOLs have specific contraindications. They should not be used if there is preexisting intraocular disease such as compromise of the corneal endothelium, iritis, significant iris abnormality, rubeosis iridis, cataract, or glaucoma.

When compared with clear lens extraction (discussed later in this chapter), the PIOL has the advantage of preserving natural accommodation and may have a lower risk of postoperative retinal detachment because of the preservation of the crystalline lens and the lack of vitreous destabilization. The anterior chamber diameter, anterior chamber depth, and pupil size must be appropriate for the specific PIOL being considered. (The anatomical requirements for the placement of each style of IOL are discussed in the next section.)

Patient evaluation

A thorough preoperative evaluation is necessary, as detailed in Chapter 3. One area that has not been well investigated is the import of IOL optic size relative to scotopic pupil size. Pupil size larger than optic size may be associated with edge glare.

Informed consent

As with any refractive procedure, an informed consent written specifically for this procedure should be obtained at least one day prior to surgery. The patient should be informed about both the potential short-term and long-term risks of the procedure and about any available alternatives. With some of the newer technologies, long-term risks and results may not yet be known. The surgeon must make sure the patient has realistic expectations about the surgical outcome of the procedure.

Ancillary tests

Specular microscopy and corneal pachymetry are both helpful for evaluating the health of the corneal endothelium. In addition, anterior chamber depth should be carefully assessed because adequate depth is critical for the safe implantation of a PIOL. If the anterior chamber depth is <3.0 mm, the risk of endothelial and iris/angle trauma from the placement of an anterior chamber, iris-fixated, or posterior chamber PIOL is increased. Anterior chamber depth can be estimated at the slit lamp by using the measured central corneal thickness as a reference. Anterior chamber depth can also be measured by ultrasound and checked with the Orbscan (Orbtek), if available. The phakic eye has a shallower anterior chamber than the aphakic eye.

Methods for IOL power selection are specific to each PIOL and manufacturer. Some manufacturers provide software for IOL power calculation. As with any IOL implant, novice surgeons should follow the guidelines prescribed by manufacturers and experienced trusted surgeons and then modify the formulas as they gain their own experience.

Surgical Technique

Topical anesthesia with intracameral supplement is suitable if the patient can cooperate and the PIOL can be inserted through a small incision. If the patient cannot cooperate for topical anesthesia or if a large incision is required, peribulbar anesthesia is preferable. Retrobulbar anesthesia should be used with caution in patients with a high axial length because of the increased risk of perforation. Pupil dilation may occur after anesthetic injection. This may be undesirable in the case of anterior chamber PIOL and iris-fixated PIOL insertion. Topical pilocarpine 1% or 2% administered preoperatively can block this dilation effect but may decenter the pupil.

A peripheral iridotomy is recommended for each of the PIOL categories in order to reduce the risk of pupillary block and angle closure. A laser iridotomy can be performed 7 to 14 days prior to the PIOL surgery, or the iridotomy can be performed as part of the implant procedure. Preoperative laser iridotomy is preferable when small-incision implant surgery is performed (eg, foldable anterior chamber or posterior chamber PIOLs). Both iridotomy and iridectomy are technically more difficult to perform through a beveled clear corneal incision. Viscoelastic should be meticulously removed at the conclusion of surgery to prevent postoperative elevation of IOP.

Anterior chamber phakic intraocular lens (ACPIOL)

An ACPIOL can be inserted through a temporal clear corneal wound or a superior scleral pocket. The larger the incision, the greater the likelihood of induced astigmatism. The wound size is dependent on the diameter of the ACPIOL optic. The effective optical diameter for some of the ACPIOLs is small, for example, the 4.5 mm NuVita (Bausch & Lomb) and the 5.0 mm 93A (Morcher). This minimizes the wound size required for insertion but increases the potential for edge glare in patients with larger pupils. The Vivarte ACPIOL (CIBA Vision) has an acrylic optic that is 5.5 mm and foldable and that can be inserted through a 3.2 mm clear corneal incision (Fig 8-1).

Sizing the ACPIOL These IOLs are generally available in lengths between 12.0 and 14.0 mm with 0.5 mm intervals. The proper length is usually estimated by measuring the white-to-white diameter with calipers between the 3 and 9 o'clock meridians. Computer topography devices such as Orbscan can provide a white-to-white measurement. High-frequency biomicroscopy may ultimately provide more accurate measurements for AC-PIOL implantation. Apple has examined autopsy eyes and found the white-to-white measurement to be an imprecise approximation of anterior chamber diameter. It is important to remember that the white-to-white measurement in the 12 o'clock meridian

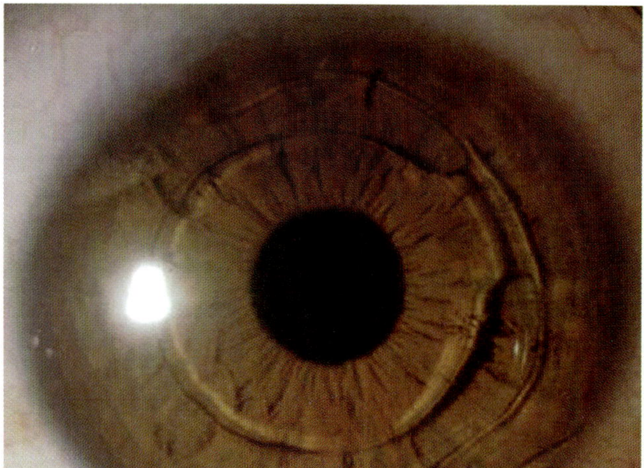

Figure 8-1 Vivarte (CIBA Vision) ACPIOL 3 months after implantation. *(Courtesy of CIBA Vision.)*

is significantly less than the same measurement between 3 and 9 o'clock. Consequently, an ACPIOL length based on the horizontal measurement may be too large for the anterior chamber if the IOL is oriented vertically. Proper sizing is critical to reduce the risk of problems such as pupil ovalization, lens decentration, chronic inflammation, and secondary glaucoma.

Iris-fixated PIOL

This type of PIOL is generally inserted through a superior limbal incision. The long axis of the PIOL is ultimately oriented perpendicular to the axis of the incision. A side port incision is made approximately 2 clock hours on either side of the center of the incision. A 12 o'clock incision will require side port incisions at 10 and 2 o'clock. The "claw" haptics are fixated to the iris by a process called enclavation. After the PIOL has been carefully centered over the pupil, it is stabilized with a forceps while a specially designed enclavation needle is introduced through one of the side port incisions and a knuckle of iris is brought up into the "claw" haptic. This is repeated on the other side. If adjustment of the PIOL position becomes necessary after fixation, the iris must first be released before the PIOL is moved. Careful wound closure will help minimize surgically induced astigmatism.

The Verisyse (Ophtec) is currently FDA approved for myopia of −5.0 to −20.0 D with recommendations for minimal preoperative endothelial cell count dependent on age.

Sizing the iris-fixated PIOL Since this PIOL is fixated to the mid-peripheral iris, not the angle or sulcus, the iris-fixated PIOL has the advantage of being a one-size-fits-all length. It is 8.5 mm in length with a 5.0 or 6.0 mm PMMA optic (Fig 8-2).

Posterior chamber phakic intraocular lens (PCPIOL)

The smaller incision used for foldable PCPIOLs offers the advantage of decreased astigmatism. The available plate-haptic PCPIOLs are made of flexible materials. The Implantable Contact Lens, or ICL (STAAR) (Fig 8-3), is made of a hydrophilic material known

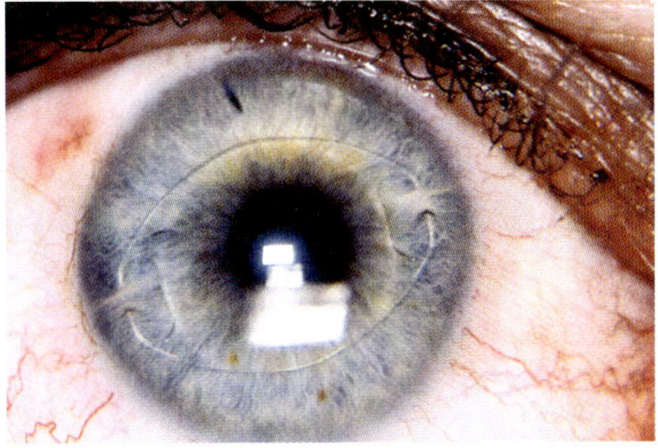

Figure 8-2 Artisan (Ophtec) iris-fixation PIOL for myopic correction. *(Courtesy of Ophtec.)*

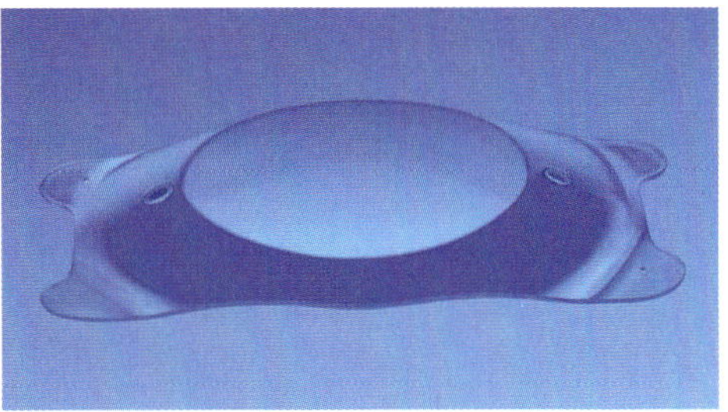

Figure 8-3 Side view of ICL (STAAR) PCPIOL. *(Courtesy of STAAR.)*

as Collamer, which is a copolymer of hema (99%) and porcine collagen (1%). The Phakic Refractive Lens, or PRL (CIBA Vision), has a silicone optic (Fig 8-4). The optic of the PCPIOL is vaulted both to avoid contact between the crystalline lens and the IOL and to allow aqueous to flow over the crystalline lens. This vaulting can be visualized with ultrasound biomicroscopy or Scheimpflug photography (Fig 8-5). The manufacturers suggest that an acceptable amount of vaulting of the PCPIOL optic over the crystalline lens is 1.0 ± 0.5 corneal thicknesses.

To perform the implantation, the pupil is first dilated preoperatively to 8.0 mm with tropicamide 1% and Neo-Synephrine (phenylephrine) 2.5%. A 3.0 to 3.2 mm temporal clear corneal incision is made. A paracentesis is made superiorly and inferiorly to aid in positioning the PCPIOL. The PCPIOL is inserted and, after it unfolds, the haptics are manipulated under the iris (Fig 8-6). The surgeon should avoid contact with the central 6.0 mm of the lens. Positioning instruments should be inserted through the paracenteses and should be kept peripheral to this central area. The surgeon must avoid touching the PCPIOL optic and possibly damaging it. The pupil is then constricted with an intracameral miotic agent such as Miochol (acetylcholine chloride).

Sizing the PCPIOL The white-to-white caliper measurement between the 3 and 9 o'clock meridians is used to select the correct IOL length.

Outcomes

The outcomes and complications of various PIOLs are analyzed in several studies (Tables 8-2 and 8-3). With improved methods for power determination, the outcomes have steadily improved. Significant postoperative gains in lines of best-corrected visual acuity over the preoperative levels likely occur as a result of a reduction in the image minification that is present with spectacle correction of myopia. A loss of best-corrected visual acuity is rare. The loss of contrast sensitivity after LASIK for high myopia does not occur after PIOL surgery. In fact, contrast sensitivity increases in all spatial frequencies when compared with preoperative contrast sensitivity with best spectacle correction.

Alió JL, de la Hoz F, Perez-Santonja JJ, et al. Phakic anterior chamber lenses for the correction of myopia: a 7-year cumulative analysis of complications in 263 cases. *Ophthalmology.* 1999;106:458–466.

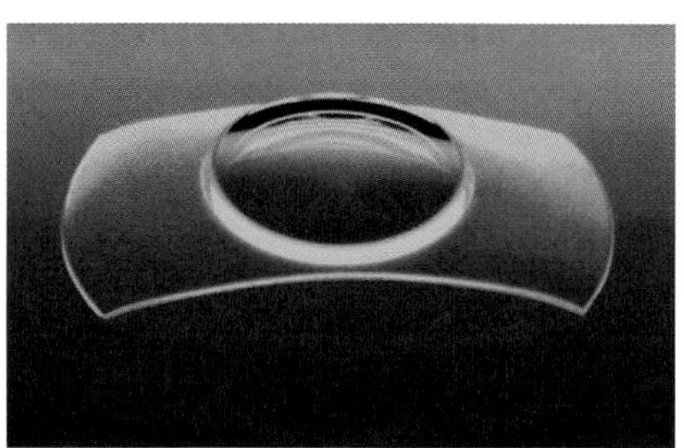

Figure 8-4 PRL (CIBA Vision) PCPIOL for myopic correction. *(Courtesy of CIBA Vision.)*

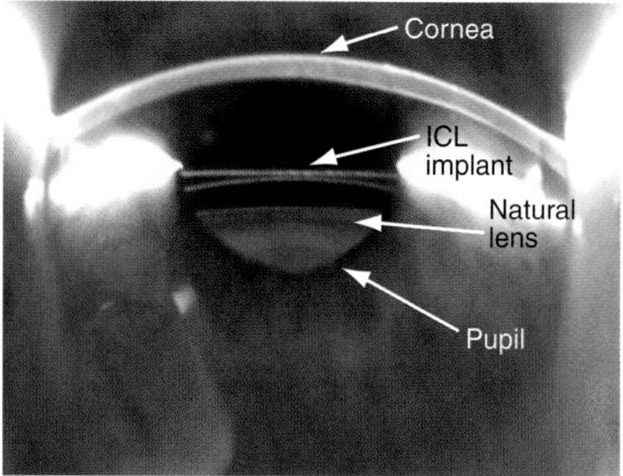

Figure 8-5 ICL (STAAR) PCPIOL within the posterior chamber, as seen with Scheimpflug photography. *(Courtesy of STAAR.)*

Allemann N, Chamon W, Tanaka HM, et al. Myopic angle-supported intraocular lenses: two-year follow-up. *Ophthalmology.* 2000;107:1549–1554.

Arne JL, Al LC. Phakic posterior chamber lenses for high myopia: functional and anatomical outcomes. *J Cataract Refract Surg.* 2000;26:369–374.

Baikoff G, Arne JL, Bokobza Y, et al. Angle-fixated anterior chamber phakic intraocular lens for myopia of −7 to −19 diopters. *J Cataract Refract Surg.* 1998;14:282–293.

Budo C, Hessloehl JC, Izak M, et al. Multicenter study of the Artisan phakic intraocular lens. *J Cataract Refract Surg.* 2000;26:1163–1171.

Davidorf JM, Zaldivar R, Oscherow S. Posterior chamber phakic intraocular lens for hyperopia of +4 to +11 diopters. *J Refract Surg.* 1998;14:306–311.

Jimenez-Alfaro I, Gomez-Telleria G, Bueno JL, et al. Contrast sensitivity after posterior chamber phakic intraocular lens implantation for high myopia. *J Refract Surg.* 2001;17:641–645.

Manche EE. The Artisan anterior chamber lens. In: Durrie DS, O'Brien TP, eds. *Refractive Surgery: Back to the Future.* San Francisco: American Academy of Ophthalmology; 2002.

Menezo JL, Cisneros AL, Rodriguez-Salvador V. Endothelial study of iris-claw phakic lens: 4-year follow-up. *J Cataract Refract Surg.* 1998;24:1039–1049.

Pérez-Santonja JJ, Alió JL, Jimenez-Alfaro I, et al. Surgical correction of severe myopia with an angle-supported phakic intraocular lens. *J Cataract Refract Surg.* 2000;26:1288–1302.

Vukich JA, Ticlittom ISG: U.S. Food and Drug Administration clinical trial of the implantable contact lens for moderate to high myopia. *Ophthalmology.* 2003;110:255–266.

Zaldivar R, Davidorf JM, Oscherow S. Posterior chamber phakic intraocular lens for myopia of −8 to −19 diopters. *J Refract Surg.* 1998;14:294.

Complications

Each manufacturer continues to modify the design of its PIOLs to improve results and to minimize complications. Older studies do not necessarily reflect the complication rate associated with more recently developed PIOLs. When experienced surgeons implant these PIOLs, the incidence of sight-threatening complications is quite low. However, since the PIOLs are used in young, active individuals, longer follow-up is needed to accurately determine their safety. Many of the most important potential complications of PIOLs, such as cataract, endothelial cell loss, and retinal detachment, may not manifest for many

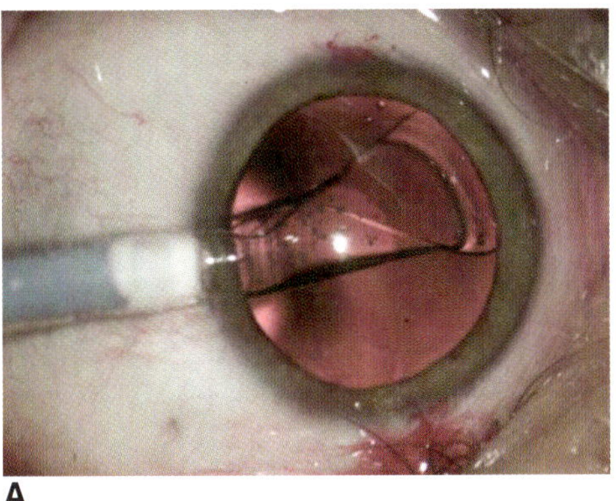

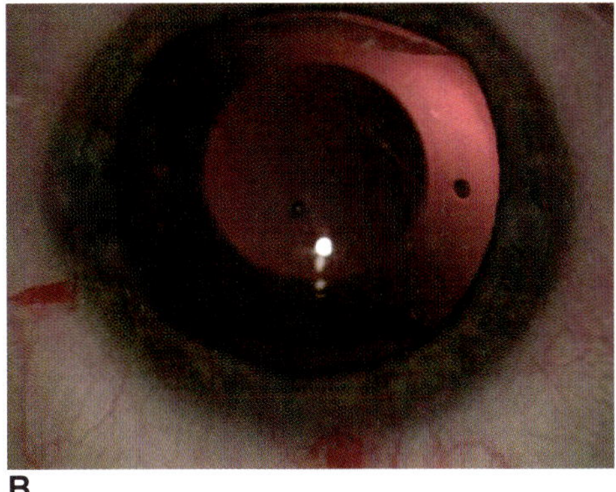

Figure 8-6 **A,** ICL (STAAR) PCPIOL unfolds in the anterior chamber after placement with the IOL inserter. **B,** ICL PCPIOL unfolded and in position in the posterior chamber anterior to the crystalline lens. *(Courtesy of STAAR.)*

years. A much longer follow-up will be needed to determine the true rate of these complications. Consequently, both the patient and the surgeon need to recognize our current inability to accurately assess the incidence of PIOL complications.

ACPIOL

The most frequent complications reported are nighttime glare and haloes, pupil ovalization, and endothelial cell loss (see Table 8-3). Ovalization of the pupil is more likely if ACPIOL is too large, while movement of an ACPIOL that is too small can cause endothelial damage and decentration. The risk of pupillary block is low because iridotomies have become part of the surgical protocol. Because complications such as endothelial cell loss and pupil ovalization may take years to develop, the true frequency of these complications can only be assessed after a follow-up of many years. A stated rate of endothelial cell loss at a particular postoperative interval is the equivalent of a snapshot view. Whether cell loss continues or the endothelium stabilizes can only be determined with long-term follow-up, and any reported complication rate should be critically evaluated with these considerations in mind (see Table 8-3). Further, direct comparison of studies of varying size using different IOL models within a given PIOL category may have limited value.

The most commonly reported symptoms following ACPIOL insertion, glare and haloes, occur in 18.8% to 20% of patients, but these symptoms appear to decrease by as much as 50% over a postoperative period of 7 years. The incidence is significantly reduced with a larger ACPIOL optic. Endothelial cell loss years after ACPIOL insertion ranges from 4.2% to 8.4%. Pupil ovalization can occur because of iris tuck during ACPIOL insertion or it can occur over time due to chronic inflammation and fibrosis around the haptics within the anterior chamber angle. The incidence of pupil ovalization ranges from 5.9% to 27.5% and is directly related to the postoperative interval studied.

ACPIOL rotation was frequently observed in one study, but not in others. Acute postoperative iritis occurred in 4.6%, and retinal detachment occurred in 3% of cases.

Table 8-2 Results of Phakic IOLs

Study	PIOL Model	Number of Eyes	Mean Preoperative Spherical Equivalent (Range)	Postoperative Result Within ±0.50 D of Emmetropia	Postoperative Result Within ±1.00 D of Emmetropia	Uncorrected Visual Acuity 20/40 or Better	Gain ≥2 Lines Best-Corrected Visual Acuity	Loss ≥2 Lines Best-Corrected Visual Acuity
ACPIOL								
Baikoff (1998)	ZB5M	134	−12.50 D (−7.00 to −18.80 D)	32%	58.8%	57%	50.7%	8.3%
Perez-Santonja (2000)	ZSAL-4	23	−19.56 D (−16.75 to −23.25 D)	56.5%	82.6%	56%	Mean increase 2 lines	0%
Allemann (2000)	NuVita	21	−18.95 D		Mean spherical equivalent −1.93 D		65%	0%
Iris-fixated IOL								
Menezo (1998)	Iris claw lens	111	−14.81 D (−8.00 to −20.00 D)		82.9%	36.3%	77%	
Budo (2000)	Artisan	249	−12.95 D (−5.00 to −20.00 D)	57.1%	78.8%	76.8%	42.6%	1.2%
FDA clinical trial Manche (2002) Interim report (6 mo.)	Artisan	498	−12.79 D (−6.5 to −19.5 D)	63%	89%	87%	20%	0%
PCPIOL								
Zaldivar (1998)	ICL	124	−13.38 D (−8.50 to −18.65 D)	44%	69%	68%	36%	0.8%
Arne (2000)	ICL	58	−13.85 D (−8.00 to −19.25 D)	Mean spherical equivalent −1.22 D	56.9%	Mean postoperative acuity 20/50	77.6% gained ≥1 line	3.4%
Vukich (2003)	ICL	258	−10.05 D (−3.00 to −20.00 D)	57.4% at 2 years	80.2% at 2 years	92.5% at 1 year	10.9%	1.2%
Davidorf (1998)	ICL (for hyperopia)	24	+6.51 D (+3.75 to +10.50 D)	58%	79%	63%	8%	4%

Table 8-3 Incidence of Complications with Phakic IOLs

Study	PIOL Model	Number of Eyes	Glare/Haloes	Pupil Ovalization	Mean Endothelial Cell Loss	Cataract	Pigment Dispersion	IOP Elevation
ACPIOL								
Alio (1999)	ZB5M/MF/ZSAL-4	263	20% at 1 year 10% at 7 years	5.9%	8.4% at 7 years			
Baikoff (1998)	ZB5M	134 35	18.8% at 1 year 12.5% at 3 years	9.9% at 1 year 27.5% at 3 years	4.6% at 3 years			
Perez-Santonja (2000)	ZSAL-4	23	26.1% at 2 years	17.4% at 2 years	4.2% at 2 years	3%	18.7%	15.6%
Iris-fixated IOL								
Menezo (1998)	Iris claw lens	111	1.8%		13.4% at 4 years		12.8%	5.3%
Manche (2002)	Artisan	228	3.5% with 5.0 mm optic 4.1% with 6.0 mm optic	2.6% at 2 years				
Budo (2000)	Artisan	518	13.7% at 3 years	2.4% at 1 year; 0.7% at 3 years	2.4%			
PCPIOL								
Vukich (2003)	ICL	257			No corneal edema from 1–24 months	6.7% anterior subcapsular cataract at 2 years		
Arne (2000)	ICL	58	54.3%		<3.9% at 1 year	3.4% anterior subcapsular cataract	15.5%	3.4%
Zaldivar (1998)	ICL	124	2.4%			2.4%		11.3%

Iris-fixated PIOL

Menezo evaluated 111 cases over a 4-year period during the 1990s. Of the patients studied, 84% had no complications. Glare occurred in 1.8%. PIOL decentration was present in 13.5%; however, in 14/15 eyes this was minimal and caused no visual impairment. Intraoperative hyphema and iris trauma each occurred in 4.5%. Iritis and elevated IOP occurred in 3.6% and 4.5%, respectively. The mean endothelial cell loss at 4 years was 13.4%; however, by 2 years the variation in cell size and the percentage of hexagonal figures had nearly returned to preoperative levels. The largest amount of change in cell density was seen by 6 months.

Manche reported interim results of the FDA clinical trials of 421 patients who had the Artisan iris-fixation PIOL (Ophtec) implanted for myopia, with 228 patients followed for 2 years. Glare and haloes were present in 3.5% of patients with the 5.0 mm optic and 4.1% with the 6.0 mm optic. Two PIOLs were exchanged for the larger-optic PIOL because of glare, and 2 PIOLs were removed because the pupil was larger than the optic. Only 2 PIOLs required repositioning. Mean endothelial cell loss in the 2-year cohort was 2.6%, significantly less than that reported by Menezo. No hyphema or iris trauma was reported. Pupillary block was rare in the presence of a patent iridotomy.

Manche EE. The Artisan anterior chamber lens. In: Durrie DS, O'Brien TP, eds. *Refractive Surgery: Back to the Future.* San Francisco: American Academy of Ophthalmology; 2002.

Menezo JL, Cisneros AL, Rodriguez-Salvador V. Endothelial study of iris-claw phakic lens: 4-year follow-up. *J Cataract Refract Surg.* 1998;24:1039–1049.

PCPIOL

In addition to creating a potential for the endothelial damage and nighttime glare and haloes seen in other types of PIOLs, the placement of a PCPIOL may increase the risk of cataract formation and pigmentary dispersion. If the PCPIOL is undersized, the vaulting will decrease, but the risk of cataract may increase; if the PCPIOL is too large, iris chafing with pigmentary dispersion could result. The concern over cataract formation was confirmed by a series published in 1999, where cataract formation was reported in 53% of eyes (9/17) at 3 months to 2 years after insertion of a silicone PCPIOL of a Fyodorov design. The majority of these cataracts were anterior subcapsular. It is not currently known if the mechanism of cataract formation is mechanical or metabolic. If a visually significant cataract develops, it is possible to remove the PCPIOL, perform cataract surgery, and implant a standard posterior chamber IOL.

Brauweiler PH, Wehler T, Busin M. High incidence of cataract formation after implantation of a silicone posterior chamber lens in phakic, highly myopic eyes. *Ophthalmology.* 1999;106:1651–1655.

The ICL (STAAR) is currently undergoing clinical trials in the United States. It is already in use in many other countries. In Zaldivar's report of 124 eyes implanted with the ICL, mean follow-up was 11 months. Glare was present in only 2.4% of eyes (3/124). In 2 years of follow-up on 58 eyes, Arne reported a 54.3% incidence of haloes and night-driving disturbance, which was less frequent when a larger optic was used. Lens opacities occurred in 2.4% (3/124) to 3.4% (2/58). The most frequent complication was PCPIOL decentration, with <1 mm in 14.5% of eyes (18/124) and visually significant decentration of >1 mm in 1.6% of eyes (2/124). In one case, recentration was performed, and in the other the PCPIOL was removed (Fig 8-7). A case of inverted PCPIOL occurred. This has been reported with the PRL silicone lens (CIBA Vision) as well. No eye had an endothelial cell loss of >3.8% at 1 year.

Arne JL, Al LC. Phakic posterior chamber lenses for high myopia: functional and anatomical outcomes. *J Cataract Refract Surg.* 2000;26:369–374.

Zaldivar R, Davidorf JM, Oscherow S. Posterior chamber phakic intraocular lens for myopia of −8 to −19 diopters. *J Refract Surg.* 1998;14:294.

Lens fluorophotometry showed a steady reduction in crystalline lens transmittance over a 2-year period with a decrease of 2.24% at the second postoperative year. Aqueous flare increased to nearly 50% in the first month after surgery and was still 27% above normal 2 years following surgery.

Jimenez-Alfaro I, Benitez del Castillo JM, Garcia-Feijoo J, et al. Safety of posterior chamber phakic intraocular lenses for the correction of high myopia: anterior segment changes after posterior chamber phakic intraocular lens implantation. *Ophthalmology.* 2001;108:90–99.

Newer models of PCPIOLs such as the V4 ICL (STAAR) have been designed with an increased vault to minimize contact with the crystalline lens. Early indications are that this has resulted in a substantially reduced incidence of cataract; this finding requires validation with long-term follow-up.

Bioptics

Bioptics is a term suggested by Zaldivar in the late 1990s to describe the combination of PCPIOL implantation followed at a later time with LASIK to treat patients with extreme myopia. The concept of first inserting a PIOL to reduce the amount of myopia correction required and then refining the residual spherical and astigmatic correction with LASIK has gained appeal, because of the limitations of the individual procedures. LASIK is typically performed approximately 1 month after the PIOL surgery.

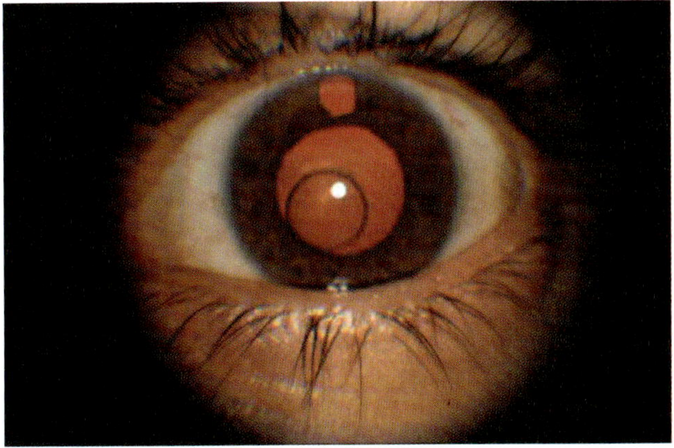

Figure 8-7 Patient with inferiorly decentered PCPIOL. *(Photograph courtesy of Jayne S. Weiss, MD.)*

Another term, adjustable refractive surgery (ARS), is also used to describe combined intraocular and corneal refractive surgery. Güell described ARS, which involves creating a corneal flap just prior to inserting an iris-fixated PIOL and then at a later time lifting the flap and performing the laser procedure. This two-stage modification is necessary to avoid the potential for endothelial trauma caused by the iris-fixated PIOL that could occur during the microkeratome pass. The bioptics concept has been used to correct high hyperopia as well. As new treatment options are developed, the possibilities for other combinations of refractive surgery will likely increase.

The ability to successfully combine refractive procedures further expands the limits of refractive surgery. The predictability, stability, and safety of LASIK may increase by treating a smaller refractive error with the corneal surgery. In addition, there is usually sufficient corneal tissue to maximize the treatment zone diameter without exceeding the limits of ablation depth. The LASIK procedure provides the feature of adjustability to the overall refractive operation. These benefits must be balanced with the combined risks of performing two surgeries rather than one.

Outcomes

In the initial reports of bioptics and ARS, the range of treatment for myopia was −18.75 to −35.00 D and −16.00 to −23.00 D, respectively (Table 8-4). If the long-term results of PIOLs prove acceptable, the use of bioptics may expand to the treatment of smaller refractive errors because of the advantages of superior optical performance and greater accuracy of refractive correction.

Güell JL, Vázquez M, Gris O, et al. Combined surgery to correct high myopia: iris claw phakic intraocular lens and laser in situ keratomileusis. *J Refract Surg.* 1999;15:529.

Güell JL, Vázquez M, Gris O. Adjustable refractive surgery: 6-mm Artisan lens plus laser in situ keratomileusis for the correction of high myopia. *Ophthalmology.* 2001;108:945–952.

Zaldivar R, Davidorf JM, Oscherow S, et al. Combined posterior chamber phakic intraocular lens and laser in situ keratomileusis: bioptics for extreme myopia. *J Refract Surg.* 1999;15:299–308.

Clear Lens Extraction (Refractive Lens Exchange)

Patient Selection

Indications

The indications for refractive lensectomy with IOL implantation are controversial. Refractive lensectomy with IOL implantation is usually considered only if alternative refractive procedures are not feasible and there is a strong reason why spectacles or contact lenses are unacceptable alternatives. If the cornea is too thin, too flat, or too steep, or the refractive error exceeds the limit of excimer laser treatment, clear lens extraction or PIOL implantation are options. Refractive lens exchange may be preferable to a PIOL in the presence of a lens opacity that is presently visually insignificant but that may eventually progress and cause visual loss.

Table 8-4 Results of Bioptics and Adjustable Refractive Surgery

Study	Number of Eyes	Mean Preoperative Spherical Equivalent (Range)	Postoperative Result Within ±0.50 D of Emmetropia	Postoperative Result Within ±1.00 D of Emmetropia	Uncorrected Visual Acuity 20/40 or Better	Gain ≥2 Lines Best-Corrected Visual Acuity	Loss ≥2 Lines Best-Corrected Visual Acuity
Zaldivar (1999) Bioptics	67	−23.00 D (−18.75 to −35.00 D)	67%	85%	69%	76%	0%
Güell (2001) Adjustable refractive surgery	26	−18.42 D (−16.00 to −23.00 D)	80.7%	100%	77%	42%	0%
Chayet (2001) ICL/LASIK or PRK	37	−17.74 D (−9.75 to −28.00 D)	83.7%	97.2%	89.1%	64.8%	3%

Informed consent

Potential candidates must be capable of understanding the short-term and long-term risks of this intraocular procedure. They must understand that performing the surgery on both eyes sequentially rather than simultaneously is recommended to decrease the potential of a devastating complication such as bilateral endophthalmitis. Younger patients must understand that unless they are left myopic or a multifocal or accommodating IOL is implanted, they will eventually incur the loss of near vision. A consent form developed specifically for this surgery should be given to the patient a minimum of one day prior to surgery to allow ample time for review and signature.

Myopia

In addition to all the risks associated with cataract surgery, the surgeon must specifically inform the patient about the substantial risk of retinal detachment associated with removal of the crystalline lens. Myopia is already a significant risk factor for retinal detachment in the absence of lens surgery, and this risk increases with the degree of nearsightedness. The risk in eyes with up to 3.0 D of myopia may be as much as 4 times as great as in emmetropic eyes. In eyes with greater than 3.0 D of myopia the risk of retinal detachment may be as high as 10 times the risk in emmetropia. In the absence of trauma, more than 50% of retinal detachments occur in myopic eyes.

Preferred Practice Patterns Committee. *Management of Posterior Vitreous Detachment, Retinal Breaks, and Lattice Degeneration.* San Francisco: American Academy of Ophthalmology; 1998.

Wilkinson CP. Retinal implications of refractive lensectomy and phakic IOLs. *Subspecialty Day Program 2001.* San Francisco: American Academy of Ophthalmology; 2001.

Hyperopia

As patients approach presbyopic age, moderate and high hyperopia become increasingly bothersome. The perceived accelerated onset of presbyopia occurs because some accommodation is expended in an effort to clarify distance vision. Many hyperopic patients have significant chronic accommodative spasm.

If the amount of hyperopia is beyond the range of alternative refractive procedures, clear lens extraction with IOL insertion might be the only available surgical option. As is the case with myopia, the patient must be informed about the risks of intraocular surgery. A patient with a crowded anterior segment from a thickened crystalline lens would not be a candidate for a PIOL and could benefit from a reduced risk of angle-closure glaucoma following clear lens extraction. The hyperopic patient has a lower risk of retinal detachment than the myopic patient.

Surgical Planning and Technique

While refractive lensectomy has similarities to cataract surgery, there are some special considerations for planning and performing the procedure. It is important to determine if the source of myopia is a steep cornea or an increased axial length. If the cornea is quite steep, corneal topography should be performed to rule out corneal ectasia. Keratoconus and pellucid marginal degeneration induce irregular astigmatism, which can affect the immediate visual outcome and can have long-term implications. When astigmatism is present in the refraction, keratometry and corneal topography will help the surgeon determine if the astigmatism is lenticular or corneal in origin. Only the corneal component of astigmatism will remain postoperatively. The patient should be informed if substantial astigmatism is expected to be present after surgery. A plan should be devised to correct it in order to optimize the visual outcome. Small amounts of corneal astigmatism (under 1.0 D) may be reduced if the incision is placed in the steep meridian. Superior clear corneal incisions are occasionally associated with large unpredictable astigmatic shifts, possibly because of the reduced distance from the superior limbus to the center of the cornea as compared with the temporal limbus. Some surgeons believe that scleral pocket incisions are preferable when a superior incision site is required.

Limbal relaxing incisions may be used to correct larger amounts of corneal astigmatism (see Chapter 4). Toric IOLs are another option. Supplemental PRK or LASIK could be considered (see the preceding discussion of bioptics). While glasses or contact lenses are an alternative for managing residual astigmatism, refractive surgery patients often reject this option.

If the patient is a high axial myope, retrobulbar injections should be avoided due to the risk of perforating the globe. Peribulbar, sub-Tenon's, topical, and intracameral anesthesia are options. In determining the preferred route of anesthetic administration, the surgeon should keep in mind that younger patients are often more anxious than older cataract patients.

In high axial myopia, an excessively deep anterior chamber may develop during surgery. A deep anterior chamber impairs surgical visualization and instrument manipulation. The patient may complain of pain, particularly when the eye is anesthetized with topical and intracameral anesthetic only. An excessively deep chamber can be minimized by avoiding a viscoelastic overfill and by lowering the irrigation bottle at the start of the operation.

In hyperopia, a small cornea may be more prone to surgical trauma, the lens may be located more anteriorly, and the crowded anterior chamber may make surgical maneuvers more difficult. In a highly hyperopic eye with an axial length of less than 18 mm, the diagnosis of nanophthalmos should be considered. These eyes are prone to uveal effusion syndrome and postoperative choroidal detachment (see BCSC Section 11, *Lens and Cataract*, Special Considerations in Cataract Surgery).

Careful and complete hydrodissection is essential to facilitate lens mobilization. In younger patients, the nucleus is too soft to turn easily with a nucleus rotator if cortical adhesions persist. The soft nucleus is likely to partially prolapse out of the capsular bag during hydrodissection and can be repositioned with viscoelastic.

The younger the patient, the more likely the lens can be aspirated with the phacoemulsification tip with vacuum and little to no ultrasound. No matter how soft, a nucleus cannot be aspirated through a 0.3 mm irrigation/aspiration tip. Techniques such as "divide and conquer" and "phaco chop" will not be possible if the lens is very soft. If the lens cannot easily be aspirated, necessitating the use of ultrasound, the power should be reduced to the lowest level needed to remove the lens. The surgeon must carefully guard against capsular rupture, as the softer lens material may aspirate abruptly, followed by the capsule.

Many surgeons believe that an IOL should always be used after clear lens extraction, even with little to no optical power in high myopia. Plano IOL power is available if indicated. The IOL acts as a barrier to anterior prolapse of the vitreous in the event that Nd:YAG laser posterior capsulotomy is required, maintaining the integrity of the aqueous–vitreous barrier. Some IOL models reduce the rate of posterior capsule opacification.

IOL Calculations in Refractive Lensectomy

High expectations for excellent uncorrected visual acuity make accurate IOL power determination even more critical here than in cataract surgery. However, IOL power formulas are less accurate at the higher levels of myopia and hyperopia. In addition, in high myopia a posterior staphyloma can make the axial length measurements inaccurate. Careful fundus examination and B-scan ultrasound can identify the position and extent of staphylomata. The SRK/T formula is generally considered to be the most accurate in moderate and highly myopic patients, while the Hoffer Q formula is more accurate for moderate and highly hyperopic eyes. Nonetheless, it is best to use several formulas to determine IOL power for the refractive patient. Software programs are now available that can give the surgeon IOL predictions calculated by several formulas. The subject of IOL power determination is covered in detail in BCSC Section 11, *Lens and Cataract.*

In the case of a highly hyperopic patient, biometry may suggest that an IOL power beyond what is commercially available is required. Most IOLs have an upper range of +30.0 to +33.0 D. A special-order IOL of a higher power may be available or may be designed, but it will usually require the approval of the institutional review board at the hospital or surgical center, delaying the surgery. Another option is a "piggyback" IOL system in which two posterior chamber IOLs are inserted. One IOL is placed in the capsular bag, while the other is placed in the ciliary sulcus. The Holladay 2, Hoffer Q, and Haigis formulas can be used for calculation of piggyback IOL power. When piggyback IOLs are used, the combined power should be increased +1.5 to +2.0 D to compensate for the posterior shift of the posterior IOL. One serious complication of a piggyback IOL is the potential for development of an interlenticular opaque membrane. These membranes cannot be mechanically removed or cleared with the Nd:YAG laser; the IOLs must be removed. Interlenticular membranes have occurred most commonly between two acrylic IOLs, especially when both IOLs are placed in the capsular bag, which is why this type of piggyback IOL implantation should be avoided.

Masket S. Refractive lensectomy for correction of hyperopia. *Subspecialty Day Program 2001.* San Francisco: American Academy of Ophthalmology; 2001.

Complications

The incidence of retinal detachment in 49 clear lens exchange patients with greater than −12 D of myopia was reported to be 2% at 4 years, increasing to 8.1% at 7 years. It is not known if the risk continues to increase with even longer follow-up; long-term follow-up will be required to answer this question. In this study population, 61% of patients required Nd:YAG laser posterior capsulotomy. Laser capsulotomy increased the risk of detached retina from 5.3% to 10% over a 7-year period. The effectiveness of prophylactic laser treatment to the retina in prevention of detachment is unproven.

Colin J, Robinet A, Cochener B. Retinal detachment after clear lens extraction for high myopia. *Ophthalmology.* 1999;106:2281–2285.

Advantages

Clear lens extraction with IOL implantation has the advantage of greatly expanding the range of refractive surgery beyond currently available methods. Clear lens extraction retains the normal corneal contour, which may enhance visual quality.

Disadvantages

The disadvantages of clear lens extraction include the risks associated with any intraocular surgery. While retinal detachment is a significant concern in the myopic patient, it is less of a risk in the hyperopic eye. Patient expectations for excellent uncorrected visual acuity are much higher in this surgery than in cataract surgery, which increases the need for attention to detail preoperatively and intraoperatively.

Toric IOL

Corneal astigmatism of ≥1.5 D is present in 15% to 29% of cataract patients. Methods of corrective surgery include arcuate keratotomy or limbal relaxing incisions during or after cataract surgery, excimer laser ablation by either LASIK or PRK after adequate healing of the incision, or, for small amounts of cylinder, placing the incision in the axis of plus cylinder. Alternatively, a toric IOL can incorporate the astigmatic correction into the spherical IOL power. Toric IOL placement after clear lens extraction has not been well studied.

Instrumentation

The STAAR toric IOL is an FDA-approved, single-piece, plate-haptic, foldable silicone IOL designed to be placed in the capsular bag using an injector through a 3 mm incision. Once in the eye it must be oriented with its long axis precisely in the steep meridian. The 6 mm optic is biconvex with a spherocylindrical anterior surface and a spherical posterior surface. The optic has a mark at either end to indicate the axis of plus cylinder. The IOL is available in a length of 10.8 mm or 11.2 mm. A 1.15 mm fenestration located at the end of each haptic is designed to maximize capsular fixation. The IOLs are available in the range of +10.0 to +28.0 D spherical powers with a choice of cylindrical powers of 2.0 D and 3.5 D. The toric surface corrects less astigmatism when measured at the corneal plane; STAAR states that the 2.0 D IOL corrects 1.4 D of corneal astigmatism and the 3.5 D IOL corrects 2.3 D.

Patient Selection

This toric IOL is designed for cataract patients with 1.5 to 3.5 D of regular corneal astigmatism. In addition to understanding the risks associated with intraocular surgery, the patient should be capable of understanding the limitations of this IOL in fully correcting astigmatism. The patient should also be informed that implantation of a toric

IOL will not eliminate the need for reading glasses (unless monovision is planned). The patient also needs to be informed that the IOL may rotate in the capsular bag shortly after surgery and may require a secondary intraocular surgery to reposition the IOL. Since the STAAR toric IOL is available only in silicone, it would not be appropriate for diabetic patients who require an acrylic IOL optic, such as patients with a history of iritis, or patients who may require silicone oil for retinal detachment repair.

Planning and Surgical Technique

The astigmatism should be measured accurately with a keratometer and confirmed if possible with corneal topography. The axis of astigmatism should be marked on the cornea with the patient in the upright position, to avoid misalignment that could result from torsional globe rotation that sometimes occurs with movement to the supine position. Cataract surgery with a wound that is astigmatism-neutral is necessary to achieve the intended benefit of a toric lens.

After the IOL is injected into the capsular bag, the viscoelastic material behind the IOL is aspirated and the IOL is rotated into position on the steep meridian. If the IOL is too short for the capsular bag diameter, it may rotate when balanced salt solution is used to re-form the anterior chamber. Since the toric IOL has a plate haptic, the surgeon should be careful when performing Nd:YAG capsulotomy. If the capsulotomy is too large, a plate-haptic IOL may prolapse posteriorly. Capsular fixation around the fenestrations helps to stabilize this IOL.

Outcomes

In clinical trials, an uncorrected visual acuity of ≥20/40 following implantation of the toric IOL occurred in 48% to 84% of patients. Postoperative astigmatism was <0.50 D in 48% of patients and <1.00 D in 75% to 81% of patients.

Complications

The major disadvantage of this IOL is the possibility of IOL rotation resulting in a misalignment of the astigmatic correction. The full correction is not achieved unless the IOL is properly aligned in the axis of astigmatism. According to the manufacturer a 10° off-axis rotation reduces the correction by approximately ⅓, a 20° off-axis rotation reduces the correction by ⅔, and an off-axis correction of >30° can actually increase the cylindrical refractive error. In the FDA clinical trials, 76% of patients were reportedly within 10° of preoperative alignment, and 95% were within 30° degrees. Till and colleagues found that 14% of 100 consecutive IOLs inserted had rotated postoperatively by more than 15°. Typically, a misaligned IOL is usually recognized within days of the surgery and should be repositioned before permanent fibrosis occurs within the capsular bag. However, waiting 1 week for some capsule contraction to occur may ultimately help stabilize the IOL.

Ruhswurm I, Scholz U, Zehetmayer M, et al. Astigmatism correction with a foldable toric intraocular lens in cataract patients. *J Cataract Refract Surg.* 2000;26:1022–1027.

Sun XY, Vicary D, Montgomery P, et al. Toric intraocular lenses for correcting astigmatism in 130 eyes. *Ophthalmology.* 2000;107:1776–1782.

Till JS, Yoder PR, Wilcox TK, et al. Toric intraocular lens implantation: 100 consecutive cases. *J Cataract Refract Surg.* 2001;28:295–301.

Multifocal IOL

A multifocal IOL has the advantage of providing the patient with functional vision at near, intermediate, and remote distances. Careful patient selection and counseling along with preoperative measurement are critically important for achieving patient satisfaction postoperatively.

Instrumentation

The Array (AMO) multifocal silicone posterior chamber IOL is the most widely available multifocal IOL in the United States. It is a flexible biconvex IOL, with a zonal progressive multifocal anterior surface, designed to be inserted through a 3.2 mm incision and implanted into the capsular bag (Fig 8-8). The Array has a 6.0 mm optic and a 13.0 mm length. While the optical design is distance-dominant with a +3.5 D add, the functional add power is approximately 2.5 D at the corneal plane. The focusing of the incoming light is divided 50% for distance, 30% for near, and 20% for intermediate. Diffractive-optic multifocal IOLs are also available outside the United States (Pharmacia) and are undergoing clinical trials in the United States (Alcon).

Patient Selection

Patients likely to be successful with a multifocal IOL after cataract surgery are adaptable, relatively easy-going people who place a high value on reducing dependence on glasses or contact lenses. They have good potential vision and are currently dependent on glasses with more than −2.0 D of myopic correction (or more than +1.0 D of preoperative hyperopic correction). They generally have less than 1.0 D of residual astigmatism. A patient's pupil should be at least 4.0 mm diameter to benefit fully from the IOL. Surgery on the fellow eye is usually performed within 1 month of the first eye.

The Array IOL has been used for presbyopic refractive lensectomy (the so-called PRELEX procedure) in which clear lens extraction is performed with multifocal IOL insertion. This may be of particular benefit to the hyperopic patient with presbyopia. As

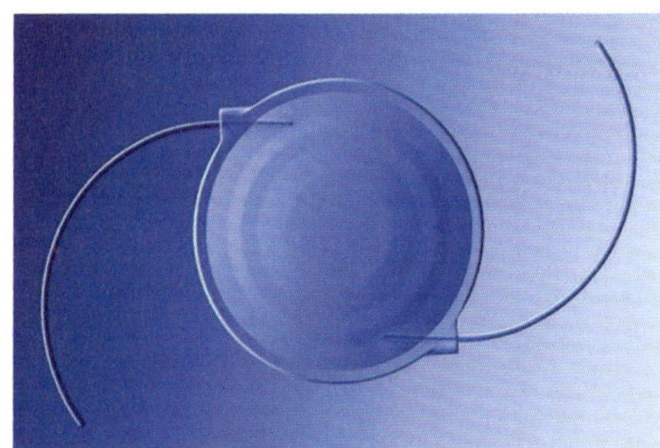

Figure 8-8 Array (AMO) multifocal IOL. Note circular zones of correction shown in lens optic. *(Courtesy of AMO.)*

with any refractive surgery procedure, careful patient selection, education, and expectation management are essential to the success of the procedure.

Surgical Technique

The surgical technique is not different from that used in standard small-incision cataract surgery with a foldable silicone IOL. The optics are dependent on good IOL centration. If the posterior capsule is not intact, IOL decentration is more likely to occur, and a multifocal IOL should not be used.

Outcomes

Patients are four times more likely to never wear glasses after bilateral sequential surgery with insertion of the Array multifocal lens as compared with insertion of a monofocal IOL (32% vs 8%). At 3 months postoperatively, binocular uncorrected distance acuity of 20/40 or better and near acuity of at least J3 was achieved in 96% of multifocal IOL patients, as compared with 65% of monofocal IOL patients. One study reported a higher postoperative satisfaction rate in multifocal IOL patients when compared with monofocal IOL patients.

As patients age, the pupillary diameter may decrease. When the pupillary diameter falls below 4.0 mm the unaided reading ability may diminish. Gentle dilation with topical mydriatic agents or laser photomydriasis may restore the near acuity. Photomydriasis may be performed with an argon or dye photocoagulator, by placing green laser burns circumferentially outside the iris sphincter, or with an Nd:YAG photodisruptor, by creating about four partial sphincterotomies.

Side Effects and Complications

Patients with the Array IOL have more glare (11% vs 1%) and more haloes (15% vs 6%) than monofocal IOL patients. Over several months the haloes tend to subside, perhaps because of the patient's ability to adapt to them. With some reduction in contrast sensitivity, the quality of vision perceived by the patient after multifocal IOL insertion may not be as good as the best-corrected quality of vision after a monofocal IOL. The tradeoff of quality of vision for the reduced dependence on glasses must be fully discussed with the patient preoperatively. It is estimated that approximately 1% of patients with the Array multifocal IOL have insisted on exchange for a monofocal IOL.

For a more detailed discussion of the surgical treatment of presbyopia, see Chapter 9 of this book.

Fine IH. Refractive lensectomy with multifocal IOL. In: Durrie DS, O'Brien TP, eds. *Refractive Surgery: Back to the Future.* San Francisco: American Academy of Ophthalmology; 2002.

Javitt JC, Steinert RF. Cataract extraction with multifocal intraocular lens implantation: a multinational clinical trial evaluating clinical, functional, and quality-of-life outcomes. *Ophthalmology.* 2000;107:2040–2048.

Javitt JC, Wang F, Trentacost DJ, et al. Outcomes of cataract extraction with multifocal intraocular lens implantation: functional status and quality of life. *Ophthalmology.* 1997;104:589–599.

Accommodating IOL

Several models of accommodating IOL are being investigated. The most widely publicized results to date are on the CrystaLens (Eyeonics) silicone accommodating IOL (see Figure 9-6), which has been approved by the FDA for improvement of near, intermediate, and distance vision. (See Accommodating IOLs in Chapter 9 for more discussion.)

Light-Adjustable IOL

The Light-Adjustable Lens, or LAL (Calhoun Vision), is a three-piece silicone-optic IOL in which the silicone matrix has been embedded with silicone subunits called macromers. When the IOL is irradiated with ultraviolet light through a slit-lamp delivery system, the macromers polymerize and are depleted. Macromers from the nonirradiated part of the IOL optic are in higher concentration and, because of the induced osmotic gradient, diffuse toward the area of irradiation, causing the IOL to swell in this region. The light is thus able to induce a change in the shape of the IOL (Fig 8-9). For myopia, irradiation of the IOL periphery causes a reduction in the central thickness of the IOL. For hyperopia, irradiation of the center of the IOL causes the IOL center to swell. Correction of astigmatism can be achieved through a toric exposure pattern. Nomograms have been developed that reportedly can correct hyperopia, myopia, and astigmatism over a 5.0 D range. Once the desired power has been achieved, the IOL optic is diffusely irradiated in a subsequent session within 1 to 2 weeks postoperatively. This causes all remaining macromers to polymerize in their current location, stopping further diffusion and "locking in" the IOL shape. After that step, the power change becomes irreversible and is no longer adjustable.

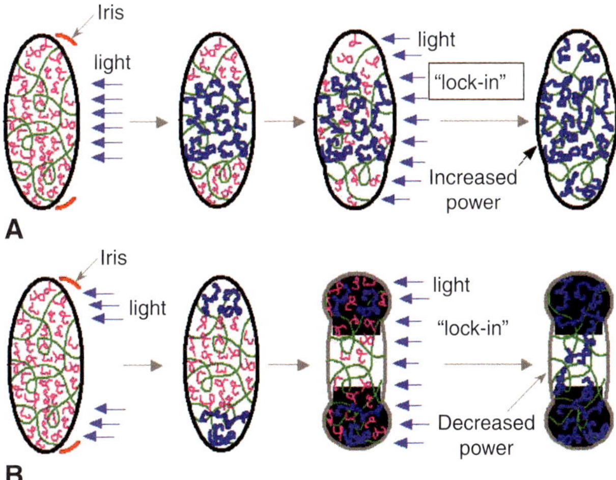

Figure 8-9 Light-adjustable IOL (Calhoun Vision). **A,** When the IOL is treated with light in the center, polymerization occurs and macromers move to the center, increasing the IOL power. **B,** When the IOL is treated with light in the periphery, macromers move to the periphery, decreasing the IOL power. *(Courtesy of Calhoun Vision.)*

Theoretically, the effect of the initial irradiation is reversible to a limited degree. If, for example, an overcorrection of residual myopia occurred and the patient became hyperopic, the previously untouched IOL center could be irradiated in a second procedure prior to the final locking-in step.

This system could hypothetically be used to induce a reversible monovision state that could be adjusted if the patient failed to adapt to it in the first week after surgery. In laboratory studies multifocal patterns have been placed in the IOL optic and could possibly be designed for specific pupil diameters. In principle, it may be possible to induce a wavefront correction on the IOL that could correct higher-order aberrations.

The IOL is foldable and is reportedly biocompatible in the rabbit model. The system has accurately induced intended power changes at specific irradiation levels in in vitro models. At the time of this writing human trials have not begun.

One disadvantage of this IOL system is the need to protect the IOL from sunlight exposure between implantation and the locking-in treatment. Further, it seems possible that if there is an error in the irradiation treatment related to centration or improper data entry, irreversible changes to the IOL could occur that could affect visual function, potentially requiring IOL exchange surgery. (See also Other IOL Innovations on the Horizon in Chapter 9.)

Schwartz DM, Jethmalani J, Sandstedt C, et al. Adjustable IOLs. In: Durrie DS, O'Brien TP, eds. *Refractive Surgery: Back to the Future.* San Francisco: American Academy of Ophthalmology; 2002.

CHAPTER 9

Accommodative and Nonaccommodative Treatment of Presbyopia

Introduction

Presbyopia, the normal progressive loss of accommodation, affects all individuals regardless of their underlying refractive error. As much as myopia, hyperopia, and astigmatism are bothersome, nothing compares with the relentless loss of near vision and the dependency on glasses that a 20/15 emmetrope feels as middle age approaches. The possibility of "curing" or reducing the effects of presbyopia remains the Holy Grail of refractive surgery.

A number of procedures intended to increase the amplitude of accommodation are being investigated. Some of these techniques rely on various types of "scleral expansion." Others involve IOLs capable of anteroposterior movement with a subsequent change in effective lens power. Still others involve the creation of a multifocal cornea. Many of the procedures are based, in part, on the rejection of the long-accepted Helmholtz theory of accommodation. Because other theories have been formulated to explain the rationale behind other proposed types of surgery for presbyopia, we begin by examining the various theories of accommodation.

Theories of Accommodation

We do not yet have a complete understanding of the relationship between the effect of ciliary muscle contraction and zonular tension on the equatorial lens. In addition, markedly different anatomical relationships have been described between the origin of the zonular fibers and the insertion of these fibers into the lens.

The Helmholtz hypothesis or "capsular theory" of accommodation states that during distance vision, the ciliary muscle is relaxed and the zonular fibers that cross the circumlental space between the ciliary body and the lens equator are under a "resting" tension. With accommodative effort, circumferential ciliary muscle contraction releases this tension on the zonules. There is also an anterior movement of the ciliary muscle annular ring during accommodation. The reduced zonular tension allows the elastic capsule of the lens to contract, causing a decrease in equatorial lens diameter and an increase in the curvatures of the anterior and posterior lens surfaces. This "rounding up" of the lens yields a corresponding increase in dioptric power of the lens necessary for near vision (Fig 9-1). When the accommodative effort ceases, the ciliary muscle relaxes and the zonular tension on the lens equator rises to its resting state. This increased tension on the lens equator causes a flattening of the lens, a decrease in the curvature of the anterior and posterior lens surfaces, and a decrease in the dioptric power of the unaccommodated eye.

In the Helmholtz theory, the equatorial edge of the lens moves away from the sclera during accommodation and toward the sclera when accommodation ends. In this theory, all zonular fibers are relaxed during accommodation and all are under tension when the accommodative effort ends. According to Helmholtz, presbyopia results from the loss of lens elasticity with age. When the zonules are relaxed the lens does not change its shape to the same degree as the young lens; therefore, presbyopia is an aging process that could only be reversed by changing the elasticity of the lens or its capsule.

Southall JPC, ed. *Helmholtz's Treatise on Physiologic Optics.* Translated from the 3rd German ed. New York: Dover Publications; 1962.

Diametrically opposed to Helmholtz is the Schachar theory of accommodation. Schachar suggests that during accommodation, ciliary muscle contraction leads to a selective increase in equatorial zonular tension rather than the uniform decrease (anterior, equatorial, and posterior) proposed by the Helmholtz theory, with a subsequent pulling of the equatorial lens outward toward the sclera (Fig 9-2). Schachar postulates that ac-

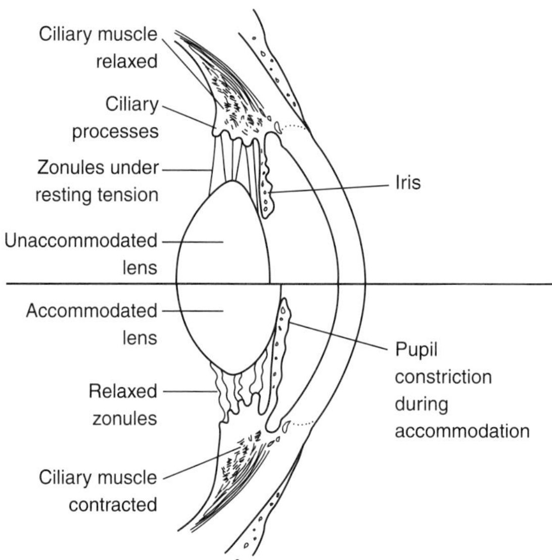

Figure 9-1 In the Helmholtz theory of accommodation, contraction of the ciliary muscle leads to a relaxation of the zonular fibers. The reduced zonular tension allows the elastic capsule of the lens to contract, causing an increase in the anterior and posterior lens curvature. *(Illustration by Jeanne Koelling.)*

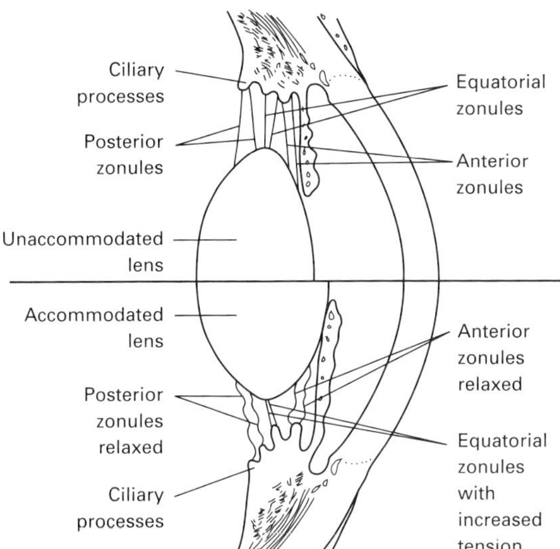

Figure 9-2 Schachar proposes that only the equatorial zonules are under tension during accommodation and that the anterior and posterior zonular fibers serve solely as passive support structures for the lens. *(Illustration by Jeanne Koelling.)*

commodation occurs through a direct effect of zonular tension (as opposed to the passive effect proposed by Helmholtz) causing an increase in lens curvature. The loss of accommodation with age in this theory is a result of the continued growth of the lens and a decrease in the lens–ciliary body distance with a resultant loss of zonular tension. Anything that increases resting zonular tension (eg, scleral expansion) should restore accommodation.

To generate this accommodative zonular tension on the equatorial lens, Schachar proposes that the equatorial zonules insert into the anterior aspect of the ciliary muscle at the root of the iris. Ciliary muscle contraction generates the movement of extralenticular structures toward the sclera at the iris root in what Schachar believes provides a net outward-directed force at the lens equator through the critical equatorial zonular fibers.

The mechanism he proposes for functional lens shape change is that equatorial stretching (by the zonules) decreases the peripheral lens volume and increases the central volume, thus producing the central steepening of the anterior central lens capsule (Fig 9-3). In the Schachar model, only the equatorial zonules transmit the ciliary muscle contraction. During accommodation and ciliary muscle contraction, tension on the equatorial zonular fibers increases while tension on the anterior and posterior zonules is reduced. That way, the lens maintains a stable position at all times even though it is undergoing changes in shape. He suggests that the anterior and posterior zonules serve as passive support structures for the lens, while the equatorial zonules are the active components in determining the optical power of the lens. To restate, in Schachar's model presbyopia is due to equatorial lens expansion during age-related growth, thus reducing

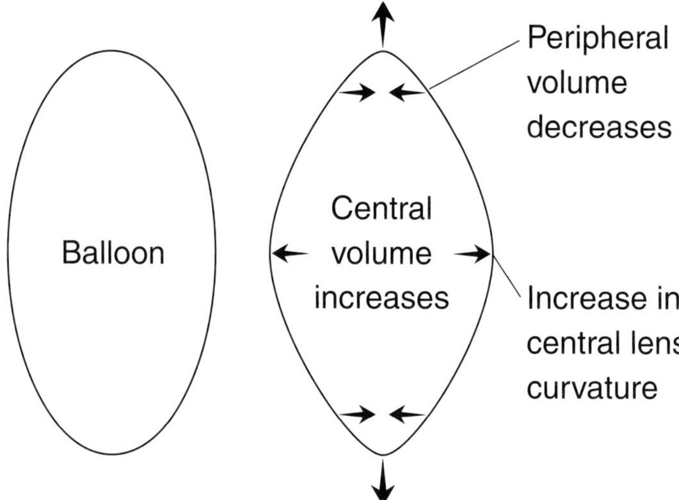

Figure 9-3 Schachar proposes that the increase in equatorial zonular tension causes a decrease in peripheral lens volume and an increase in central lens volume, thus producing an increase in central lens curvature. *(Illustration by Jeanne Koelling.)*

the resting tension of the zonular fibers, which in turn reduces the effect of ciliary muscle contraction on the equatorial zonules across the shortened circumlental distance.

Schachar RA. Cause and treatment of presbyopia with a method for increasing the amplitude of accommodation. *Ann Ophthalmol.* 1992;24:445–452.

Evidence from recent studies on both human and nonhuman primates disputes Schachar's theories on accommodation and presbyopia. Investigations in human tissues and with scanning electron microscopy reveal no zonular insertions (equatorial or otherwise) at the iris root or anterior ciliary muscle. Various imaging techniques consistently indicate that the diameter of the crystalline lens *decreases* with accommodation. In vitro laser scanning imaging shows that the crystalline lens does not change focal length when increasing and decreasing radial stretching forces are applied. This runs contrary to Schachar's proposal that the lens remains pliable with age and that presbyopia is due solely to lens growth and crowding that prevents optimum ciliary muscle action.

Glasser A, Kaufman PL. The mechanism of accommodation in primates. *Ophthalmology.* 1999;106:863–872.

Objective measures of accommodation using a dynamic infrared optometer have shown no evidence of increased amplitude after scleral expansion implant surgery. Subjective improvement in some patients has not been completely explained. Factors other than accommodation must be considered including depth of focus, patient effort, test learning, and nonlenticular optical shifts.

Mathews S. Scleral expansion surgery does not restore accommodation in human presbyopia. *Ophthalmology.* 1999;106:873–877.

The catenary, or hydraulic support, theory proposed by Coleman and Fish suggests that the lens, zonules, and anterior vitreous form a functional diaphragm between the anterior and posterior chambers of the eye. Contraction of the circular ciliary muscle generates a pressure gradient between the anterior and posterior chambers, causing anterior movement of this lens–zonule diaphragm and steepening of the anterior central lens curvature. Studies done by Coleman with differential IOP transducers in nonhuman primate eyes have revealed a rise in posterior chamber IOP relative to the anterior chamber during accommodation. The catenary model shares with the Helmholtz theory the concept that zonular fibers are under tension in the unaccommodated eye and are relaxed in the accommodated state. The lax zonular fibers during accommodation may allow for some of the forward translational movement of the lens during accommodation that is proposed by this theory.

In this model, presbyopia is due to increasing lens volume with age that causes a reduced response of the anterior lens curvature to the posterior chamber pressure gradient generated by ciliary body contraction. Of note, decreased strength/contractility of the ciliary muscle with age is not implicated in this theory.

Coleman DJ, Fish SK. Presbyopia, accommodation, and the mature catenary. *Ophthalmology.* 2001;108:1544–1551.

The premise of "vitreous support" and the lens–zonule diaphragm role in accommodation is important in the theoretical functioning of some of the new IOL models for reversal of presbyopia that will be discussed later. None of the above three theories fully accounts for all the physiologic and optical events that occur during accommodation. A complete understanding of the process of accommodation and presbyopia remains elusive.

Agarwal A. *Presbyopia: A Surgical Textbook.* Thorofare, NJ: Slack Publishing; 2002.

Nonaccommodative Treatment of Presbyopia

Monovision

Currently, presbyopia modification in phakic individuals is limited to monovision, in which the refractive power of one eye is adjusted to improve near vision (see also Chapter 3). This involves intentionally undercorrecting a myope, overcorrecting a hyperope, or inducing mild myopia in an emmetrope. Historically, the term *monovision* was typically applied to patients who wore a distance contact lens in one eye and a near lens in the other. Often the power difference between the two eyes was significant (1.25 to 2.50 D), because the patient always had the option of replacing the near lens with a distance lens when the activity demanded. This obviously is not possible with refractive surgery so many refractive surgeons routinely target mild myopia (−0.50 to −1.50 D) for the near eye in the presbyopic and peripresbyopic population. The term "modified monovision" is probably more appropriate for this lower level of myopia. While not affecting the accommodative amplitude, this level of myopia is associated with only a mild decrease in distance vision, retention of good stereopsis, and a significant increase in the intermediate zone of functional vision. The intermediate zone is where many activities of daily life occur (eg, seeing a computer screen, store shelves, or a car dashboard). Patients retain good distance vision in their distance eye and an increase in near and intermediate vision in their near eye. For many patients, this compromise between good distance vision in both eyes with a loss of near vision as opposed to good distance vision in one eye with an increase in near visual function is an attractive alternative to constantly reaching for a pair of reading glasses. Selected patients who expect better near vision may prefer higher amounts of monovision correction (−1.50 to −2.50 D) despite the accompanying decrease in distance vision and stereopsis.

Patient selection

Appropriate patient selection is important in determining the overall success of the treatment. The monovision correction can be demonstrated with trial lenses but often a contact lens trial is useful. Patients who are not presbyopic or approaching presbyopia are typically not good candidates for modified monovision. A 25-year-old myope will not appreciate the long-term benefit of mild myopia in one eye. Young myopic individuals are usually looking for the best possible distance vision in both eyes.

The best candidates for modified monovision are myopes over the age of 40 who, because of their refractive error, retain some useful near vision. This group is able to understand the importance of near vision, and these patients have always experienced adequate near vision simply by removing their glasses. Patients who do not have useful near vision preoperatively (myopia >4.50 D, high astigmatism, or contact lens wearers) may be more accepting of the need for reading glasses when their refractive error is treated. In addition, it has long been accepted that in order for most patients to function free of spectacles, a minimum of 20/25 or better uncorrected visual acuity is required. Individuals whose correction is high have a decreased likelihood of achieving a final uncorrected visual acuity of 20/25 or better. It is typically better to attempt to obtain distance correction in both eyes in order to increase the chance of obtaining adequate distance vision. Finally, most hyperopic patients are typically bothered by their loss of near vision (this is why they seek refractive surgery) and a planned overcorrection in their nondominant eye should be considered.

Many refractive surgeons routinely aim for a minimal undercorrection (−0.50 to −0.75 D) in the nondominant eye. Other surgeons may demonstrate monovision with trial lenses or give the patient a trial with contact lenses to ascertain patient acceptance and the degree of near vision desired. While higher amounts of ametropia (>1.50 D) are not typically used, some patients are willing to accept a decrease in stereopsis and depth perception for the greater improvement in near vision.

Monovision may be accomplished with LASIK, PRK, conductive keratoplasty, or even cataract surgery. In carefully selected patients it has a high degree of acceptance and affords the potential of greater spectacle-free functional vision.

Conductive Keratoplasty

As discussed earlier (Chapter 7), conductive keratoplasty (CK) is a nonablative, collagen-shrinking procedure approved for the correction of low levels of hyperopia (+0.75 to +3.00 D). CK is based on the delivery of radiofrequency energy through a fine conducting tip inserted into the peripheral corneal stroma. CK is now FDA approved for the treatment of presbyopia in hyeropic and emmetropic individuals. The treatment obviously does not restore accommodation, but instead induces mild myopia (modified monovision) in one eye. Relative to the degree of near visual gain, the decrease in distance vision is relatively mild. Initial data reported that 79% of patients could read J2, 94% could read J3, and 95% maintained >20/25 binocular distance vision. The gain in near vision appears to be greater than expected for the amount of myopia induced and may be caused by the multifocal nature of the post-CK cornea. CK is a relatively simple, noninvasive procedure that spares the central corneal visual axis and has a high safety profile. While not increasing accommodative amplitude, CK for presbyopia is capable of increasing the range of functional vision in the presbyopic population.

IOL Implants

Currently, individuals undergoing cataract surgery can have a standard monofocal IOL with a refractive target of either emmetropia, mild myopia, or monovision (one eye distance, one eye near), or they can choose a multifocal IOL (discussed here) or an accommodating IOL (discussed later in this chapter).

The Array lens (Advanced Medical Optics) is a multifocal IOL that simulates accommodation by allowing pseudophakic patients to visualize images at different focal distances without relying on capsular mechanics or ciliary body function. The lens is a zonally progressive, flexible, silicone posterior chamber IOL with five concentric zones on its anterior surface. It has a 6.0 mm silicone optic, 13 mm diameter PMMA haptics, and the IOL can be placed through a 3.25 mm incision. It is an aspheric design that uses 100% of incoming light: 50% for distance, 30% for near, and 20% for intermediate. The IOL has an effective add of approximately +2.5 D at the corneal plane. While some loss of contrast sensitivity was noted when the IOL was tested monocularly, no loss was noted when Array IOLs were placed and tested bilaterally.

Capsular opacification is of greater concern with multifocal IOLs because minimal peripheral changes in the capsule can cause early deterioration in vision. While capsular opacification is not frequent, future changes in IOL design (eg, edge design) will attempt to reduce the incidence of lens epithelial migration/ingrowth with the objective of limiting posterior capsular opacification.

Because multifocal IOLs cause an increased incidence of glare and haloes around lights at night, careful selection of motivated, well-informed patients is prudent. Most of these symptoms are found to decrease over time. They can be further reduced when nighttime driving glasses are used or 0.15% topical brimonidine drops are instilled to reduce scotopic pupil size (see also Chapter 8).

Other types of multifocal IOLs are available outside the United States. Pharmacia markets a multifocal IOL that is based on diffractive optics, and many other companies have multifocal IOLs under investigational trials.

Custom or Multifocal Ablations

Similar to conductive keratoplasty or corneal inlays, the approach to presbyopia with the excimer laser relies on creating a multifocal cornea as opposed to restoring accommodation. The potential for improving near vision without significantly compromising distance vision was investigated after noting that many patients after hyperopic PRK or LASIK had an improvement in uncorrected near vision in excess of what would have been expected. Hyperopic ablations induce central steepening in a relatively small optical zone and have a large peripheral blend zone (Fig 9-4).

Attempts at correcting both distance and near vision use a variation of this multifocal approach. A number of ablation patterns are being evaluated and include the following:

- A small central steep zone, where the central portion of the cornea is used for near and the midperiphery is used for distance
- An inferior near-zone ablation pattern
- An inferiorly decentered hyperopic ablation
- A central distance ablation with an intermediate/near midperipheral ablation

Some of these patterns rely on simultaneous vision (similar to some bifocal contact lenses or the Array IOL); others use the pupil constriction that occurs with the near reflex (accommodative convergence) to concentrate light rays through the steeper central ablation.

The safety and efficacy of multifocal ablations was recently examined in a clinical study at the University of Ottawa Eye Institute. This study found that multifocal correction for presbyopia did not compromise the accuracy of distance correction. According to preliminary results, 100% of the eyes had 20/40 or better uncorrected visual acuity after 3 months for distance, and 80% had 20/40 or better for near vision.

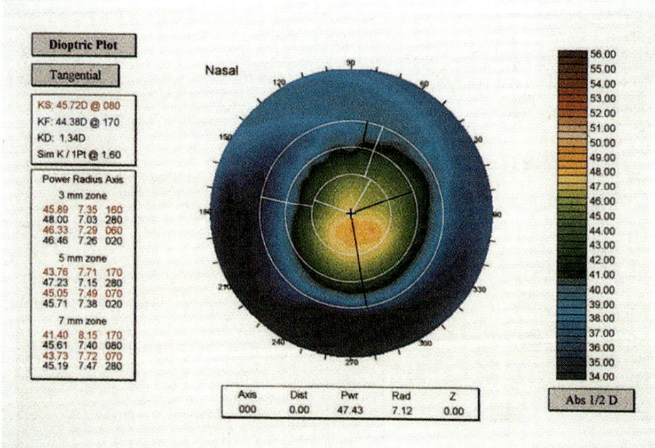

Figure 9-4 Multifocal ablation. Corneal topographic map showing multifocal ablation after hyperopic LASIK in a 62-year-old with preoperative hyperopia of +4.00. Postoperatively the uncorrected visual acuity at distance is $20/25^{-2}$ and the uncorrected visual acuity at near is J1. Manifest refraction of −0.25 +0.75 × 20 yields 20/20. Corneal topography demonstrates central hyperopic ablation *(green)* with relative steepening in the lower portion of the pupillary axis *(orange)*, which provides the near add for reading vision. *(Photograph courtesy of Jayne S. Weiss, MD.)*

Some investigators are approaching the multifocal ablation for presbyopia by correcting the central optical zone for distance and the successive concentric zones for intermediate and near. These ablations use a 10 mm optical zone under a very large flap but supposedly result in a final overall aspheric curvature to the cornea.

While the data are limited, the excimer laser offers some potential advantages over other methods to manage presbyopia. The procedure is less invasive than scleral expansion or an accommodating IOL, although more invasive than a corneal inlay, which can be removed. It can concomitantly correct the near and distance refractive error. Continued improvement of the multifocal pattern, using computer modeling that considers a patient's pupil size, treatment diameter, and corneal shape, along with data from long-term studies, may further improve this treatment.

Corneal Inlays

Originally, experimental intracorneal lenses were placed deep in the stroma. These lenses relied on the intrinsic refractive power of the insert for their effect as there was little or no change in the anterior corneal curvature. The lenses had a high index of refraction and were made of material such as polysulfone (used by Choyce and Lindstrom). These materials, however, were not permeable to water and metabolites, and opacification and corneal necrosis were major complications. (See also Chapter 5 under Alloplastic Corneal Inlays.)

The further development of intracorneal lenses has depended upon the use of permeable polymer materials that are able to transmit both fluid and nutrients from the aqueous through the endothelium and corneal stroma to the epithelium. PermaVision lenses (Anamed) are made of an optically clear hydrogel material called Nutrapore. While hydrogels have a long history of ophthalmic use, this new material has improved biocompatibility and optical properties. Clarity and permeability are both improved because the water content of the polymer exceeds 70%. In addition, the PermaVision lens's meniscus shape is 6 to 9 times thinner than previous hydrogel implants, further improving its permeability. The inlay has a refractive index nearly identical to that of the cornea (1.376). It therefore lacks a refractive power of its own and relies on altering the anterior corneal curvature to induce its refractive effect. Long-term animal studies have confirmed the safety and biocompatibility of the implant, and early human trials have demonstrated stable induced corneal topographic changes, although inlay decentrations and intrastromal deposits remain problematic.

While the current use of intracorneal lens implants is principally for the correction of hyperopia, multifocal versions are in development that offer hope for presbyopia correction. Most of the newer implants are placed in the corneal stroma beneath a planar microkeratome flap (similar to that made for LASIK). The implant acts as a refractive prosthesis and yields a refractive power change to the eye by changing the anterior curvature of the cornea. The degree of curvature change, and thus the refractive power, is partly dependent on the predictability of the flap dimensions (both diameter and thickness).

Another approach being used to obtain a multifocal or bifocal effect with the intracorneal inlay lens is the center-surround or bull's eye optic. The patient uses the outer portion of the pupillary area for distance, and a small, round, central optical area for near vision. This concentric design has been used previously in contact lenses and IOLs. In a small group of patients who underwent the procedure in the mid-1990s, the 5-year follow-up data of a majority of cases revealed a mean uncorrected visual acuity at distance of 20/25 and J2 at near.

A key advantage with all corneal inlays is that essentially no tissue is removed to obtain the refractive correction. Because the implants are removable, the effect is theoretically reversible or modifiable when results are less than satisfactory. Because of the small optical zone, however, problems exist with lens centration, lens movement after insertion, and quality of vision.

Accommodative Treatment of Presbyopia

Scleral Surgery

A number of scleral surgical procedures are being evaluated for the reversal of presbyopia. They all share the objective of attempting to increase zonular tension by weakening or altering the sclera over the ciliary body in order to allow for its passive expansion. Thornton first proposed weakening the sclera by creating 8 or more scleral incisions over the ciliary body (anterior ciliary sclerotomy, or ACS). Results were mixed and any positive effect appeared short-lived, but numerous studies to advance the technique and understand its effect continue. A recent prospective study of ACS using a 4-incision technique was discontinued because of significant adverse events, including anterior segment ischemia. In 2001, the American Academy of Ophthalmology stated that ACS was ineffective and a potentially dangerous treatment for presbyopia.

Hamilton DR, Davidorf JM, Maloney RK. Anterior ciliary sclerotomy for treatment of presbyopia. *Ophthalmology.* 2002;109:1970–1977.

In an attempt to limit the regression associated with ACS, Fukasaku and Marron inserted silicone plugs into the scleral incisions. The surgery was also limited to 4 radial incisions in the oblique quadrants. Experience and data with this technique are limited.

Fukasaku H, Marron JA. Anterior ciliary sclerotomy with silicone expansion plug implantation: effect on presbyopia and intraocular pressure. *Int Ophthalmol Clin.* 2001;41:133–141.

PresVIEW scleral expansion bands (Refocus Group) are small PMMA bands, 5.5 mm × 1.3 mm, that are placed in scleral tunnels over the ciliary body parallel to the limbus in the 4 oblique quadrants (Fig 9-5). The bands act as stents to pull on the sclera and actively expand the space between the ciliary body and the lens equator. This procedure has been shown to temporarily improve near vision in some patients; however, there are safety concerns. Postoperative complications include anterior segment ischemia with residual iris atrophy and lens opacities, monocular diplopia, infection, late-onset mild iritis, progressive scleral thinning over the band, and dry eye. Malecaze and colleagues reported that the scleral bands showed inconsistent results, limited if any effect, and poor patient acceptance.

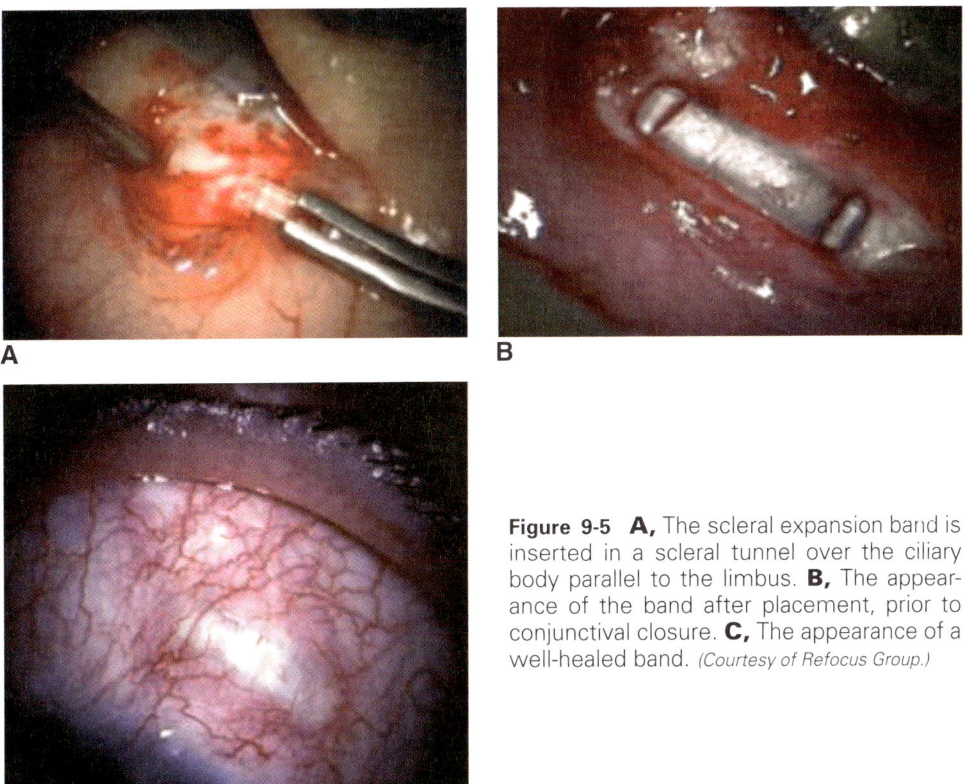

Figure 9-5 **A,** The scleral expansion band is inserted in a scleral tunnel over the ciliary body parallel to the limbus. **B,** The appearance of the band after placement, prior to conjunctival closure. **C,** The appearance of a well-healed band. *(Courtesy of Refocus Group.)*

Malecaze FJ, Gazagne CS, Tarroux MC, et al. Scleral expansion bands for presbyopia. *Ophthalmology.* 2001;108:2165–2171.

Mathews S. Scleral expansion surgery does not restore accommodation in human presbyopia. *Ophthalmology.* 1999;106:873–877.

Further efforts at scleral expansion have been attempted with an erbium:YAG infrared laser (SurgiLight). Using a fiberoptic handpiece, the surgeon makes four 80%-depth scleral incisions (400 to 500 μm) radially in the oblique quadrants over the ciliary body.

It is unclear whether any of these "expansion" procedures produce real and lasting results with an acceptable safety profile. The Schachar theory of accommodation is not generally accepted and has been questioned by modern scientific studies. Specifically, any temporal improvement in near vision has not been shown to result from a restoration of true accommodation of the lens. Although the basis for the surgical procedures may be dubious, it does not necessarily follow that the surgery is ineffective. Indeed, some type of "pseudoaccommodation" may be responsible. Further investigations are needed to determine the clinical applications of scleral expansion (including a possible reduction of IOP in glaucoma patients).

Accommodating IOLs

While scleral expansion surgery is designed for phakic patients, the accommodating IOL attempts to restore a significant amount of true accommodation to the surgically induced pseudophake. Accommodating IOLs were designed after observing that some patients, when fitted with a silicone-plate IOL, reported a return of their near vision beyond what would be expected from their refractive result. Investigations found that during ciliary muscle contraction there was a forward displacement of the IOL, leading to an increase in the effective power of the IOL and an increase in near vision. (Anterior chamber IOLs have lower A-constants than posterior chamber IOLs for the same reason.) Recent studies have questioned the amplitude of true accommodation that can be expected based solely on the anterior displacement of the IOL optic. Other factors, such as pupil size, with-the-rule astigmatism, and mild myopia may also contribute to unaided near visual acuity.

Findl O, Kiss B, Petternel V, et al. Intraocular lens movement caused by ciliary muscle contraction. *J Cataract Refract Surg.* 2003;29:669–676.

Langenbucher A, Huber S, Nguyen NX, et al. Measurement of accommodation after implantation of an accommodating posterior chamber intraocular lens. *J Cataract Refract Surg.* 2003;29:677–685.

Two IOLs that use this accommodative approach are the CrystaLens and the Akkommodative 1CU. The CrystaLens (Eyeonics) is approved by the FDA for improvement of near, intermediate, and distance vision after cataract extraction (Fig 9-6). The Akkommodative 1CU IOL (HumanOptics AG) is undergoing clinical trials (Figs 9-7, 9-8).

The CrystaLens was designed to maximize anterior movement of the IOL. While the exact cause of the movement is unclear, it appears to be a combination of posterior chamber pressure on the back surface of the IOL and pressure of the ciliary body on the IOL haptics, vaulting the optic forward. A forward movement of the entire ciliary body may also carry the IOL anteriorly. The IOL, made of third-generation silicone, is designed with grooved "hinges" within the optic plate and haptics. The use of atropine drops postoperatively facilitates the posterior seating of the IOL in the capsular bag until fibrosis occurs. Oversized polyamide haptics are attached to the ends of the plate lens to prevent rotation of the IOL in the bag and to maintain constant contact with the ciliary body. As the ciliary body contracts, it thickens, causing increased pressure on the polyamide haptics. The compression between the haptics causes the IOL to bow forward. The exaggerated anterior displacement is postulated to result in an effective increase in optical power and near vision. Although this mechanism was not definitively proven in clinical trials, there was an average of 1 D of power generated at near.

The FDA clinical trials investigated the 4.5 mm CrystaLens for primary implantation at the time of cataract surgery. Immersion ultrasound is critical for determining accurate IOL power. Because the accommodative effect is dependent on IOL placement posterior to an intact capsulorrhexis, this IOL is not indicated for secondary IOL placement. While most patients had excellent uncorrected distance and intermediate vision, only 57% of patients could read a newspaper without spectacles. This reflects the average of 1 D of power generated by the IOL at near. Contrast sensitivity for the CrystaLens was better than standard posterior chamber IOLs, despite the 4.5 mm optic. The use of this IOL in younger patients with larger pupils has not been investigated. In laboratory experiments,

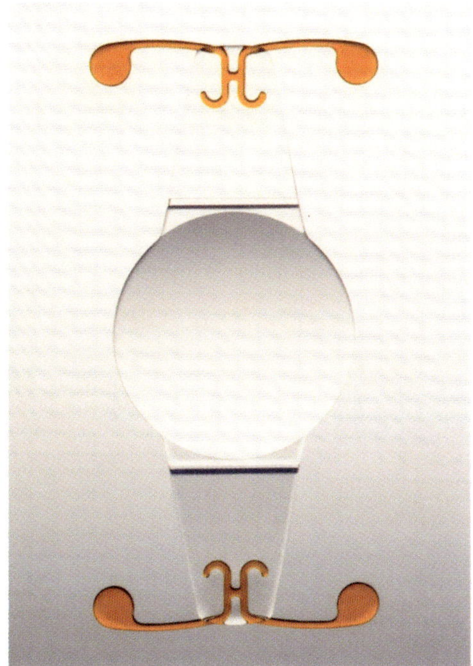

Figure 9-6 The CrystaLens is designed with a flexible hinge in the haptic at the proximal end and a polyamide foot plate at the distal end. The foot plate functions to maximize contact with the capsule and ciliary body, and the hinge transfers the horizontal force into an anteroposterior movement of the optic. *(Courtesy of Eyeonics.)*

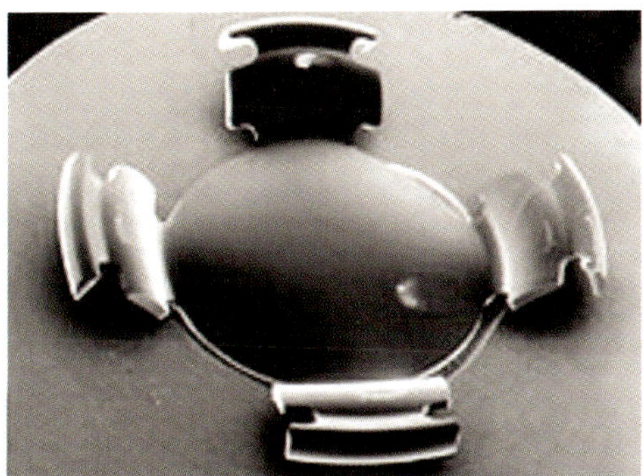

Figure 9-7 The Akkommodative 1CU is a foldable acrylic IOL with four haptics with flexible transition zones. *(Courtesy of HumanOptics AG.)*

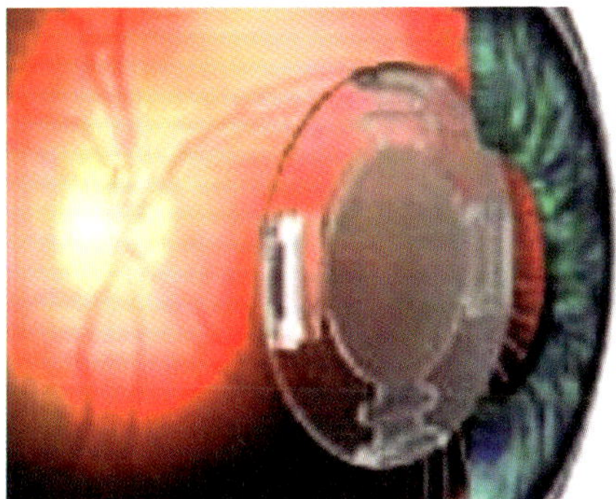

Figure 9-8 Schematic representation of the Akkommodative 1CU in contact with the capsular bag and its relationship to the zonular fibers. *(Courtesy of HumanOptics AG.)*

the IOL was flexed 1,000,000 times without mechanical failure. It is not known how many times the CrystaLens flexes in a patient's eye on a yearly basis nor whether there is a risk of mechanical failure of the haptics in the patient's lifetime.

The Akkommodative 1CU is a foldable acrylic IOL with a 5.5 mm optic and four haptics with flexible transition zones. It is designed for capsular placement and to transform the contracting forces of the ciliary muscle into anterior movement of the IOL optic. Preliminary reports suggest an anterior shift of approximately 0.60 mm with accommodation and an accompanying myopic shift of 1.3 to 1.7 D. Clinically, however, accommodative amplitudes of less than 1.0 D are more commonly seen. Similar to the CrystaLens, the Akkommodative 1CU requires the continued functioning of the ciliary body and relies on forward movement of the optic for its refractive effect.

An important observation on the preliminary success of these IOLs in restoring accommodative facility in older patients is the apparent maintenance of effective ciliary muscle function despite years without a "normal" accommodative effort. The impact of long-term capsular fibrosis on the dynamic functioning of these IOL designs is not yet known, but regression does not seem to be a problem after more than 2 years of follow-up.

Besides holding promise for cataract patients, the accommodating IOL may allow for greater acceptance of clear lens extraction as a refractive procedure for moderate to high hyperopia. While clear lens extraction for high myopia is associated with a number of possible serious complications, many of these are infrequently seen in hyperopic patients. Nevertheless, the loss of accommodation in a hyperope who normally has a large accommodative amplitude for his or her age is a substantial and often undesirable surgical trade-off in clear lens extraction. The accommodating IOL offers, at least in part, the promise for the pseudophake of emmetropia without presbyopia.

Other IOL Innovations on the Horizon

A number of other experimental IOLs are undergoing clinical investigation (see Chapter 8). The SmartLens (Medennium), currently in laboratory studies, involves a thermoplastic acrylic gel that can be customized to any size, shape, or power specified by the physician. After compression to a small rod at room temperature, it inserts into the capsular bag and reconfigures into a crystalline lens–sized, flexible IOL in the aqueous at body temperature. When placed into the capsule, its designers believe it may restore accommodation by increasing its surface curvature in response to zonule-induced changes in the lens capsule.

The Light-Adjustable Lens (LAL, Calhoun Vision) involves a macromer silicone matrix with smaller embedded photosensitive molecules that will allow for postoperative customization of the power by means of tunable ultraviolet light treatment (see Figure 8-9). Finally, flexible polymers are being designed for injection into a nearly intact capsular bag, after extraction of the crystalline lens through a tiny laterally placed capsulorrhexis.

PART III

Refractive Surgery in the Setting of Other Conditions

CHAPTER 10

Refractive Surgery in Ocular and Systemic Disease

Introduction

While many ophthalmologists viewed the field of refractive surgery with skepticism only a few decades ago, refractive surgery is now highly accepted and much practiced. As refractive surgery has evolved from the controversial to the routine, the spectrum of indications has enlarged. The success of refractive surgery has been so magnified by the media that some of the public has even come to believe that these procedures are trivial. Increasingly, ophthalmologists are confronted with refractive surgical candidates who also have ocular or systemic disease.

In some cases, it may not be clear whether refractive surgery may pose an unacceptable risk. Patients with many ocular or systemic diseases were excluded from the clinical trials leading to FDA approval for excimer lasers. As the field of refractive surgery evolves, some former absolute contraindications may change to relative contraindications.

The surgeon must always remember that refractive surgery is entirely elective and does involve risks. Refractive surgery is typically contraindicated in the monocular patient. The adverse effect of even small risks may be markedly magnified in the monocular patient because any postoperative visual loss may prove devastating.

On the other hand, the envelope is constantly being stretched and refractive surgery is successfully being performed in patients who were previously considered poor candidates. Some of the categories of patients with relative contraindications to refractive surgery are addressed below. Although many refractive modalities are available, most of the discussion will concentrate on the most common procedures performed, PRK and LASIK.

As with other surgeries, ophthalmologists should never go beyond their comfort zone when performing refractive surgery. The surgeon may want to obtain a second opinion for a difficult case or refer some patients to more experienced colleagues. In addition, the process of consent should be altered not only to inform the patient but also to document the patient's understanding of the additional risks and limitations of postoperative results because of the associated ocular or systemic diseases. The refractive surgeon may want to supplement the written consent and include these additional risks.

The ophthalmologist should assiduously avoid the high-risk refractive surgery patient who volunteers to sign any preoperative consent because "they know these complications won't happen to them." This patient has not heard or understood the informed consent.

Preferred Practice Patterns Committee. *Refractive Errors.* San Francisco: American Academy of Ophthalmology; 2002.

Ocular Conditions

Dry Eye

Many patients seek refractive surgery because underlying dry eye has resulted in contact lens intolerance. However, refractive surgery may be problematic in dry eye because a normal tear film layer is important for wound healing of the corneal stroma and epithelium. Epidermal growth factor, vitamin A, and IgA in the tears help prevent postoperative infection and help potentiate wound healing. Consequently, severe dry eye has previously been thought to be a relative contraindication to refractive surgery.

Any refractive surgery candidate with signs or symptoms of dry eyes should be thoroughly evaluated. Patient history should include questions about connective tissue diseases and conjunctival cicatrizing disorders, because these are relative contraindications to any refractive procedure and would need to be addressed prior to any surgical consideration (see Chapter 3).

External examination should include evaluation of the blink reflex for such conditions as incomplete blink or lagophthalmos. On slit-lamp examination, notation should be made of blepharitis, meibomitis, tear film quantity and quality, and keratitis. Ancillary testing for dry eyes, such as Schirmer testing and tear break-up time, can be performed.

Preferred Practice Patterns Committee. *Dry Eye Syndrome.* San Francisco: American Academy of Ophthalmology; 1998.

If connective tissue diseases or cicatrizing diseases are suspected, appropriate referral or laboratory testing should be performed to rule out these conditions prior to consideration of refractive surgery. Preexisting abnormalities should be treated. Topical tear replacement and/or punctal occlusion can be performed. In appropriate cases, a preoperative course of topical anti-inflammatories such as topical corticosteroids or cyclosporine may be indicated prior to refractive surgery. Blepharitis and/or meibomitis should be treated.

A series of 21 eyes in 13 patients found PRK to be safe when performed for contact lens intolerance from dry eye, as long as there was reflex tearing noted (as checked by Schirmer test with nasal stimulation).

LASIK may result in a temporary dry eye postoperatively, because corneal nerves are severed when making the flap. In a series of 543 eyes of 290 patients after LASIK, no significant differences were found in uncorrected or best-corrected visual acuity among eyes with or without preoperative dry eye. There was no increased incidence of epithelial defects in the patients with preoperative dry eye. However, the dry eye group did manifest a slower recovery of corneal sensation, more vital staining of the ocular surface, lower tear function, and more severe dry eye symptoms until 1 year after LASIK.

Consequently, while excimer laser ablation may be performed in selected patients with dry eye, these patients must be cautioned about their increased risk of postoperative dry eye, which may result in discomfort and/or visual decrease. Proper ocular surface management by means of topical tear replacement therapy and/or punctal occlusion must be provided in the perioperative and postoperative period.

Toda I, Asano-Kato N, Hori-Komai Y, et al. Laser-assisted in situ keratomileusis for patients with dry eye. *Arch Ophthalmol.* 2002;120:1024–1028.

Toda I, Yagi Y, Hata S, et al. Excimer laser photorefractive keratectomy for patients with contact lens intolerance caused by dry eye. *Br J Ophthalmol.* 1996;66:755–763.

Herpesvirus

Many surgeons avoid excimer laser ablation in patients with herpetic keratitis because of the concern that this exposure may increase viral shedding and recurrence. The role of excimer laser ablation in inciting recurrence of herpetic keratitis has been investigated in the laboratory. Rabbits infected with herpes simplex virus (HSV) type 1 had viral reactivation after exposure of the corneal stroma to 193 nm ultraviolet radiation during PRK and after LASIK. Pretreatment with valacyclovir prior to laser treatment, however, decreased the rate of recurrence in the rabbit model.

Reactivation of HSV keratitis has been reported in humans after RK, phototherapeutic keratectomy, PRK, and LASIK. Fagerholm and colleagues reported a 25% incidence of postoperative herpes simplex keratitis in patients who underwent phototherapeutic keratectomy 17 months prior for surface irregularities from prior herpetic infections, compared with an 18% recurrence rate in the same time period prior to treatment. They concluded that the procedure does not seem to increase the incidence of recurrences.

A retrospective review of 13,200 PRK-treated eyes with no primary history of HSV revealed a 0.14% incidence of HSV keratitis. Of these, 16.5% occurred within 10 days, which the authors postulated could indicate a direct effect of the excimer ultraviolet laser. In 78%, HSV keratitis occurred within 15 weeks, which could be an effect of the corticosteroid therapy.

Corneal perforation after LASIK has been reported in a patient who had a prior penetrating keratoplasty for herpetic disease and had resultant high myopia and astigmatism. The HSV recurred 10 days after the LASIK with corneal thinning and subsequent perforation. Reactivation of herpes zoster ophthalmicus has also been reported after LASIK, with excellent recovery of vision after topical and oral antiviral treatment.

There is insufficient information to determine conclusively whether surface ablation or LASIK increases the risk of recurrence in the patient with prior HSV keratitis. Because recurrences have occurred months after excimer laser treatment, some authors have concluded that the recurrence simply reflected the natural course of the disease and was not reactivation as a result of the excimer laser ablation. Others, however, have postulated that trauma from the lamellar dissection or exposure to the excimer laser reactivates the virus and causes recurrent keratitis.

Because of the potential for visual loss from herpetic recurrence, some refractive surgeons consider prior herpetic keratitis a contraindication to refractive surgery. Caution should be exercised in making the decision to perform PRK, phototherapeutic keratectomy, or LASIK in a patient with a history of prior ocular herpetic infection. Patients with pronounced corneal anesthesia, vascularization, and/or recent herpetic attacks should not be considered candidates for refractive surgery.

Some surgeons will consider LASIK in a patient with a past history of HSV keratitis who has not had any recent recurrences, has good corneal sensation, has minimal to no corneal vascularization or scarring, and has normal best-corrected visual acuity. Preoperative and postoperative prophylaxis with systemic and/or topical antivirals should be strongly considered. Any patient with a history of herpes simplex or zoster keratitis must be counseled about the continued risk of recurrence and its concomitant potential for visual loss after excimer laser vision correction.

Asbell PA. Valacyclovir for the prevention of recurrent herpes simplex virus eye disease after excimer laser photokeratectomy. *Trans Am Ophthalmol Soc.* 2000;98:285–303.

Fagerholm P, Ohman L, Orndahl M. Phototherapeutic keratectomy in herpes simplex keratitis: clinical results in 20 patients. *Acta Ophthalmol.* 1994;72:457–460.

Nagy ZZ, Keleman E, Kovacs A. Herpes simplex keratitis after photorefractive keratectomy. *J Cataract Refract Surg.* 2003;29:222–223.

Keratoconus

Keratoconus is a contraindication to LASIK and PRK. Performance of LASIK may result in loss of best-corrected visual acuity and may increase the need for penetrating keratoplasty in such cases. In a series of 16 eyes of 9 patients with keratoconus who underwent LASIK, 5 eyes lost 1 or more lines of best-corrected visual acuity and 3 eyes required penetrating keratoplasty.

Often, the refractive surgeon is the first physician to inform a refractive surgery patient that she or he has form fruste keratoconus. The patient may have excellent vision with glasses or contact lenses and may be seeking the convenience of a more permanent correction through LASIK. Often the patient is shocked to learn about an eye disease that contraindicates refractive surgery. It is important that the ophthalmologist clearly convey that refractive surgery should not be performed because of the potential for unpredictable results and loss of vision. Otherwise, some patients may be tempted to seek out another refractive surgeon in the hope of having surgery performed.

Intrastromal corneal ring segments (Intacs) have been FDA approved under HDE for keratoconus (see Chapter 5). Epikeratoplasty has also been attempted to change corneal curvature, to permit contact lens wear in keratoconic corneas. One study reported 7-year results after epikeratoplasty in a series of 36 keratoconus eyes that were contact lens intolerant and had no central scarring. Mean refractive power decreased 6 D and astigmatism decreased 7 D from preoperative values. The authors concluded that epikeratoplasty should be considered as an alternative to penetrating keratoplasty in contact lens intolerant keratoconus in the absence of corneal scarring. However, epikeratoplasty has mostly been abandoned in the United States because of poor predictability.

Buzard KA, Tuengler A, Febbraro JL. Treatment of mild to moderate keratoconus with laser in situ keratomileusis. *J Cataract Refract Surg.* 1999;25:1600–1609.

Spitznas M, Eckert J, Frising M, et al. Long-term functional and topographic results seven years after epikeratophakia for keratoconus. *Graefes Arch Clin Exp Ophthalmol.* 2002;240:639–643.

Post–Penetrating Keratoplasty

Despite successful penetrating keratoplasty (PKP), patients may have poor vision because of the high residual refractive error. Anisometropia may result if there is a large change in corneal curvature. High astigmatism may be difficult to correct adequately with spectacles. Irregular astigmatism can only be corrected with gas-permeable contact lenses. Between 10% and 30% of patients require contact lens correction after PKP. However, contact lens fitting may not be possible because of the abnormal corneal curvature.

Refractive surgery can be performed to reduce refractive error after PKP in patients who are contact lens intolerant. Often the attainment of excellent postoperative uncorrected visual acuity is not a realistic goal. Depending on the original refractive error, refractive surgery may allow the patient to be fitted successfully with a contact lens or may permit use of spectacles.

Previously, relaxing incision and/or wedge resection were the most common procedures used to reduce post-PKP astigmatism. In one series of 20 patients with excessive corneal astigmatism after PKP, arcuate keratotomy and compression sutures reduced the corneal astigmatism by 56% with an average cylinder reduction of 5.5 D. Corrected visual acuity improved in 75% of patients, declined in 15%, and was unchanged in 10%. Although incisional surgery was effective, results were sometimes unpredictable because of differences in individual wound healing. Consequently, LASIK is increasingly being used to correct post-PKP refractive errors (Fig 10-1). PRK can be used to correct refractive errors after PKP but has disadvantages associated with epithelial removal in a corneal transplant and the potential for corneal haze when high refractive errors are treated

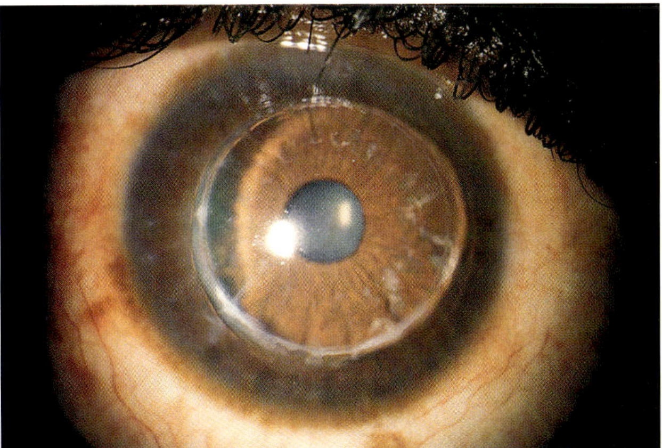

Figure 10-1 A LASIK flap in a patient who had previously undergone penetrating keratoplasty for keratoconus. Pre-LASIK manifest refraction −9.00 +6.00 × 85 20/25; pre-LASIK uncorrected visual acuity 20/400; post-LASIK manifest refraction −2.50 +1.25 × 25 20/20^{-2}; post-LASIK uncorrected visual acuity 20/25. *(Photograph courtesy of Jayne S. Weiss, MD.)*

(mitomycin can be used prophylactically in such cases). PRK does not have the risk of wound dehiscence that LASIK has with its suction ring placement for the microkeratome.

It is important to remember that there are no FDA-approved procedures to treat irregular astigmatism. Patients with irregular astigmatism whose corneal curvature prevents contact lens fitting need to be clearly told that the goal of the LASIK is solely to allow a comfortable fit with a gas-permeable contact lens postoperatively.

Preoperative examination of the post-PKP patient who is considering refractive surgery should include investigation of the reasons for the PKP. Herpetic keratitis is a relative contraindication as is connective tissue disease.

Gas-permeable contact lenses should be discontinued for at least 2 to 3 weeks prior to performing refraction. Refraction and corneal topography should be stable as documented by two consecutive readings on separate visits. LASIK should not be performed if there appear to be signs of corneal decompensation. Areas of neovascularization should be noted and areas of suspected ectasia should be confirmed with pachymetry to avoid perforation. The surgeon should confirm that there is sufficient scarring/healing in the graft/host interface. Refractive surgery should be avoided if the corneal graft has evidence of inflammation, diffuse vascularization, ectasia, inadequate healing of the graft/host interface, refractive instability, or signs of rejection or decompensation.

The timing of surgical intervention is controversial. Sutures should be removed and refraction should be stable. In order to avoid wound dehiscence, many surgeons wait at least 1 year after PKP and an additional 6 months after all sutures are removed. An interval of 18 to 24 months after PKP provides sufficient wound healing in most cases.

Because patient alignment under the laser is critical to accurately treat astigmatism, some surgeons like to mark the vertical or horizontal axis of the cornea at the slit lamp prior to placing the patient under the laser. Suction time should be minimized to decrease stress on the corneal wound and to lessen the potentially devastating complication of wound dehiscence. If the corneal curvature is very steep, cutting a thicker flap may decrease the possibility of buttonhole formation during the microkeratome pass. PRK can also be considered in steep corneas to avoid flap complications, although late-developing corneal haze has been reported.

Because the creation of a lamellar flap may itself cause a change in the amount and axis of the astigmatism, some surgeons perform LASIK as a two-stage procedure. The flap is first cut and laid back down. One or more weeks later, after the refractive error has stabilized, the flap is lifted and the laser ablation is performed. Other surgeons prefer to perform LASIK in one step to avoid increasing the potential complications (including infection and graft rejection associated with performing two separate procedures).

Mean percentage reduction of astigmatism after LASIK following PKP ranges from 54% to 87.9%. Although most series report an improvement in uncorrected visual acuity, up to 42.9% of patients require enhancement due to cylindrical undercorrection. In addition, up to 35% of patients are reported to lose 1 line of best-corrected visual acuity. Corneal graft rejection has been described after PRK. Higher and more prolonged dosing of topical corticosteroids should be prescribed in the post-PKP LASIK patient in order to avoid graft rejection, because short-lasting anterior chamber flare has been reported in these patients after LASIK. Although one earlier study reported a rate of endothelial cell loss of up to 4.11% for LASIK after PKP, this finding has not been confirmed by other reports.

Forseto AS, Francesconi CM, Nose RA, et al. Laser in situ keratomileusis to correct refractive errors after keratoplasty. *J Cataract Refract Surg.* 1999;25:479–485.

Kwitko S, Marinjo DR, Rymer S, et al. Laser in situ keratomileusis after penetrating keratoplasty. *J Cataract Refract Surg.* 2001;27:374–379.

Lam DSS, Leung AT, Wu JT, et al. How long should one wait to perform LASIK after PKP? *J Cataract Refract Surg.* 1998;24:6–7.

Rashad KM. Laser in situ keratomileusis for correction of high astigmatism after penetrating keratoplasty. *J Refract Surg.* 2000;16:701–710.

Tuunanen TH, Ruusuvaara PJ, Uusitalo RJ, et al. Photoastigmatic keratectomy for correction of astigmatism in corneal grafts. *Cornea.* 1997;16:48–53.

Ocular Hypertension and Glaucoma

Between 9% and 28% of myopic patients have primary open-angle glaucoma (POAG). The frequency of myopia in the glaucomatous population has been reported at between 6.6% and 37.8% as compared with 3% to 25% in the normal population. Consequently, it is likely that some patients with glaucoma will request refractive surgery.

Of particular concern in the patient with ocular hypertension or POAG is the effect of the acute IOP rise to more than 65 mm Hg when suction is applied to cut the corneal flap for LASIK. While the normal optic nerve seems to tolerate this IOP elevation, we do not yet fully know the resultant effect on the compromised optic nerve. There have been few reports of new visual field defects immediately after LASIK attributed to mechanical compression or ischemia of the optic nerve head from the increase of IOP.

Evaluation of the patient with ocular hypertension or POAG includes a complete history and ocular examination with peripheral visual field testing and corneal pachymetry. A history of poor IOP control, noncompliance with treatment, maximal medical therapy, or prior surgical interventions may suggest progressive disease, which may contraindicate refractive surgery. As part of the complete dilated examination, the surgeon should note the status of the angle, the presence and amount of optic nerve cupping, and the degree of visual field loss.

Central corneal thickness must be considered in the evaluation of IOP as measured by the applanation tonometer (see Chapter 11). The principle of applanation tonometry assumes a corneal thickness of 0.52 mm. For example, the IOP is underestimated by 5.2 mm Hg in a cornea of 0.45 mm thickness. Corneal curvature can also influence IOP readings, with an estimated 1 mm Hg IOP increase for every 3 D increase in corneal curvature.

There are publications that document the inaccuracy of IOP measurements after PRK or LASIK because of apparent lowering of the reading. These inaccurately low central applanation tonometry measurements have been reported to obscure the diagnosis of corticosteroid-induced glaucoma after PRK or LASIK, resulting in optic nerve cupping, visual field loss, and decreased visual acuity (Fig 10-2). Because of the difficulty interpreting IOP measurements after PRK or LASIK, these procedures should not be considered when the IOP is poorly controlled. The patient should be referred to a glaucoma specialist when indicated.

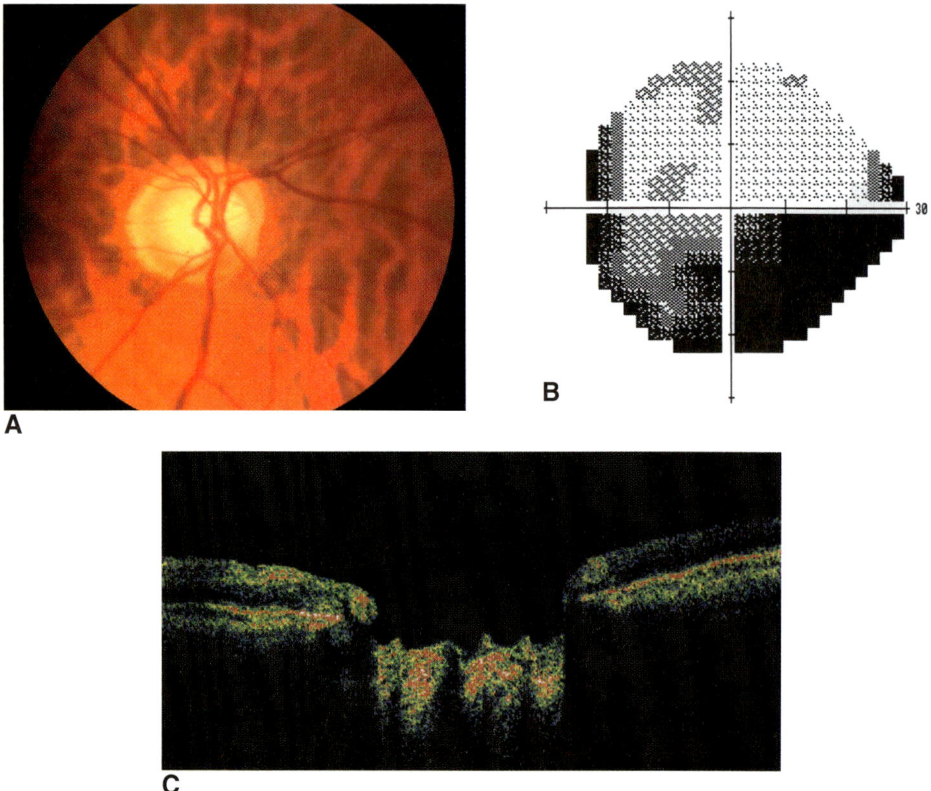

Figure 10-2 Glaucomatous optic nerve atrophy in a patient with "normal IOP" after LASIK. **A,** Increased cup/disc ratio in a patient diagnosed with glaucoma 1 year after LASIK. Patient had decreased vision with best-corrected visual acuity of 20/40 and IOP of 21 mm Hg. **B,** 24-2 visual field with extensive inferior arcuate visual field loss corresponds to thinning of the superior optic nerve rim. **C,** Ocular CT demonstrates marked optic nerve cupping. *(A, B, and C courtesy of Jayne S. Weiss, MD.)*

Patients with ocular hypertension can often have refractive surgery. Such a patient must be counseled preoperatively that the LASIK only treats the refractive error and not the natural history of the ocular hypertension, which can sometimes progress to glaucoma with optic nerve cupping and visual field loss. Particular attention should be paid to risk factors for progression to glaucoma, including age, corneal thickness, cup/disc ratio, and IOP. The patient needs to understand that refractive surgery will make it more difficult to accurately assess the IOP after excimer laser ablation.

The decision as to whether to perform refractive surgery in a patient with glaucoma is controversial. There are no long-term studies on refractive surgery in this population. LASIK is contraindicated in any patient with marked optic nerve cupping, visual field loss, or visual acuity loss. The refractive surgeon may want the patient to sign an ancillary consent form documenting the understanding that POAG may result in progressive visual loss independent of any refractive surgery.

The surgeon should be aware that placement of a suction ring may not be possible if there is a functioning filtering bleb. Typically, the glaucoma should be well controlled before refractive surgery is even considered. In the rare case in which filtering surgery and LASIK are both being planned, it is preferable that the LASIK be performed before placement of the filter. Suction time should be minimized to decrease the chance of optic nerve damage from the transient increase of IOP. Alternatively, surface ablation may be preferable because it eliminates the IOP rise associated with use of the microkeratome. The surgeon must be careful with the use of postoperative corticosteroids because of the potential for elevation of the IOP. The patient should be informed about when he or she can resume postoperative topical medications for glaucoma.

In order to avoid trauma to the flap, the IOP should not be checked for at least 72 hours. The patient should be told to inform a subsequent ophthalmologist of the prior LASIK as well as of the preoperative refractive error in order to more accurately assess the post-LASIK IOP.

Bushley DM, Parmley VC, Paglen P. Visual field defect associated with laser in situ keratomileusis. *Am J Ophthalmol.* 2000;129:668–671.

Hamilton DR, Manche EE, Rich LF, et al. Steroid-induced glaucoma after laser in situ keratomileusis associated with interface fluid. *Ophthalmology.* 2002;109:659–665.

Kass MA, Heuer DK, Higginbotham EJ, et al. The Ocular Hypertension Treatment Study. *Arch Ophthalmol.* 2002;120:701–713.

Lewis RA. Refractive surgery and the glaucoma patient: customized corneas under pressure. *Ophthalmology.* 2000;107:1621–1622.

Morales J, Good D. Permanent glaucomatous visual loss after photorefractive keratectomy. *J Cataract Refract Surg.* 1998;24:715–718.

Shaikh NM, Ahsikh S, Singh K, et al. Progression to end-stage glaucoma after laser in situ keratomileusis. *J Cataract Refract Surg.* 2002;28:356–359.

Retinal Disease

All patients undergoing refractive surgery should have a dilated preoperative examination. Retinal referral and/or a scleral depression exam of the retinal periphery should be performed if indicated. The patient should be informed of the significance, treatment, and prognosis of vitreoretinal pathology.

High myopia

A highly myopic patient is at increased risk for retinal tears and detachment. The yearly incidence of retinal detachments has been estimated as 0.015% in patients with less than 4.75 D of myopia and increases to 0.07% in patients with ≥5.00 D of myopia. A study of 1000 patients with myopia greater than −6.00 D revealed a 3.20% incidence of retinal detachment. Scleral depression exam and referral to a retina specialist should be performed as indicated in the highly myopic refractive surgery candidate. Symptomatic retinal tears or subclinical retinal detachments should be treated. Asymptomatic lattice degeneration with or without atrophic holes generally does not require prophylactic treatment, with absence of other risk factors. Asymptomatic retinal flap tears or holes usually do not require treatment (see BCSC Section 12, *Retina and Vitreous*); tears or holes associated with high myopia and other risk factors should be considered for treatment. In a study of 29,916 myopic and hyperopic eyes undergoing LASIK, 1.5% required preoperative treatment of retinal pathology.

High myopes should be counseled that refractive surgery corrects only the refractive aspect of the high myopia and not the natural history of the myopic eye with its known complications. Highly myopic patients will remain at risk for retinal tears and detachment despite refractive surgery.

Although no causal link has been established between retinal detachment and excimer laser refractive surgery, the potential adverse effects should be considered. The rapid increase and then decrease of IOP could theoretically stretch the vitreous base, and the acoustic shock wave from the laser could play a role in the development of a posterior vitreous detachment. Current data, however, suggest that RK, PRK, and LASIK do not appear to increase the incidence of retinal detachment. The actual risk to eyes with high myopia or preexisting retinal pathology has not been determined through well-controlled, long-term studies. The occurrence of retinal detachment after LASIK has been reported to range from 0.034% to 0.25%. In a series of 1554 eyes that were undergoing LASIK for myopia with a mean refractive error of -13.52 ± 3.38 D, 4 eyes (0.25%) developed retinal detachments at 11.25 ± 8.53 months after the procedure. Three of the eyes had flap tears and 1 eye had an atrophic hole. There was no statistically significant difference in the best-corrected visual acuity before and after conventional retinal reattachment surgery. A myopic shift did result from the scleral buckle, however.

Another study of 38,823 eyes with a mean myopia of −6.00 D had a 0.8% frequency of rhegmatogenous retinal detachments at a mean of 16.3 months after LASIK. The eyes that developed retinal detachments had a mean preoperative myopia of −8.75 D. Final best-corrected visual acuity after conventional scleral buckling procedures in such patients is usually good.

Using retrospective review, Blumenkranz reported that the frequency of retinal detachment after excimer laser was similar to the frequency in the general population, averaging 0.034% over 2 years. The operating retinal surgeon must be informed that LASIK has previously been performed because of the potential for late flap dehiscence during retinal detachment surgery during epithelial scraping.

The risk of retinal detachment after cataract surgery is well described (see BCSC Section 11, *Lens and Cataract*). Cataract surgery is the intraocular surgical procedure that is most commonly complicated subsequently by retinal detachment. Highly myopic eyes undergoing phakic IOL procedures are at risk for retinal detachment from the underlying high myopia in addition to the intraocular surgery. A retinal detachment rate of 4.8% was reported in a study of phakic IOLs to correct high myopia. Clear lens extraction has also been associated with retinal detachment. Longer-term follow-up is needed to determine whether these surgeries increase morbidity in the highly myopic eye.

Arevalo JF, Ramirez E, Suarez E, et al. Incidence of vitreoretinal pathologic conditions within 24 months after laser in situ keratomileusis. *Ophthalmology.* 2000;107:258–262.

Arevalo JF, Ramirez E, Suarez E, et al. Retinal detachment in myopic eyes after laser in situ keratomileusis. *J Refract Surg.* 2002;18:708–714.

Blumenkranz MS. LASIK and retinal detachment: should we be concerned? [editorial]. *Retina.* 2000;5:578–581.

Loewenstein A, Goldstein M, Lazar M. Retinal pathology occurring after excimer laser surgery or phakic intraocular lens implantation: evaluation of possible relationship. *Surv Ophthalmol.* 2002;47:125–135.

Ruiz-Moreno JM, Alio JL, Perez-Santonja JJ, et al. Retinal detachment in phakic eyes with anterior chamber intraocular lenses to correct severe myopia. *Am J Ophthalmol.* 1999;127:270–275.

Ruiz-Moreno JM, Perez-Santonja JJ, Alio JL. Retinal detachment in myopic eyes after laser in situ keratomileusis. *Am J Ophthalmol.* 1999;128:588–594.

Sakurai E, Okuda M, Nozki M, et al. Late-onset laser in situ keratomileusis (LASIK) flap dehiscence during retinal detachment surgery. *Am J Ophthalmol.* 2002;134:265–266.

Retinal detachment surgery

Patients who have had prior scleral buckle surgery or vitrectomy may desire refractive surgery because of resultant myopia. Prior retinal detachment surgery can result in a myopic shift because of axial elongation of the eye from indentation of the scleral buckle. Refractive surgery can be considered in selected cases if there is anisometropia with good best-corrected visual acuity.

The retina should be extensively evaluated preoperatively. Referral to a retinal specialist should be made when indicated. The surgeon should determine whether the scleral buckle will interfere with placement of the suction ring during the microkeratome pass. If so, PRK may be considered instead of LASIK.

The patient must be informed that the role of the surgery is solely to treat the refractive error to correct anisometropia or to make her or him less dependent on corrective eye wear. Preoperative pathology, including preexisting macular pathology, will continue to limit the uncorrected and best-corrected visual acuity after refractive surgery. There are no published long-term series of the results of excimer laser vision correction in patients who have had prior retinal detachment surgery. Both the patient and the doctor should realize that the final visual results may not be as predictable as after other refractive surgeries. Unexpected corneal steepening has been reported in patients undergoing LASIK with previously placed scleral buckles.

Panozzo G, Parolini B. Relationships between vitreoretinal and refractive surgery. *Ophthalmology.* 2001;108:1663–1668.

Amblyopia and Strabismus in the Adult and Child

Amblyopia and anisometropic amblyopia

The prevalence of amblyopia is 2.5% of the population, with 0.6% representing anisometropic amblyopia. Anisometropia of more than 3.0 D between the two eyes will induce amblyopia. This form of amblyopia may be more resistant to traditional amblyopia therapy such as glasses, contact lenses, patching, or atropine 1% because of the large aniseikonia induced.

Assessment of the amblyopic patient should include a thorough history to identify any known cause of amblyopia, a history of ocular disease or surgery, assessment of ocular alignment and motility, and a thorough dilated exam. Referral to a strabismologist should be made when indicated. Preoperative counseling of an amblyopic patient must emphasize that even after LASIK the vision in the amblyopic eye will not be as good as in the normal eye. The patient should understand that the best-corrected visual acuity will be the same with or without refractive surgery.

LASIK has been successfully performed in the higher-myopic amblyopic eye in patients with anisometropic amblyopia. The performance of refractive surgery in the normal eye of the adult amblyopic patient is controversial. The decision depends on many factors, including the level of best-corrected visual acuity in the amblyopic eye and the normal eye and the ocular alignment. To increase safety, unilateral surgery in the amblyopic eye followed by surgery in the nonamblyopic eye can be considered. However, ocular deviation has been reported after unilateral LASIK for high myopia because of focus disparity resulting in esodeviation and impairment of fusion.

In many U.S. states, 20/40 visual acuity is needed in at least one eye to obtain an unrestricted driver's license. Once the best-corrected visual acuity is below 20/40 in the amblyopic eye, the patient is dependent on the normal eye for driving vision. In suburban or rural areas where driving is a necessary daily function, the loss of 20/40 vision in both eyes can be devastating. Consequently, some ophthalmologists may choose to only perform refractive surgery in the normal eye if the best-corrected visual acuity in the fellow amblyopic eye is 20/40 or better.

A patient with anisometropic amblyopia, for example, who is corrected to 20/40 with −7.0 D in the right eye and to 20/20 with −1.0 D in the left eye may be an excellent candidate for LASIK in the amblyopic right eye. This patient cannot tolerate glasses to correct the anisometropic amblyopia and may not want contact lenses. Even if the post-LASIK uncorrected visual acuity was less than 20/40 in the amblyopic eye, it would be better than the pre-LASIK uncorrected visual acuity of counting fingers.

If the post-LASIK uncorrected visual acuity in the amblyopic right eye improved to 20/40, the patient could request LASIK in the left eye for −1.0 D. However, if the patient was presbyopic, many surgeons would discourage further intervention and discuss potential advantages of the myopia. In a younger patient with accommodation, some surgeons would inform the patient of the potential risks associated with treating the better eye, but would perform the excimer laser vision correction.

If the best-corrected visual acuity in the amblyopic eye is 20/200 or worse, the patient is considered legally blind. In such cases, refractive surgery in the amblyopic eye may not offer much benefit and refractive surgery in the nonamblyopic eye is absolutely contraindicated.

Kim SK, Lee JB, Han SH, et al. Ocular deviation after unilateral laser in situ keratomileusis. *Yonsei Med J.* 2000;41:404–406.

Persistent diplopia has been reported after bilateral LASIK in a patient with anisometropic amblyopia and a history of intermittent diplopia in childhood. Preoperatively, this type of patient can adjust to the disparity of the retinal image sizes with spectacle correction. Refractive surgery can result in a dissimilar image size that the patient cannot fuse, resulting in diplopia because the patient lacks adequate fusion ability. This diplopia cannot be treated by prisms or muscle surgery.

Holland D, Amm M, de Decker W. Persisting diplopia after bilateral laser in situ keratomileusis. *J Cataract Refract Surg.* 2000;26:1555–1557.

Nemet P, Levinger S, Nemet A. Refractive surgery for refractive errors which cause strabismus. *Binocul Vis Strabismus Q.* 2002;17:187–190.

The use of excimer laser vision correction in children is controversial because their eyes and refractive state continue to change. More studies on the growing eye and the effect of excimer laser on the pediatric corneal endothelium are needed before the effect of refractive surgery in the pediatric age group can be fully understood. Consequently, these procedures are typically contraindicated in children.

There are numerous reports outside the United States of the "successful" performance of PRK and LASIK in children, mostly age 8 years and older, when conventional therapies failed. Most of these children underwent treatment in the more myopic eye to treat anisometropic amblyopia. Amblyopia can typically only be treated by age 8 or before. The refractive error was decreased and the visual acuity was maintained or improved in moderately amblyopic eyes. Refractive surgery did not improve the best-corrected visual acuity in older children with densely amblyopic eyes, and stereopsis did not improve. The limited effect on visual acuity was frequently attributable to the fact that the children were beyond amblyogenic age. Many authors have reported a myopic shift and haze after PRK or LASIK, possibly related to a more vigorous wound healing response that occurs in children.

General anesthesia was used to perform PRK in 40 children ages 1 to 6 years who were unable to wear glasses or contact lenses for high myopia or anisometropic amblyopia from myopia. Patients were treated for existing amblyopia. The mean best-corrected visual acuity improved from 20/70 to 20/40. The study found that 60% of eyes developed posttreatment corneal haze, with most patients demonstrating "increasing corneal clarity" within 1 year, although 2 of 27 patients required phototherapeutic keratectomy for the corneal haze. Regression of effect was attributed to the vigorous healing response and to axial myopic shift associated with growth.

Agarwal A, Agarwal A, Agarwal T, et al. Results of pediatric laser in situ keratomileusis. *J Cataract Refract Surg.* 2000;26:684–689.

Astle WF, Huang PT, Ells AL, et al. Photorefractive keratectomy in children. *J Cataract Refract Surg.* 2002;28:932–941.

Nassaralla BRA, Nassaralla JJ. Laser in situ keratomileusis in children 8–15 years old. *J Refract Surg.* 2001;17:519–524.

Nucci P, Drack AV. Refractive surgery for unilateral high myopia in children. *J AAPOS.* 2001;5:348–351.

Accommodative esotropia

Uncorrected hyperopia causes an increase in accommodation leading to accommodative convergence. In accommodative esotropia, esotropia results because of insufficient fusional divergence. Traditional optical treatment includes correction of hyperopia with glasses or contact lenses and muscle surgery for any residual esotropia (see BCSC Section 6, *Pediatric Ophthalmology and Strabismus*). While glasses or contact lenses are being worn, the esotropia is usually kept in check. Hyperopia typically decreases in adolescence, so emmetropia and resolution of the accommodative esotropia may occur with age. If significant hyperopia persists, glasses or contact lenses continue to be needed to control the esotropia.

It is extremely important to perform an adequate cycloplegic refraction on patients younger than 35 years of age who have intermittent strabismus or phoria. The surgeon must determine the accurate refraction to avoid inducing postoperative hyperopia. Otherwise, the postoperative hyperopia may result in new onset of an esotropia with an accommodative element.

There have been reports outside the United States of PRK and LASIK for adults with accommodative esotropia. Orthophoria or microesotropia was achieved after LASIK for hyperopia in accommodative esotropia in a series of 9 patients over 18 years of age. However, another study of LASIK in accommodative esotropia in patients from 10 to 52 years of age found that 42% of patients had no reduction in their esotropia and these patients could not be predicted on the basis of preoperative sensorimotor testing.

Hoyos JE, Cigales M, Hoyos-Chacon J, et al. Hyperopic laser in situ keratomileusis for refractive accommodative esotropia. *J Cataract Refract Surg.* 2002;28:1522–1529.

Stidham DB, Borissova O, Borissov V, et al. Effect of hyperopic laser in situ keratomileusis on ocular alignment and stereopsis in patients with accommodative esotropia. *Ophthalmology.* 2002;109:1148–1153.

Systemic Conditions

Human Immunodeficiency Virus

Little has been written on the performance of refractive surgery in patients with known human immunodeficiency virus (HIV) infection. Many surgeons counsel these patients against refractive surgery because of concerns about postoperative complications, including increased risk of infection associated with their immunosuppression. If the patient has progressed to acquired immunodeficiency syndrome (AIDS), the underlying severe immunosuppression must be the paramount consideration. More importantly, these patients should be monitored for vision-threatening diseases such as cytomegalovirus retinitis (see BCSC Section 12, *Retina and Vitreous*). Most ophthalmologists consider AIDS an absolute contraindication to refractive surgery.

As HIV-infected patients have begun to live productive lives for longer periods before the onset of AIDS, the question of the appropriateness of refractive surgery in this "healthier" population has become relevant. Uniform precautions must always be applied because the refractive surgeon may operate on patients who do not know they have been infected with viruses such as HIV or hepatitis. One concern is the vaporization of the corneal tissue and the potential for aerosolizing live virus during laser ablation, which could pose a risk to laser suite personnel.

In one study, excimer ablation of pseudorabies virus, a porcine-enveloped herpes virus similar to HIV and HSV, did not appear capable of causing infection by transmission through the air. The authors concluded that excimer laser ablation of the cornea in a patient infected with HIV is unlikely to pose a health hazard to the surgeon or the assistants. In another study, after excimer laser ablation of infected corneal stroma, polymerase chain reaction did not detect viable varicella virus (200 nm) but did detect viable polio particles (70 nm).

Whereas inhaled particles ≥5 μm are deposited in the bronchial, tracheal, nasopharyngeal, or nasal walls, particles smaller than 2 μm are deposited in the bronchioles and alveoli. Even if viral particles are not viable, the excimer laser plume produces particles of a mean diameter of 0.22 μm that are able to be inhaled. The health effects of inhaled particles from the plume have not yet been determined. There are anecdotal reports of respiratory ailments such as chronic bronchitis in laser surgeons. Canister filter masks can filter particles down to 0.1 μm and may be more protective than conventional surgical masks. In addition, evacuation of the laser plume may potentially decrease the amount of breathable debris.

Because of the many unknowns involved, most surgeons consider patients with known HIV to be poor candidates for refractive surgery. If a surgeon is considering performing excimer laser ablation in a "healthy" HIV-infected patient with a normal eye exam and excellent best-corrected vision, extra precautions should be exercised. The patient should be extensively counseled preoperatively concerning the visual risks of HIV and the lack of long-term follow-up of refractive surgery in this population. The surgeon should consider additional precautions for the operating room staff, such as wearing filter masks during the procedure and evacuating the laser plume.

Hagen KB, Kettering JD, Aprecia RM, et al. Lack of virus transmission by the excimer laser plume. *Am J Ophthalmol.* 1997;124:206–211.

Taravella MJ, Viega J, Luiszer F, et al. Respirable particles in the excimer laser plume. *J Cataract Refract Surg.* 2001;27:604–607.

Diabetes Mellitus

Diabetes mellitus affects 4% to 8% of Americans. Diabetic patients who are considering refractive surgery should have a thorough preoperative history and examination. The diabetic's blood sugar must be under good control at the time of examination to ensure an accurate refraction. A history of laser treatment for proliferative diabetic retinopathy or cystoid macular edema indicates visually significant diabetic complications that typically contraindicate refractive surgery. Any patient who has preexisting visually significant diabetic ocular complications is not a good refractive surgery candidate. Ocular examination should include inspection of the corneal epithelium to check the health of the ocular surface, detection of cataract formation, and detailed retinal examination.

There are few long-term studies of refractive surgery in the diabetic. A retrospective review of 30 eyes of diabetic patients who had LASIK 6 months earlier revealed a complication rate of 47% compared with a complication rate in the control group of 6.9%. The most common problems were related to epithelial healing and included epithelial defects and erosions. Although the uncorrected visual acuity was worse in the diabetic group than in controls, the difference was not statistically significant. There was a loss of 2 or more lines of best-corrected visual acuity in less than 1% of both the diabetic group and the control group. However, 6 diabetic eyes (6/30) required a mean time of 4.3 months to heal because of persistent epithelial defects. The authors concluded that the high complication rate in diabetics was explained by unmasking subclinical diabetic keratopathy.

The refractive surgeon should exercise caution in the selection of diabetic patients for refractive surgery. Intraoperative technique should be adjusted to ensure maximal epithelial health. In order to minimize corneal toxicity, the surgeon should use the minimal amount of topical anesthetic immediately before doing the procedure. Tears, not anesthetic, are used during the microkeratome pass.

Diabetic patients should be counseled preoperatively that there is an increased risk of postoperative complications and that there may be prolonged healing time after LASIK. In addition, the patient needs to be told that the procedure only treats the refractive error and not the natural history of the diabetes, which can lead to future diabetic ocular complications and associated visual loss.

Fraunfelder FW, Rich LR. Laser-assisted in situ keratomileusis: complications in diabetes mellitus. *Cornea.* 2002;21:246–248.

Connective Tissue Disease

Most surgeons consider active, uncontrolled connective tissue diseases such as systemic lupus erythematosus, polyarteritis nodosa, and so on to be contraindications to surface laser ablation because of reports of postoperative corneal melt and perforation. Late corneal scarring has been reported after PRK in a patient with systemic lupus erythematosus.

Cua IY, Pepose JS. Late corneal scarring after photorefractive keratectomy concurrent with development of systemic lupus erythematosus. *J Refract Surg.* 2002;18:750–752.

CHAPTER 11

Considerations After Refractive Surgery

The number of patients who have had refractive surgery continues to increase yearly. Ophthalmologists are beginning to be confronted with the management of other conditions, such as glaucoma and contact lens fitting, in patients who have had refractive surgery. In addition, the performance of IOL calculations or retinal detachment surgery presents additional challenges in this population. Finally, corneal transplantation may occasionally be needed later. A discussion of all these considerations after refractive surgery follows.

IOL Calculations After Refractive Surgery

The difficulties inherent in obtaining accurate IOL calculations after refractive surgery become more important as the population of patients who have undergone refractive surgery ages. Numerous formulas are available to calculate the IOL power prior to cataract surgery, which rely primarily on axial length, keratometric measurements, and desired postoperative refraction. While measurement of axial length after refractive surgery should still be accurate, determining the actual keratometric power of the post–refractive surgery cornea is problematic. The difficulty most likely arises from several factors. Small central optical zones after refractive surgery (especially after RK) can lead to inaccurate measurements, because keratometers and corneal topography units measure the corneal curvature several millimeters away from the center of the cornea. Also, the anterior and posterior corneal curvatures can be very different from each other after refractive surgery (especially after PRK, LASEK, or LASIK), leading to inaccurate results. Generally, if standard keratometry readings are used to calculate IOL power, the postoperative refraction will be hyperopic because the keratometry readings are higher than the real corneal power. It is not uncommon for IOL exchanges to be necessary in these cases due to refractive surprises.

A variety of methods to better estimate the central corneal power after refractive surgery have been developed. None of these methods is perfectly accurate, and different methods can lead to rather disparate values. The techniques are classified by whether they require information about refraction prior to or after refractive surgery or keratometry prior to refractive surgery. As many methods as possible to calculate the corneal power should be performed and these estimations should be compared with each other and with standard keratometric readings and corneal topographic central power and simulated K readings.

With Pre–Refractive Surgery Refraction and Keratometry and Post–Refractive Surgery Refraction

The most accurate IOL power calculation method is probably the "clinical history method," where pre–refractive surgery information is available. The precise calculation depends on exactly what clinical information is available. If preoperative refraction and keratometry readings are available, the change in spherical equivalent can be calculated at the spectacle plane or, better yet, at the corneal plane. The postoperative refraction used must be a stable refraction obtained several months after the refractive surgery but before any potential onset of induced myopia from a nuclear sclerotic cataract.

For example:

Preoperative average keratometry: 44.00 D
Preoperative spherical equivalent refraction (vertex distance 12 mm): -8.00 D
Preoperative refraction at the corneal plane:
$-8.00 \text{ D}/(1 - [0.012 \times -8.00 \text{ D}]) = -7.30 \text{ D}$
Postoperative spherical equivalent refraction (vertex distance 12 mm): -1.00 D
Postoperative refraction at the corneal plane:
$-1.00 \text{ D}/(1 - [0.012 \times -1.00 \text{ D}]) = -0.98 \text{ D}$
Change in manifest refraction at the corneal plane:
$-7.30 \text{ D} - (-0.98 \text{ D}) = -6.32 \text{ D}$
Postoperative estimated keratometry: $44.00 - 6.32 \text{ D} = 37.68 \text{ D}$

With Pre–Refractive Surgery Refraction and Keratometry

Another method, used when preoperative keratometry and refraction information is known, is to perform the IOL power calculation based on the pre–refractive surgery numbers, using the preoperative refraction (assuming the patient was plano after refractive surgery) as the desired refraction after cataract surgery.

For example:

Preoperative average keratometry: 44.0 D
Preoperative axial length: 25 mm
Preoperative spherical equivalent refraction: -8.0 D
IOL power using IOL calculation formula (A-constant 118.4): 25.0 D

With Pre–Refractive Surgery Refraction and Post–Refractive Surgery Refraction

When preoperative and postoperative refraction information is available after PRK or LASIK, but not preoperative keratometry information, one method is to simply subtract 20% of the spherical equivalent refractive change from the measured postoperative keratometry reading.

For example:

Preoperative spherical equivalent refraction: −8.0 D
Postoperative spherical equivalent refraction: −1.0 D
20% of change in spherical refraction: 0.2 × (−8.0 D − [−1.0 D]) = −1.4 D
Postoperative keratometry reading: 40.0 D
"New" postoperative keratometry reading: 40.0 D − 1.4 D = 38.6 D

With Pre–Refractive Surgery Refraction Only

Feiz and associates describe a theoretical nomogram for adjusting the IOL power after LASIK when the only preoperative data available is the refraction. The IOL calculation is performed with current manual keratometric measurements. The IOL power is then adjusted per their nomogram (Table 11-1).

With No Preoperative Information

When no preoperative information is available, the "hard contact lens method" can be used to calculate the corneal power. The best-corrected visual acuity needs to be at least 20/80 for this approach to work. First perform a manifest refraction. Then place a plano hard contact lens of known base curve (power) on the eye and perform another manifest refraction. If the manifest refraction does not change, then the cornea has the same power as the contact lens. If the refraction is more myopic, the contact lens is steeper (more

Table 11-1 Nomogram of IOL Power Adjustment for Emmetropia

AFTER MYOPIC LASIK:	
When the change in spherical equivalent induced by LASIK (D) is	Increase the IOL power (D) by
1.0	0.36
2.0	0.96
3.0	1.55
4.0	2.15
5.0	2.74
6.0	3.34
7.0	3.93
8.0	4.53
9.0	5.12
10.0	5.72
AFTER HYPEROPIC LASIK:	
When the change in spherical equivalent induced by LASIK (D) is	Decrease the IOL power (D) by
1.0	0.00
2.0	0.97
3.0	1.84
4.0	2.70
5.0	3.56
6.0	4.42

(From Feiz V, Mannis MJ, Garcia-Ferrer F, et al. Intraocular lens power calculation after laser in situ keratomileusis for myopia and hyperopia. *Cornea.* 2001;20:792–797.)

powerful) than the cornea by the amount of change in the refraction; the reverse holds true if the refraction is more hyperopic.

For example:

Current spherical equivalent manifest refraction: −1.0 D
Place a hard contact lens of known base curve (8.7 mm) and power (37.0 D)
Overrefraction: +2.0 D
Change in refraction: +2.0 D − (−1.0 D) = +3.0 D
Calculation of corneal power: 37.0 D + 3.0 D = 40.0 D

Conclusion

Randleman and associates found that either refractive history or hard contact lens overrefraction or an average of these two methods is the most accurate. They noted that the Feiz nomogram was not as accurate as these other methods.

In general, after calculations by several different methods are compared, the lowest corneal power obtained should be used. Whenever the postoperative refractive error is used to calculate IOL power, it should represent a stable refraction done several months after the refractive surgery so as not to be influenced by a myopic shift due to nuclear sclerosis.

The modern third-generation theoretical optical formulas (eg, Holladay 2, Hoffer Q, SRK/T, Haigis) tend to be better for post–refractive surgery IOL calculations than the empirical regression formulas (eg, SRK I, SRK II). The results of more than one IOL power formula should be compared and the highest IOL power selected.

Cataract surgery that is done after RK often induces the cornea to swell somewhat, causing excess flattening and a hyperopic shift. An IOL exchange should not be performed until the cornea and refraction stabilize, which may take several weeks. As corneal curvature does not tend to change much when cataract surgery is done after PRK or LASIK, it may be possible to examine a patient by retinoscopy or refraction immediately after the cataract surgery, and if the IOL power is not correct, to perform an IOL exchange right away. Preoperatively, patients need to be informed that IOL calculations are not as accurate if performed after refractive surgery and that additional surgery to attain a better refractive result may be required.

Feiz V, Mannis MJ, Garcia-Ferrer F, et al. Intraocular lens power calculation after laser in situ keratomileusis for myopia and hyperopia. *Cornea.* 2001;20:792–797.

Gimbel HV, Sun R. Accuracy and predictability of intraocular lens power calculation after laser in situ keratomileusis. *J Cataract Refract Surg.* 2001;27:571–576.

Kim JH, Lee DH, Joo CK. Measuring corneal power for intraocular lens power calculation after refractive surgery: comparison of methods. *J Cataract Refract Surg.* 2002;28:1932–1938.

Odenthal MT, Eggink CA, Melles G, et al. Clinical and theoretical results of intraocular lens power calculation for cataract surgery after photorefractive keratectomy for myopia. *Arch Ophthalmol.* 2002;120:431–438.

Randleman JB, Loupe DN, Song CD, et al. Intraocular lens power calculations after laser in situ keratomileusis. *Cornea.* 2002;22:751–755.

Seitz B, Langenbucher A. Intraocular lens calculations status after corneal refractive surgery. *Curr Opin Ophthalmol.* 2000;11:35–46.

Speicher L. Intraocular lens calculation status after corneal refractive surgery. *Curr Opin Ophthalmol.* 2001;12:17–29.

Retinal Detachment Repair After LASIK

Patients need to be informed that highly myopic eyes are still at increased risk of retinal detachment, even if they are made emmetropic after refractive surgery. The vitreoretinal surgeon should ask the patient if she or he has had prior refractive surgery. Eyes undergoing retinal detachment repair after LASIK are prone to flap problems, including flap dehiscence and micro- and macrostriae (see Table 6-1). The retinal surgeon may want to mark the edge of the flap prior to surgery to aid in flap replacement should it become dehisced. The risk of flap problems dramatically increases if the epithelium is debrided during the retinal detachment repair. Should a flap dehiscence occur, the flap needs to be carefully repositioned and the interface irrigated. A bandage soft contact lens may be placed at the end of surgery. Postoperatively, the patient should be followed closely for flap problems such as epithelial ingrowth and diffuse lamellar keratitis, especially if an epithelial defect was present in the flap. While the IOP needs to be monitored carefully in all patients after retinal detachment repair, especially when an intraocular gas bubble is used, several issues about IOP need to be kept in mind in post-LASIK patients. First, IOP measurements may be falsely low due to corneal thinning. Second, elevated IOP can cause a diffuse lamellar keratitis–like picture or even a fluid cleft between the flap and the stroma (resulting in an extremely low IOP measurement).

Corneal Transplantation After Refractive Surgery

Penetrating keratoplasty is, unfortunately, occasionally required after refractive surgery. Reasons for needing a corneal graft after refractive surgery include significant corneal scarring, irregular astigmatism, corneal ectasia, and corneal edema. Issues unrelated to refractive surgery, such as trauma or corneal edema after cataract surgery, can also necessitate penetrating keratoplasty surgery. Each refractive surgical procedure has unique reasons why a graft may be required and ways to avoid problems with the corneal transplant.

After RK, a graft may be required secondary to an incision into the visual axis; central scarring not responsive to phototherapeutic keratectomy with or without mitomycin; irregular astigmatism; contact lens intolerance; or progressive hyperopia. The RK incisions can gape or dehisce during penetrating keratoplasty trephination, preventing an even, uniform, and deep trephination. One method used to avoid RK wound gape/dehiscence is to mark the cornea with the trephine and then to reinforce the RK incisions outside the trephine mark with interrupted sutures, prior to trephination. The RK incisions may also gape peripheral to the graft/host margin, causing difficulty in obtaining a watertight seal at the end of surgery. X, mattress, or lasso sutures may be required to close these "stellate" wounds.

After PRK or LASEK, a corneal graft may be necessary due to central haze or an irregularity not responsive to phototherapeutic keratectomy with or without mitomycin;

irregular astigmatism; or rarely corneal ectasia. Fortunately, the corneal periphery is generally not thinned with the 6 to 8 mm ablation zones typically used, so corneal transplantation after PRK or LASEK is usually routine.

After LASIK, corneal transplantation may be required due to central scarring (eg, after infection, buttonhole) not responsive to phototherapeutic keratectomy with or without mitomycin; irregular astigmatism; or corneal ectasia. The main problem is that most LASIK flaps are larger than a typical trephine size (8 mm). Trephination through the LASIK flap increases the risk that the flap peripheral to the penetrating keratoplasty wound will dehisce. This complication may be avoidable by careful trephination and gentle suture technique that incorporates the LASIK flap under the penetrating keratoplasty suture.

There have been a few case reports of inadvertent use of donor tissue that had undergone prior LASIK. The risk of this untoward event will increase as the donor pool undergoes more LASIK. Eye banks need to develop better screening techniques to screen out such donor corneas. Should a post-LASIK eye inadvertently be used for corneal transplantation, the patient should be informed. A regraft may be required to address significant anisometropia.

Corneal transplantation after placement of intrastromal corneal ring segments is rarely required. The PMMA ring segments are typically near the edge of a standard penetrating keratoplasty, so the ring segments should be removed prior to penetrating keratoplasty, ideally well before the corneal transplant to allow the cornea to heal.

Penetrating keratoplasty is also rarely required after laser thermokeratoplasty or conductive keratoplasty. Trephination should be routine in such cases and the thermal scars should generally be incorporated in the corneal button. Even if they are not, they should not significantly affect wound architecture, graft healing, or corneal curvature.

Prior phakic IOL implants should generally not affect penetrating keratoplasty surgery. However, an important issue with phakic IOLs is the need to monitor for progressive endothelial cell loss, especially with anterior chamber IOLs. The IOL should probably be removed prior to development of corneal edema if progressive cell loss is noted.

Contact Lens Use After Refractive Surgery

Indications

Contact lenses can be employed as an adjunctive treatment in the management of the refractive surgery patient before, during, and after the procedure. Hydrophilic soft contact lenses can give a presbyopic patient an experience of monovision prior to refractive surgery, in order to avoid postoperative dissatisfaction. Years after refractive surgery, a presbyopic patient with excellent distance acuity may also find a contact lens helpful. Contact lenses can also be used preoperatively in a patient with a motility abnormality to simulate what the vision might be like following refractive surgery and to make certain there is no troublesome diplopia.

In the perioperative period hydrophilic soft contact lenses can be used to promote epithelialization, provide patient comfort, and perhaps reduce the risk of epithelial ingrowth and flap dehiscence in the case of a free cap. A soft contact lens can be used following a flap relift for enhancement, interface debridement, or removal of striae if the epithelial edge is irregular. Soft contact lenses can also relieve problems related to unexpected myopia or hyperopia after refractive surgery.

Rigid gas-permeable (RGP) lenses may be used to improve vision that is reduced because of irregular astigmatism. In this case RGP lenses may be more effective than soft lenses. Night vision symptoms may be reduced by using contact lenses if the symptoms are caused by uncorrected refractive error or irregular astigmatism. If the symptoms are caused by pupil dilation in the dark beyond the diameter of the treatment zone or by higher-order aberration, the symptoms may persist despite contact lens use.

General Principles

Obtaining the past ocular history, including any previous history of contact lens intolerance, can be helpful in predicting a patient's likelihood of success with contact lenses postoperatively. A history of conditions such as dry eye, blepharitis, atopic keratoconjunctivitis, giant papillary conjunctivitis, and infectious or sterile keratitis may adversely affect a patient's ability to tolerate contact lenses.

Contact lenses for refractive purposes should not be fitted until surgical wounds and serial refractions are stable. A trial fitting technique with overrefraction is the most practical approach to fitting an RGP lens after refractive surgery.

The clinician needs to discuss with the patient in lay terms the challenges of contact lens fitting after refractive surgery and, if possible, needs to align the patient's expectations with reality. A patient who successfully wore contact lenses prior to refractive surgery is more likely to be a successful contact lens wearer postoperatively than a patient who never wore contact lenses.

Contact Lenses After RK

Contact lens fitting is a practical solution following RK when further refractive surgery is contraindicated. Examples of useful situations include the presence of irregular astigmatism, fluctuating vision, corneal contour instability, or abnormalities of incisions or incision pattern.

Centration is a challenge in fitting contact lenses following RK because the corneal apex is displaced to the midperiphery. Popular fitting techniques involve referring to the preoperative keratometry and basing the initial lens trial on the flatter curvature. Contact lens stability is achieved by adjusting the lens diameter. In general larger-diameter lenses take advantage of the eyelid to achieve stability. However, they also increase the effective steepness of the lens due to increased sagittal depth. If preoperative keratometry is not available, the ophthalmologist can use a paracentral or midperipheral curve, as measured with postoperative computer-assisted topography, as a starting place.

When a successful fit cannot be obtained with a standard RGP lens, a reverse-geometry lens can be used. In contrast to the standard RGP lens, the reverse-geometry lens is flatter in the center and steeper in the periphery. The secondary curves can be designed as steep as necessary to achieve a stable fit. The larger the optical zone the flatter the fit.

Once a stable lens fit is obtained, overrefraction is performed to identify the optimal refractive correction. The tear film will fill the gap between the lens and the central cornea and result in a dramatic increase in refractive ametropia in the preoperative direction.

Hydrophilic soft lenses are also part of the contact lens armamentarium for RK. Toric soft lenses can be helpful when regular astigmatism is present. Soft lenses will be less helpful in cases of irregular astigmatism, because they are less able to mask an irregular surface. Soft lenses that typically drape the limbus may stimulate corneal neovascularization, especially when the lens is fitted more tightly. Neovascular proliferation may progress centrally, tracking along the corneal incisions.

Bacterial keratitis is always a risk in the contact lens user. A corneal infection near a deep RK scar may more rapidly progress posteriorly. Because of diurnal variation that occurs after RK, an adequate lens correction in the early morning may be inadequate later in the day. The patient may require lenses of a different power later in the day.

Contact Lens Fitting After PRK

Immediately following PRK, a soft contact lens is placed on the cornea as a bandage to help promote epithelialization and reduce discomfort. The lens is worn on an extended-wear basis until the corneal epithelium has healed. Healing time is dependent on the size of the epithelial defect created, which is determined by the treatment zone; the epithelial defect is usually closed within 3 to 7 days. A tight-fitting lens with evidence of corneal hypoxia (such as edema, folds in Descemet's membrane, or iritis) should be removed. In some cases, the lens will need to be exchanged for a properly fitting lens if an epithelial defect is still present. However, the patient should be warned that once the lens is removed there may be a marked increase in discomfort despite the lens replacement.

The PRK patient should preferably not be fitted in a contact lens for refractive purposes until the surface is well healed and the refractive correction and corneal contour have stabilized. The corneal contour after hyperopic correction may not stabilize for up to 6 months following surgery. Topical corticosteroids are often used for months following PRK. Ideally the patient should be off topical corticosteroids prior to lens fitting to reduce the risk of infectious keratitis, and there should be little or no subepithelial haze.

Contact lens fitting after PRK may be less challenging than after RK because the disparity between the central and peripheral curves may not be as dramatic. There are no risks related to deep incisions in PRK. Long-term stability may never be achieved in some RK patients; in contrast, once the refractive error stabilizes after PRK, it tends to remain stable.

In the absence of irregular astigmatism and significant haze after PRK, a soft contact lens can provide a comfortable, stable fit resulting in good visual function. Toric soft lenses can be used to treat regular astigmatism, and bifocal lenses are available for the presbyopic post-PRK patient.

An RGP lens is a better option when irregular astigmatism is present. When the contour disparity between the central and midperipheral cornea is great, reverse-geometry fitting may be helpful. An appropriate goal for fitting an RGP lens is slight clearance of the central cornea, good alignment over the midperipheral cornea, and minimal peripheral lift-off. Aspheric RGP lenses may be better than standard RGP lenses at distributing lens contact in the midperiphery.

Contact Lens Fitting After LASIK

The indications for contact lens fitting after LASIK are similar to those following other types of refractive surgery. The corneal contour following LASIK for myopia is usually stable by 3 months postoperatively; following LASIK for hyperopia, however, it can take up to 6 months for the cornea to stabilize. Retreatment is relatively easy to perform for at least 1 year following LASIK surgery, because the flap can easily be relifted. In many cases the flap can be relatively easy to lift even several years following the initial procedure. Contact lens fitting following initial surgery is generally not considered until a decision has been made regarding retreatment. If a large over- or undercorrection has occurred, a contact lens can be used to provide adequate visual function. However, most surgeons prefer not to have the patient inserting a contact lens into an eye with a newly created flap.

After LASIK surgery, topical corticosteroids are usually used for up to 1 week, in contrast to PRK, where anti-inflammatory medication may be used for months. Thus, the use of corticosteroids in LASIK usually does not prevent contact lens use for refractive purposes. A soft contact lens may be used immediately after LASIK surgery to promote epithelialization and to prevent epithelial ingrowth. It is generally used for a day or two on an extended-wear basis and then removed by the surgeon. Daily wear contact lenses for refractive purposes should not be considered until the surgeon feels the risk of flap displacement is low. Just as with PRK the patient can be fitted with hydrophilic soft lenses, soft toric lenses, standard or aspheric RGP lenses, bifocal lenses, or reverse-geometry lenses.

Contact Lens Assisted, Pharmacologically Induced Keratosteepening (CLAPIKS)

CLAPIKS is a means for treating consecutive hyperopia following PRK or LASIK. Overcorrected myopia and undercorrected hyperopia have both been treated. The patient is given a tight-fitting soft contact lens to use on an extended-wear basis and ketorolac tromethamine 0.5% (Acular) to administer 4 times per day. The patient is followed on a weekly basis until the desired refractive error is obtained. Treatment is continued for an additional 2 weeks to reduce the tendency for regression. The ketorolac is increased to 6 times per day if no effect is noted.

The theory behind this treatment is that the contact lens wear increases drug penetration into the cornea by inducing hypoxia, which reduces epithelial metabolism, decreases cell mitosis, and reduces tight junctions between cells. Upon penetration, the medication should theoretically induce corneal steepening by causing anterior stromal thickening and basal epithelial pleomorphism. It is also possible that the contact hypoxia alone may induce increased corneal steepening.

McDonald and Mertins reported an improvement in visual acuity in 12 of 14 eyes tested. Patients were treated starting from 1 to 36 weeks following refractive surgery. The average change in refractive power overall was 1.05 D. The mean number of weeks to achieve a measurable effect was 1.71. Posttreatment follow-up ranged from 8 to 72 weeks.

Potential risks of using a tight-fitting lens on an extended-wear basis are corneal edema, iritis, sterile or infectious keratitis, and corneal neovascularization. While the ketorolac may reduce inflammation associated with the contact lens, the patient should be watched closely for signs of contact lens intolerance. Long-term use of any preserved topical medication can be associated with toxicity. Further study of large series of patients with adequate follow-up will reveal the long-term benefit of this procedure and determine whether it becomes a well-accepted technique for managing postoperative hyperopia.

Augustine JM, Gonzalez K. Manage overcorrected LASIK with CLAPIKS. *Prim Care Optom News.* 2001;10:21.

McDonald JE, Mertins A. Contact lens assisted, pharmacologically induced keratosteepening (CLAPIKS). In: Durrie DS, O'Brien TP, eds. *Refractive Surgery: Back to the Future.* San Francisco: American Academy of Ophthalmology; 2002.

Scheid TR. Contact lens fitting and management after refractive surgery. In: Scheid TR, ed. *Clinical Manual of Specialized Contact Lens Prescribing.* Boston: Butterworth-Heinemann; 2002:127.

Glaucoma After Refractive Surgery

The force required for applanation of a Goldmann tonometer is proportional to the central corneal thickness. As a result, an eye that has a thin central cornea may have an artifactually low IOP as measured by Goldmann tonometry. Patients with normal-tension glaucoma have significantly thinner corneas than patients with primary open-angle glaucoma. When a correction factor based on corneal thickness is applied, over 30% of these patients will demonstrate abnormally high IOP. The correction factor may be less with both the Tono-Pen and the pneumotonometer.

An artifactual IOP reduction occurs following PRK and LASIK for myopia, both of which reduce central corneal thickness. Similar inaccuracies of IOP measurement can occur with PRK and LASIK for hyperopia. The mean fall in IOP measurement following excimer laser refractive surgery is 0.63 mm Hg per diopter of correction with fairly wide variation. Postoperatively, some patients may experience no change in IOP measurement, while for others an increase may occur. In general the reduction of IOP is greater for LASIK than for PRK. PRK patients with a preoperative refractive error <-5.00 D may have a negligible decrease in IOP.

Measuring IOP from the nasal side following LASIK surgery has been shown to reduce the artifactual IOP reduction by half (3.9 to 2.0 mm Hg). These data support the use of the Tono-Pen or pneumotonometer from the side (ie, over the uninvolved cornea) to minimize the artifactual IOP reduction after excimer laser refractive surgery. While some refractive surgeons cautiously measure IOP as soon as a week after LASIK, others wait a month or more because of concerns about disrupting the flap.

When topical corticosteroids are used after refractive surgery, it is important to recognize the serious risk posed by corticosteroid-induced IOP elevation, particularly because accurate IOP measurement is difficult to obtain. By 3 months postoperatively, up to 15% of PRK patients may develop an IOP above 22 mm Hg. Men appear to be more vulnerable than women to the corticosteroid effect. If the actual elevation of IOP is not detected, optic nerve damage and visual field loss can occur.

In patients with diffuse lamellar keratitis following LASIK, aqueous fluid may accumulate in the flap interface and falsely lower IOP measurement. Glaucomatous optic nerve damage and visual field loss has been reported in this setting. A syndrome of diffuse lamellar keratitis (with onset after the first postoperative week) associated with elevated IOP has been described. The syndrome does not respond to increased corticosteroids, but rather resolves upon lowering of the IOP.

When prolonged topical corticosteroids are used postoperatively, periodic careful disc evaluation is essential. Stereo disc photographs may facilitate the evaluation. Periodic visual fields may be more effective than IOP measurement for identifying at-risk patients before severe visual field loss occurs (see Figure 10-2).

Refractive surgery patients who develop glaucoma are initially treated with IOP-lowering medications along with careful measurement of the IOP. If medications or laser are insufficient for lowering IOP, glaucoma surgery may be recommended. Patients who have had refractive surgery should be warned prior to glaucoma surgery of the potential for transient vision loss from inflammation, hypotony, or change in refractive error. The glaucoma surgeon should be made aware of the patient's previous LASIK in order to avoid trauma to the corneal flap.

Belin MW, Hannush SB, Yau CW, et al. Elevated intraocular pressure-induced interlamellar stromal keratitis. *Ophthalmology.* 2002;109:1929–1933.

Brandt JD, Beiser JA, Kass MA. Central corneal thickness in the Ocular Hypertension Treatment Study (OHTS). *Ophthalmology.* 2001;108:1779–1788.

Copt RPTR, Mermoud A. Corneal thickness in ocular hypertension, primary open-angle glaucoma, and normal tension glaucoma. *Arch Ophthalmol.* 1999;117:14.

Dietze PJ, Oram O, Kohnen T, et al. Visual function following trabeculectomy: effect on corneal topography and contrast sensitivity. *J Glaucoma.* 1997;6:99–103.

Dohadwala AAMR, Damji KF. Positive correlation between Tono-Pen intraocular pressure and central corneal thickness. *Ophthalmology.* 1998;105:1849.

Ehlers NBT, Sperling S. Applanation tonometry and central corneal thickness. *Acta Ophthalmol.* 1975;53:34.

Gimeno JA, Munoz LA, Valenzuela LA, et al. Influence of refraction on tonometric readings after photorefractive keratectomy and laser assisted in situ keratomileusis. *Cornea.* 2000;19:512–516.

Hamilton DRME, Rich LF, Maloney RK. Steroid-induced glaucoma after laser in situ keratomileusis associated with interface fluid. *Ophthalmology.* 2002;109:659.

Kass MA, Heuer DK, Higginbotham EJ, et al. The ocular hypertension study: a randomized trial determines that topical ocular hypotensive medication delays or prevents the onset of primary open-angle glaucoma. *Arch Ophthalmol.* 2002;120:701–713.

Lee GA, Khaw PT, Ficker LA, et al. The corneal thickness and intraocular pressure story: where are we now? *Clin Exper Ophthalmol.* 2002;30:334–337.

Pang G, Wang Z, Zheng W, et al. [Glucocorticoid-induced ocular hypertension after photorefractive keratectomy]. *Zhongguo Yi Xue Ke Xue Yuan Xue Bao.* 1995;17:115–119.

Park HJ, Uhm KB, Hong C. Reduction in intraocular pressure after laser in situ keratomileusis. *J Cataract Refract Surg.* 2001;27:303–309.

Whitacre MMSR, Hassanein K. The effect of corneal thickness on applanation tonometry. *Am J Ophthalmol.* 1993;115:1993.

Basic Texts

Refractive Surgery

Azar DT. *Refractive Surgery.* New York: McGraw-Hill; 1997.

Boyd BF, ed. *LASIK and Beyond LASIK: Wavefront Analysis and Customized Ablation.* Panama and Bogota: Highlights of Ophthalmology, Inc; 2001.

Hardten DR, Lindstrom RL, Davis EA. *Phakic IOLs.* Thorofare, NJ: Slack; 2004.

Probst LE, ed. *LASIK: Advances, Controversies, and Custom.* Thorofare, NJ: Slack; 2004.

Troutman RC, Buzard KA. *Corneal Astigmatism: Etiology, Prevention, and Management.* St Louis: Mosby-Year Book; 1992.

Related Academy Materials

Focal Points: Clinical Modules for Ophthalmologists

Koch DD. Cataract surgery after refractive surgery (Module 5, 2001).
Lawless MA. Surgical correction of hyperopia (Module 4, 2004).
L'Esperance FA. Choosing the appropriate PRK patient (Module 9, 1998).
Price, Jr. FW. Lasik (Module 3, 2000).
Sher NA. Postoperative management of the PRK patient (Module 10, 1998).

Multimedia

Eye Care Skills on CD-ROM (all seven titles from the Eye Care Skills for the Primary Care Physician Series) (2001).
Lane SS, Hardten DR, Probst LE, et al. *LEO Clinical Update Course on Refractive Surgery* (CD-ROM, 2001).
Sher NA, ed. *External Disease and Cornea: A Multimedia Collection With Refractive Surgery Supplement* (1994, 2000).

Ophthalmic Technology Assessments

Ophthalmic Technology Assessment Committee. *Excimer Laser Photorefractive Keratectomy (PRK) for Myopia and Astigmatism* (1994).
Ophthalmic Technology Assessment Committee. *Intrastromal Corneal Ring Segments for Low Myopia* (2001).
Ophthalmic Technology Assessment Committee. *Laser In Situ Keratomileusis for Myopia and Astigmatism: Safety and Efficacy* (2002).
Ophthalmic Technology Assessment Committee. *Laser In Situ Keratomileusis for Hyperopia, Hyperopic Astigmatism, and Mixed Astigmatism* (2004).

Preferred Practice Patterns

Preferred Practice Patterns Committee, Refractive Errors Panel. *Refractive Errors* (2002).

LEO Specialty Clinical Update Online

Lindstrom RL, ed. *Refractive Management/Intervention,* Volume 1 (2004).

To order any of these materials, please call the Academy's Customer Service number at (415) 561-8540, or order online at www.aao.org.

Credit Reporting Form

Basic and Clinical Science Course, 2005–2006
Section 13

The American Academy of Ophthalmology is accredited by the Accreditation Council for Continuing Medical Education to provide continuing medical education for physicians.

The American Academy of Ophthalmology designates this educational activity for a maximum of 30 category 1 credits toward the AMA Physician's Recognition Award. Each physician should claim only those hours of credit that he/she actually spent in the activity.

The American Medical Association has determined that non-US licensed physicians who participate in this CME activity are eligible for AMA PRA category 1 credit.

If you wish to claim continuing medical education credit for your study of this section, you may claim your credit online or fill in the required forms and mail or fax them to the Academy.

To use the forms:

1. Complete the study questions and mark your answers on the Section Completion Form.
2. Complete the Section Evaluation.
3. Fill in and sign the statement below.
4. Return this page and the required forms by mail or fax to the CME Registrar (see below).

To claim credit online:

1. Log on to the Academy website (www.aao.org).
2. Go to Education Resource Center; click on CME Central.
3. Follow the instructions.

Important: These completed forms or the online claim must be received at the Academy within 3 years of purchase.

I hereby certify that I have spent _____ (up to 30) hours of study on the curriculum of this section and that I have completed the Study Questions.

Signature: ____
Date

Name: ____

Address: ____

City and State: ______________________________ Zip: ____________

Telephone: (________) ____________________ Academy Member ID# ____________________
area code

Please return completed forms to:
American Academy of Ophthalmology
P.O. Box 7424
San Francisco, CA 94120-7424
Attn: CME Registrar, Customer Service

Or you may fax them to: 415-561-8575

2005–2006
Section Completion Form

Basic and Clinical Science Course

Answer Sheet for Section 13

Question	Answer	Question	Answer	Question	Answer
1	a b c d e	17	a b c d	33	a b c d e
2	a b c d e	18	a b c d	34	a b c d e
3	a b c d e	19	a b c d	35	a b c d e
4	a b c d	20	a b c d	36	a b c d
5	a b c d	21	a b c d	37	a b c d
6	a b c d	22	a b c d	38	a b c d
7	a b c d	23	a b c d	39	a b c d
8	a b c d	24	a b c d	40	a b c d
9	a b c d	25	a b c d	41	a b c d e
10	a b c d	26	a b c d e	42	a b c d e
11	a b c d	27	a b c d	43	a b c d e
12	a b c d e	28	a b c d e	44	a b c d
13	a b c d	29	a b c d e	45	a b c d
14	a b c d	30	a b c d	46	a b c d
15	a b c d	31	a b c d e	47	a b c d e
16	a b c d	32	a b c d e	48	a b c d e

Section Evaluation

Please complete this CME questionnaire.

1. To what degree will you use knowledge from BCSC Section 13 in your practice?
   - ☐ Regularly
   - ☐ Sometimes
   - ☐ Rarely

2. Please review the stated objectives for BCSC Section 13. How effective was the material at meeting those objectives?
   - ☐ All objectives were met.
   - ☐ Most objectives were met.
   - ☐ Some objectives were met.
   - ☐ Few or no objectives were met.

3. To what degree is BCSC Section 13 likely to have a positive impact on health outcomes of your patients?
   - ☐ Extremely likely
   - ☐ Highly likely
   - ☐ Somewhat likely
   - ☐ Not at all likely

4. After you review the stated objectives for BCSC Section 13, please let us know of any additional knowledge, skills, or information useful to your practice that were acquired but were not included in the objectives. [Optional]

5. Was BCSC Section 13 free of commercial bias?
   - ☐ Yes
   - ☐ No

6. If you selected "No" in the previous question, please comment. [Optional]

7. Please tell us what might improve the applicability of BCSC to your practice. [Optional]

Study Questions

Although a concerted effort has been made to avoid ambiguity and redundancy in these questions, the authors recognize that differences of opinion may occur regarding the "best" answer. The discussions are provided to demonstrate the rationale used to derive the answer. They may also be helpful in confirming that your approach to the problem was correct or, if necessary, in fixing the principle in your memory. Where relevant, additional references are given.

1. Which of the following is true regarding keratoconus?
   a. Patients with keratoconus have corneal thinning in the paracentral region.
   b. LASIK should be avoided in keratoconus.
   c. Topography is helpful in diagnosing keratoconus in the absence of clinical findings.
   d. All of the above are true.
   e. None of the above are true.
2. Which of the following is true after conventional laser ablations for myopia (LASIK, LASEK, or PRK)?
   a. Lower-order (second-order) aberrations are generally reduced.
   b. Higher-order aberrations often increase.
   c. The central corneal curvature is flattened and the corneal apical radius of curvature is increased.
   d. Corneal asphericity changes often accompany myopic laser ablations.
   e. All of the above are true.
3. Which of the following is correct based on Munnerlyn's approximation of the depth of ablation after PRK for myopia?
   a. The ablation depth is proportional to the treatment circumference.
   b. For the same amount of intended dioptric correction, increasing the size of the ablation zone results in deeper treatment.
   c. The ablation depth is proportional to the square of the intended dioptric correction.
   d. All of the above are true.
   e. None of the above are true.
4. Contact lenses should not be worn for at least what period of time before the refraction and treatment?
   a. Soft contact lenses, 3 days; rigid gas-permeable contact lenses, 7 days
   b. Soft contact lenses, 3 days; rigid gas-permeable contact lenses, 10 days
   c. Soft contact lenses, 7 days; rigid gas-permeable contact lenses, 10 days
   d. Soft contact lenses, 3–14 days; rigid gas-permeable contact lenses, 14–21 days

5. Important aspects of the preoperative refractive surgery evaluation include all the following *except:*
   a. Social history
   b. Past ocular history
   c. Past and current medical history
   d. None of the above
6. Required parts of the preoperative refractive surgery examination include all of the following *except:*
   a. Slit-lamp examination
   b. Measurement of corneal curvature
   c. Specular microscopy
   d. Corneal thickness measurement
7. Important issues when considering monovision include all of the following *except:*
   a. Patient age
   b. Degree of myopia
   c. Success with monovision in the past
   d. Ocular dominance
8. LASIK and PRK are both commonly used to treat which refractive range?
   a. –14 to +8 D
   b. –8 to +4 D
   c. –6 to +2 D
   d. –5 to +5 D
9. Thermokeratoplasty (laser thermal keratoplasty and/or conductive keratoplasty):
   a. Is best for patients over 40 years of age
   b. Is not associated with significant refractive regression
   c. Creates a multifocal cornea, giving most patients good uncorrected distance and near vision
   d. Is effective at treating astigmatism
10. All of the following are true about radial keratotomy (RK) except which statement?
    a. RK is not a commonly performed refractive surgical procedure.
    b. Diurnal fluctuations occur after RK because the cornea is flatter upon awakening and steepens during waking hours.
    c. In the Prospective Evaluation of Radial Keratotomy (PERK) study, 43% of eyes showed a change of ≥1 D in the hyperopic direction between 6 months and 10 years postoperatively.
    d. Intersecting radial and astigmatic incisions are sometimes performed in order to enhance the surgical outcomes.

11. Which of the following is true regarding arcuate keratotomy (AK) and/or limbal relaxing incisions (LRIs)?
    a. LRIs are used in the management of high degrees of postkeratoplasty astigmatism.
    b. LRIs and AK correct astigmatism without inducing a substantial change of the spherical equivalent of the preoperative refraction.
    c. LRIs and AK are placed in the peripheral cornea just anterior to the limbus.
    d. Coupling, a hallmark of LRIs and AK, results in flattening of the surgical meridian and concomitant flattening of the orthogonal meridian.
12. In the previously normal cornea, all of the following are complications of incisional keratotomy (radial and astigmatic) *except:*
    a. Corneal ectasia
    b. Corneal perforation
    c. Traumatic rupture of the globe through the keratotomy incision
    d. Bacterial keratitis
    e. Loss of best spectacle-corrected visual acuity
13. The mechanism for necrosis of the stroma overlying a corneal inlay made of an impermeable substance such as glass can best be described as
    a. Reflection of ultraviolet light from the inlay, causing keratocyte death
    b. Hypoxia of the overlying stroma
    c. Lack of nutrients from the underlying cornea
    d. Trauma at the time of surgery
14. Epikeratoplasty to treat myopia is seldom performed today primarily because of which reason?
    a. The refractive results were disappointing when compared with other procedures.
    b. Central scarring often caused a loss of vision.
    c. The incidence of accidental perforation into the anterior chamber during the procedure was considered too high.
    d. The lens material was made of a special copolymer that was difficult to lathe into the proper shape.
15. All of the following are relative advantages of intrastromal corneal ring segments (Intacs) *except:*
    a. The refractive result is potentially reversible.
    b. The central clear zone is not violated.
    c. Astigmatism is easily corrected.
    d. The ring segments can be replaced with segments of a different size.
16. Compared with thinner corneal ring segments (Intacs), the 0.35 mm ring segments
    a. Correct lower levels of myopia
    b. Are not removed as often
    c. Cause more visual disturbances
    d. Are more likely to result in better uncorrected vision

17. Corneal ring segments (Intacs) have been used on an off-label basis (not FDA approved) to treat all the following conditions *except:*
    a. Mild keratoconus
    b. Aphakia
    c. Ectasia after LASIK
    d. Myopia after LASIK
18. The laser–tissue interaction by which the excimer laser reshapes the cornea is
    a. Photocoagulation
    b. Photodisruption
    c. Photoablation
    d. Photodynamic
19. Overcorrection in PRK has been associated with de-epithelialization using which technique?
    a. Dilute absolute alcohol
    b. A slow and precise manual scraping
    c. A rotary brush
    d. Laser scrape
20. Compared with scanning lasers, broad-beam lasers are associated with a higher incidence of which complication?
    a. Persistent epithelial defects
    b. Central islands
    c. Dry eyes
    d. Haze
21. Larger-diameter flaps are associated with which of the following?
    a. Steep corneal curvature
    b. Low microkeratome suction
    c. Thicker corneas
    d. Reused blades
22. The LASIK flap adheres to the cornea on the first postoperative day because of which of the following?
    a. The endothelial pump
    b. Re-epithelialization of the gutter
    c. Sutures
    d. A bandage soft contact lens
23. LASIK enhancements are most commonly performed by which of the following methods?
    a. Performing PRK on the flap surface
    b. Cutting a new flap
    c. Lifting the original flap
    d. Reducing the remaining stromal bed to less than 250 μm

24. Dry eye after LASIK is attributed to which of the following?
    a. De-innervation of the flap
    b. Phototoxicity to the conjunctival goblet cells
    c. Lacrimal gland insufficiency
    d. Medicamentosa

25. Diffuse lamellar keratitis
    a. Is infectious
    b. Occurs only in primary LASIK procedures
    c. Is usually treated with topical NSAIDs
    d. Can cause corneal melting if undertreated

26. Which one of the following types of lasers was approved for laser thermokeratoplasty by the FDA in the 1990s?
    a. Holmium:yttrium-aluminum-garnet
    b. Cobalt magnesium fluoride
    c. Argon fluoride
    d. Argon
    e. CO_2

27. Which of the following is true regarding conductive keratoplasty?
    a. Conductive keratoplasty uses a probe to directly heat only the corneal stroma.
    b. Conductive keratoplasty is approved for the temporary treatment of 0.75 to 3.00 D of hyperopia with astigmatism of 0.75 D or less.
    c. Conductive keratoplasty is contraindicated for patients with a decentered corneal apex.
    d. After conductive keratoplasty there is a gradual drift of the refractive error toward increasing myopia.

28. How is heat applied to the cornea during conductive keratoplasty?
    a. A probe delivers localized laser pulses to surrounding tissue.
    b. The tip of the probe applies heat directly to the corneal stroma.
    c. The tip of the probe applies heat directly to both the corneal epithelium and the stroma.
    d. Radiofrequency energy flows through the conducting tip to the eyelid speculum.
    e. None of the above are true.

29. Which of the following statements regarding laser thermokeratoplasty is false?
    a. The laser emits light in the infrared region.
    b. A high degree of treatment regression was observed.
    c. The laser leads to corneal shrinkage by creating a thermal gradient, in which the epithelial surface is hotter than the deeper stroma.
    d. Laser thermokeratoplasty is approved for treatment of up to 4.00 D of hyperopia with less than 1.00 D of astigmatism.
    e. None of the above are false.

30. Which one of the following statements is false?

    a. Conductive keratoplasty is approved for treatment of patients with a spherical equivalent of +0.75 to +3.00 D and up to 0.75 D of astigmatism.
    b. Laser thermokeratoplasty is approved for treatment of patients with a spherical equivalent of +0.75 to +2.50 D and less than 1.00 D of astigmatism.
    c. Laser thermokeratoplasty can involve placement of 8 treatment spots simultaneously, whereas conductive keratoplasty involves placement of treatment spots individually.
    d. Potential off-label use of conductive keratoplasty for a patient with +1.50 D of astigmatism at axis 180 would involve placing treatment spots at the 180° meridian.

31. Which of the following statements about PIOLs is true?

    a. The PIOL is inserted after the cataract has been removed.
    b. PIOLs are used in conjunction with clear lens extraction.
    c. PIOLs can correct myopia and hyperopia.
    d. A PIOL cannot be used if the cornea is thin.
    e. A PIOL should not be used if the cornea is flat.

32. Which of the following is not an advantage of bioptics?

    a. Bioptics extends the range of refractive error that can be treated.
    b. Bioptics has the benefit of being adjustable.
    c. Bioptics has the benefit of being less limited by corneal thickness than LASIK.
    d. Bioptics can be performed with a PCPIOL or an iris claw lens.
    e. Bioptics corrects the need for reading glasses in the presbyopic patient by virtue of its dual lens capability.

33. Which of the following statements about PIOLs is false?

    a. Since the optic of all PIOLs is foldable, astigmatism is not a significant problem.
    b. Endophthalmitis is a risk of this procedure.
    c. If the patient develops a cataract at a later time, the PIOL will need to be removed.
    d. No matter which model of PIOL is used, a stable cycloplegic refraction obtained after discontinuing contact lens wear is necessary.
    e. A healthy corneal endothelium is a requirement for PIOL use.

34. The ideal candidate for a multifocal IOL has which of the following characteristics?

    a. The patient has >1.5 D of astigmatism upon cycloplegic refraction.
    b. The pupil is <4 mm diameter.
    c. The patient has good potential vision.
    d. The patient seeks to minimize glare.
    e. The patient requests unilateral surgery.

35. Which of the following statements about clear lens extraction is true?
    a. The risk of retinal detachment peaks within 3 months of surgery and then remains stable.
    b. There is a decreased risk of retinal detachment following Nd:YAG laser posterior capsulotomy.
    c. Clear lens extraction in the high myope is similar to surgery in the high hyperope.
    d. If the predicted IOL power is very low, an IOL should not be used in order to minimize the surgical risk.
    e. One advantage of clear lensectomy over LASIK in the very high myope is that clear lensectomy does not significantly alter the corneal contour.
36. Recent studies contradicting the Schachar theory of accommodation include all of the following *except:*
    a. Scanning electron microscopy in human eye tissues reveals no zonular insertions at the anterior ciliary muscle.
    b. Improved near vision in some patients after scleral expansion surgery is due to small changes in accommodative amplitude shown on infrared optometry.
    c. Crystalline lens diameter decreases with accommodation on various imaging techniques.
    d. Scanning laser imaging shows that the focal length of the crystalline lens remains unchanged with application of equatorial radial stretching forces.
37. Which person would be the least appropriate candidate for conductive keratoplasty treatment for presbyopia?
    a. A 47-year-old long-haul truck driver with a distance manifest refraction of +1.25 sphere OU
    b. A 56-year-old emmetropic nurse supervisor
    c. A 44-year-old lawyer with a manifest refraction of +1.75 OU
    d. A 36-year-old librarian with a manifest refraction of +0.50 OU
38. Presbyopia progression theories are associated with all of the following physiologic findings *except:*
    a. A decreased response of the anterior lens curvature to a posterior vitreous pressure gradient generated by ciliary body contraction
    b. A decrease in ciliary muscle strength of approximately ⅓ by age 85
    c. A decrease in lens capsule elasticity
    d. An increase in lens volume and anteroposterior (axial) lens thickness
39. Which of the following (surgical) approaches to presbyopia reversal involve an actual increase in accommodative amplitude with accommodative effort?
    a. Scleral expansion bands
    b. Pupillary constriction with near effort after multifocal corneal ablation
    c. Hinged IOL placement after clear lens extraction
    d. Anterior ciliary sclerotomy with the erbium:YAG laser

40. Which of the following statements regarding the catenary theory of accommodation is true?
    a. Zonular fibers are under tension during the accommodated state.
    b. In this model, presbyopia involves age-related increasing lens volume with reduced curvature response of the anterior lens surface to posterior pressure on the lens.
    c. This theory helps explain the reduced accommodative amplitude typically seen after posterior vitrectomy.
    d. Ciliary body contraction during accommodation generates an increased anterior chamber pressure relative to that of the vitreous cavity.

41. Which of the following conditions is an absolute contraindication to refractive surgery?
    a. Dry eyes
    b. Glaucoma
    c. Scleral buckle
    d. Herpes virus
    e. Amblyopia with vision <20/200

42. Which of the following refractive surgery procedures is under clinical investigation for treatment of keratoconus?
    a. PRK
    b. LASIK
    c. Holmium laser
    d. Conductive keratoplasty
    e. Intrastromal corneal ring segments (Intacs)

43. Which of the following is false concerning LASIK and glaucoma?
    a. IOP increases to more than 65 mm Hg when suction is applied.
    b. Central corneal thickness must be considered in evaluation of applanation IOP.
    c. Ocular hypertension is not a contraindication to LASIK.
    d. The medical regimen should always be determined after LASIK is performed so that the post-LASIK IOP can be measured before instituting therapy.
    e. LASIK is contraindicated in any patient with marked optic nerve cupping, visual field loss, or loss of visual acuity.

44. Important pieces of information when attempting to calculate IOL power after refractive surgery include all the following *except:*
    a. Preoperative axial length
    b. Preoperative keratometry readings
    c. Preoperative manifest refraction
    d. Degree of attempted and achieved corrections

45. What is the most important reason that IOL calculation is less accurate after refractive surgery?
    a. Inability to obtain accurate central corneal power measurements
    b. Myopic shift due to nuclear sclerotic cataract
    c. Diurnal variation in corneal curvature
    d. None of the above

46. Retinal detachments after LASIK are
    a. Much more common than after PRK
    b. Much less common than after PRK
    c. Much harder to repair than after PRK
    d. None of the above
47. Contact lenses can be used after refractive surgery to do which of the following?
    a. Prevent regression
    b. Prevent astigmatism
    c. Improve visual acuity in cases of irregular astigmatism
    d. Reduce the chance of ectasia
    e. Test a patient's candidacy for monovision
48. Excimer laser keratorefractive surgery does which of the following?
    a. Induces a form of glaucoma
    b. Falsely elevates IOP
    c. Can damage the optic nerve without affecting IOP
    d. Falsely lowers IOP
    e. Leads to corticosteroid-induced glaucoma

Answers

1. **d.** Patients with keratoconus have corneal thinning in the paracentral area. This can be diagnosed using slit-lamp biomicroscopy and optical or ultrasonic pachymetry. Topographic changes in keratoconus include central corneal steepening, hemimeridional asymmetry, and a high inferior–superior (I–S) number. LASIK should be avoided in keratoconus to prevent progressive ectasia of the cornea.
2. **e.** In conventional non–wavefront-guided laser treatment of myopia, the central cornea is flattened. Defocus (a second-order aberration) is corrected at the expense of induced spherical (high-order) aberrations.
3. **b.** Munnerlyn's approximation of the ablation depth per diopter of correction = diameter^2/3, where the diameter is in mm and the depth is in μm. Thus the ablation depth is proportional to the square of the diameter. The depth of tissue ablation per diopter of correction is greater for wider ablation zones.
4. **d.** Contact lens wear can change the shape of the cornea and affect refractive error. In extreme cases, it can significantly distort the corneal curvature (a condition called corneal warpage). Removal of contact lenses prior to the refractive surgery evaluation and surgery is important to allow the corneal curvature to return to normal. While recommendations vary, soft contact lenses are generally discontinued for at least 3–14 days and rigid gas-permeable contact lenses for 14–21 days. A stable refraction and a normal-appearing corneal curvature are important prior to any refractive surgery. Repeat examinations after discontinuation of contact lenses should be performed in patients who do not have stable refractions and normal corneal curvatures.
5. **d.** Social history, past ocular history, and past and current medical history are all important in the preoperative refractive surgery evaluation. Social history includes important information about visual requirements and the likelihood of ocular trauma. Past ocular history might alert the surgeon to recurrent erosion syndrome. Medical history is important to determine whether there are conditions that might affect ocular healing, such as diabetes or a connective tissue disorder.
6. **c.** The slit-lamp examination, including looking carefully for evidence of epithelial basement membrane dystrophy, is important to make certain the cornea is healthy. Measurement of corneal curvature with corneal topography is important to make sure the cornea is regular and without evidence of ectasia (such as with keratoconus or pellucid marginal degeneration). Also, excessively steep or flat corneas increase the risk of flap complications from the microkeratome. Corneal thickness measurements are necessary to determine whether there is adequate corneal thickness to perform certain keratorefractive procedures, especially LASIK. Specular microscopy is not routinely performed prior to refractive surgery. If an endothelial abnormality is suspected, then specular microscopy can be performed.
7. **b.** Patients under age 35 are generally not interested in monovision. Success with monovision in the past indicates that the patient is likely to have success in the future. Ocular dominance is tested, because most patients are happiest with the nondominant eye corrected for near. However, monovision should be demonstrated in trial spectacles and/or contact lenses to assess the patient's preoperative satisfaction with this approach. Both low and high myopes can enjoy successful monovision.

8. **b.** LASIK is generally used to correct from −10 to +4 D and PRK from −8 to +4 D. Unlike LASIK, PRK for higher levels of myopia is associated with a greater incidence of postoperative corneal haze. Consequently, most surgeons prefer LASIK to PRK for higher levels of myopia (above −6 D). If LASIK is contraindicated for reasons such as insufficient corneal thickness, some surgeons will perform PRK with "prophylactic" mitomycin to attempt to decrease the possibility of corneal haze postoperatively.
9. **a.** Thermokeratoplasty is associated with refractive regression, does not correct astigmatism, and does not create a multifocal cornea that results in good uncorrected distance and near vision. The best answer is a.
10. **d.** All statements are true except d. Intersecting radial and astigmatic incisions result in irregular corneal topographical changes and in undesirable visual disturbances.
11. **b.** AK incisions are placed in the midperipheral cornea and are helpful in treating postkeratoplasty astigmatism. LRIs are more useful to correct astigmatism during or after phacoemulsification and IOL implantation. Coupling is a hallmark of LRIs and AK and results in concomitant steepening of the orthogonal meridian.
12. **a.** Unlike LASIK, where corneal tissue is removed, there is no removal of corneal tissue in incisional keratotomy. While LASIK may result in corneal ectasia if excessive tissue is removed, corneal ectasia should not result after radial or astigmatic keratotomy. However, corneal incisions may cause corneal instability with diurnal fluctuation of vision and/or continued effect of surgery over time. Any type of refractive surgery performed on a cornea with abnormal preoperative topography such as forme fruste keratoconus or pellucid marginal degeneration may be associated with unpredictable postoperative results.
13. **c.** The inlay impedes the flow of nutrients to the overlying stroma and can result in necrosis. Reflection of ultraviolet light from the inlay is not a recognized cause of necrosis. The epithelium and superficial stroma rely on diffusion from the tear film for oxygen. Trauma at the time of surgery can damage the stroma but is not generally responsible for the necrosis seen after inlay implantation.
14. **a.** The clinical results of myopic epikeratoplasty were not as favorable as radial keratotomy in the 1980s. In addition, IOLs for aphakia had a higher degree of refractive predictability than aphakic epikeratoplasty. Because of the disappointing results, commercial production of lenticules was halted. Scarring over the visual axis after epikeratoplasty was not a common cause of loss of vision. Accidental perforation during epikeratoplasty was a remote risk because only a limited lamellar dissection was required in the peripheral cornea; the lenticule was sewn directly onto Bowman's layer. The lens material was derived from donor cornea tissue.
15. **c.** The PMMA corneal ring segments can be removed, making the refractive results potentially reversible. Unlike most other forms of keratorefractive surgery, surgery is not performed on the cornea overlying the pupil. The ring segments can be replaced to alter the refractive result. Intacs are not approved to treat astigmatism.
16. **c.** The 0.35 mm ring segments correct higher levels of myopia. These ring segments have a lower level of refractive predictability and are less likely to result in 20/20 uncorrected vision compared with the thinner ring segments. The 0.35 mm ring segments have been found to cause more visual disturbances, which is why they are removed more often than the thinner ring segments.

17. **b.** Intacs have been used to treat mild keratoconus and ectasia after LASIK. In addition, the ring segments have been used to correct residual myopia after LASIK where there is an insufficient residual stromal bed to perform additional excimer laser surgery. The ring segments cannot be used to treat aphakia.

18. **c.** Photoablation. The high-energy photons emitted by the 193 nm excimer laser rupture the collagen peptide backbone of the cornea and eject the protein fragments into the air, ablating the desired cornea.

19. **b.** A slow and precise manual scraping. Dehydration of the stroma with any prolonged technique results in more tissue removal per pulse and therefore may cause overcorrection.

20. **b.** The dynamics of the large exposure area of broad-beam lasers are associated with central islands because the laser beam may have inhomogeneous energy.

21. **a.** A steep cornea protrudes higher above the suction ring and therefore more corneal surface area is exposed to the microkeratome.

22. **a.** The endothelial pump creates a negative suction pressure in the corneal stroma.

23. **c.** In most cases, the surgeon can lift the original flap for at least several years after the original procedure. A residual stromal bed of at least 250 μm is recommended to avoid postoperative ectasia.

24. **a.** The transection of the corneal nerves in the creation of the flap leads to a neurotrophic epitheliopathy.

25. **d.** Diffuse lamellar keratitis is a nonspecific inflammatory response to a variety of toxic insults and is usually noninfectious. While diffuse lamellar keratitis may be associated with primary or enhancement LASIK procedures, it may also occur in other settings such as after corneal epithelial erosion. Diffuse lamellar keratitis is treated primarily with topical corticosteroids. Severe cases of diffuse lamellar keratitis (stage 4) are at risk for collagenase release and corneal melting.

26. **a.** The holmium:yttrium-aluminum-garnet (Ho:YAG) laser was approved by the FDA for use in thermokeratoplasty in the 1990s.

27. **b.** The probe heats the corneal epithelium as well as the stroma. Although a decentered corneal apex may have less than optimal results, it is not a contraindication to conductive keratoplasty. There is regression toward increasing hyperopia after conductive keratoplasty.

28. **d.** Radiofrequency energy is used during conductive keratoplasty, and the resistance to the current creates localized heat.

29. **d.** Laser thermokeratoplasty is approved for the temporary treatment of 0.75 D to 2.50 D of hyperopia with less than 1.00 D of astigmatism.

30. **d.** Potential treatment of astigmatism with conductive keratoplasty would involve placing treatment at the flatter axis; therefore, in a patient with astigmatism of +1.50 D at axis 180, the treatment spots would be placed in the 90° meridian.

31. **c.** PIOLs can correct a wide range of refractive error from high myopia to high hyperopia. PIOLs are inserted over the clear lens. They have the advantage of not being dependent on corneal thickness or steepness.

32. **e.** Patients who have bioptics will still require reading glasses unless the treatment is adjusted for monovision. The other statements are all true.

33. **a.** The optics of PCPIOLs, such as ICL (STAAR) and PRL (CIBA Vision), are foldable, but the iris-fixated IOL optic and most ACPIOLs are made of PMMA and cannot fold. This increases the risk of surgically induced astigmatism. The other statements are true.

34. **c.** The ideal candidate for a multifocal IOL has <1 D of astigmatism, has a pupil >4.0 mm in diameter in order to fully benefit from the multifocal effect, has less concern about glare, requires bilateral surgery, and has good potential vision.

35. **e.** Retinal detachment risk is 4 times higher 7 years postoperatively than 4 years after surgery. Nd:YAG laser posterior capsulotomy doubles the retinal detachment risk over a 7-year period. The technique of clear lensectomy is significantly different in the myope than in the hyperope. The anterior chamber tends to become very deep in the myopic eye and is somewhat shallow in the hyperopic patient. Most retinal surgeons would prefer to have an IOL placed even when the power is near 0; the barrier of the IOL is felt to reduce the risk of retinal detachment.

36. **b.** Subjective improvement in near vision is experienced by some patients after they undergo any of the various methods of scleral expansion surgery. These improvements have not been completely explained, are usually transient, and are possibly the result of depth of focus changes, patient effort, test learning, and nonlenticular optical shifts. Dynamic testing with infrared optometers has revealed no increase in the amplitude of accommodation after scleral expansion surgery.

37. **d.** All of these patients may benefit somewhat from the induction of mild myopia (modified monovision) in the nondominant eye. The truck driver could regain the ability to see the dashboard clearly while having a 95% chance of maintaining better than 20/25 binocular distance vision. The nurse and the lawyer could both gain uncorrected near vision in their nondominant eye. The librarian, whose day is spent in constant close-in work, would probably not tolerate the induced myopia—even in her nondominant eye—due to her young age and her intact ability for full accommodation.

38. **b.** A reduction in the overall mobility of the ciliary muscle fibers is seen with advancing presbyopia, a reduction believed to be due to an increase in connective tissue between the fibers. In cross-section, the ciliary body changes with age from a lenticular-shaped structure to one more triangular. A number of recent studies, however, reveal that little if any contractile strength of the ciliary muscle fibers is lost in the normal aging process of the eye. (Without the preserved strength/function of the muscle, the recent success seen with the new accommodating IOLs would not be possible.)

39. **c.** Of all the various modes of presbyopia "reversal," only the so-called accommodating IOLs, used in surgically induced pseudophakes, restore some amount of true accommodation (the ability to change one's focal range at will). Their mechanism involves a forward displacement of the IOL in the eye, leading to an effective increase in the IOL's optical power and a subsequent increased ability for near vision. A combination of vitreous pressure on the posterior IOL surface, contracting ciliary body pressure on the IOL haptics to vault the optic forward, and a forward movement of the entire ciliary body that carries the IOL forward is believed to be responsible for the accommodative amplitude increase.

40. **b.** The catenary, or hydraulic support, theory of accommodation proposes that the lens, zonules, and anterior vitreous act as a functional diaphragm between the vitreous cavity and the anterior chamber. Contraction of the ciliary body generates an elevated posterior pressure in the vitreous cavity, causing anterior movement of the lens–zonule diaphragm. Like the Helmholtz theory, this contraction also results in a relaxation of the zonular fibers during accommodation. Presbyopic changes are believed to be due to a reduced response of anterior lens curvature to the vitreous pressure generated by ciliary body contraction in accommodation.

41. **e.** A patient who is legally blind in one eye should not consider refractive surgery in the better eye. Dry eyes should be effectively treated before refractive surgery. Some patients with controlled glaucoma may be candidates for refractive surgery. A patient who has a history of retinal detachment or herpes virus may qualify for refractive surgery.

42. **e.** Ring segments are undergoing investigational studies in keratoconus. No refractive surgery procedure is approved by the FDA for keratoconus. Refractive surgery is typically contraindicated in keratoconus because of unpredictable results and loss of vision.

43. **d.** Optimal topical IOP-lowering therapy should be determined before LASIK is considered in the glaucoma patient. Because of the difficulty in interpreting IOP measurements, PRK and LASIK should not be considered until the IOP is well controlled.

44. **a.** One of the most accurate methods to determine the power of the IOL after refractive surgery is the historical method, which uses the preoperative keratometry readings, preoperative manifest refraction, and attempted and achieved corrections. The preoperative axial length does not change significantly after refractive surgery. New axial length measurements are also accurate after refractive surgery.

45. **a.** While both myopic shift due to nuclear sclerosis and diurnal variation in corneal curvature do occur, the primary difficulty in obtaining accurate IOL calculations after refractive surgery is from the inability to obtain accurate central corneal power measurements from our instruments, which were developed to measure curvature in "normal" eyes.

46. **d.** There is no convincing evidence that retinal detachments are more or less frequent after LASIK than after PRK (when the degree of preoperative myopia is controlled for). While the surgeon should avoid trauma to the LASIK flap to decrease the risk of flap dehiscence and epithelial defect, retinal detachment surgery is no more difficult in LASIK than in PRK.

47. **c.** Contact lenses will not prevent anatomical changes or reduce their occurrence in the cornea postoperatively. If monovision is being considered, it should be done before refractive surgery. Contact lenses can improve visual function in cases of irregular astigmatism.

48. **d.** After laser surgery for myopia, the measured IOP is lower than the actual IOP. This can result in glaucomatous damage despite normal IOP readings. IOP should be measured from the side of the cornea and the optic nerve should be carefully evaluated on an ongoing basis to reduce the likelihood of glaucomatous damage going undetected.

Index

(*i* = image; *t* = table)